Biomedical Concerns in Persons with Down Syndrome

Biomedical Concerns in Persons with Down Syndrome

edited by

Siegfried M. Pueschel, M.D., Ph.D., M.P.H.
Professor of Pediatrics
Brown University School of Medicine
and
Director
Child Development Center
Rhode Island Hospital
Providence, Rhode Island

and

Jeanette K. Pueschel
Child Development Center
Rhode Island Hospital
Providence, Rhode Island

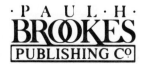

·P A U L·H·
BROOKES
PUBLISHING CO

Baltimore • London • Toronto • Sydney

Paul H. Brookes Publishing Co.
P.O. Box 10624
Baltimore, Maryland 21285-0624

Typeset by Brushwood Graphics, Inc., Baltimore, Maryland.
Manufactured in the United States of America by
The Maple Press Company, York, Pennsylvania.

Library of Congress Cataloging-in-Publication Data
Biomedical concerns in persons with Down syndrome / [edited by]
    Siegfried M. Pueschel and Jeanette K. Pueschel.
        p.   cm.
    Includes bibliographical references and index.
    ISBN 1-55766-089-1
    1. Down's syndrome—Pathophysiology.   2. Down's syndrome—
Patients—Medical care.   I. Pueschel, Siegfried M.   II. Pueschel, Jeanette K., 1970–
    [DNLM: 1. Down's Syndrome.   WS 107 B6155]
RC571.B56   1992
DNLM/DLC
for Library of Congress   91-43420
                                                                                      CIP

British Library Cataloguing-in-Publication data is available from the British Library.

Contents

Contributors

Göran Annerén, M.D., Ph.D.
Associate Professor
Department of Pediatrics
University of Uppsala
751 85 Uppsala
SWEDEN

Ilana Ariel, M.D.
Senior Lecturer in Pathology
The Hebrew University—Hadassah Medical School
Head, Pediatric Pathology Unit
Department of Pathology
Hadassah University Hospital Mount Scopus
P.O. Box 24035
91240 Jerusalem
ISRAEL

Patricia A. Baird, M.D., C.M.
Professor
Department of Medical Genetics
University of British Columbia
226-6174 University Boulevard
Vancouver, British Columbia V6T 123
CANADA

Robert L. Baldwin, M.D., F.A.C.S.
Director
Birmingham Otology Center
Suite 502
2700 10th Avenue South
Birmingham, Alabama 35205

Paul M. Benson, M.D.
Assistant Chief
Dermatology Service
Walter Reed Army Medical Center
Washington, D.C. 20307

G. Roberto Burgio, M.D.
Professor of Pediatrics
University of Pavia
Clinica Pediatrica
IRCCS Policlinico S. Matteo
27100 Pavia
ITALY

Jo-Ann Blaymore Bier, M.D., M.S.
Assistant Professor of Pediatrics
Brown University School of Medicine
Director of Pediatrics
Child Development Center
Rhode Island Hospital
593 Eddy Street
Providence, Rhode Island 02903

Sarah Cahn
Quincy House 306
Harvard College
Cambridge, Massachusetts 02138

Robert A. Catalano, M.D.
Vice President for Medical Affairs
Olean General Hospital
515 Main Street
Olean, New York 14760

Christine E. Cronk, Sc.D.
Research Associate
Division of Gastroenterology and Nutrition
Children's Hospital of Philadelphia
Route 1, Box 49
Makanda, Illinois 62958

Arthur J. Dahle, Ph.D.
Professor
Department of Biocommunication
University of Alabama at Birmingham
Sparks Center
P.O. Box 313, UAB Station
Birmingham, Alabama 35294

Thomas E. Elkins, M.D.
Associate Professor
Chief of Gynecology
Department of Obstetrics and Gynecology
University of Michigan Medical Center
Room D2234 MPB
Ann Arbor, Michigan 48109-0718

Jesús Flórez, M.D., Ph.D.
Professor of Pharmacology
Chairman
Department of Physiology and Pharmacology
University of Cantabria
39011 Santander
SPAIN

Michelle S. Howenstine, M.D.
Assistant Clinical Professor of Pediatrics
University of South Florida
Director, Section Pediatric Pulmonology
All Children's Hospital
801 6th Street S
St. Petersburg, Florida 33701

Florence Lai, M.D.
Neurologist
Eunice Kennedy Shriver Center
200 Trapelo Road
Waltham, Massachusetts 02254

Joseph Levy, M.D.
Chief
Division of Pediatric Gastroenterology and Nutrition
Cornell Medical Center
New York Hospital
525 East 68th Street
New York, New York 10021

Bertram H. Lubin, M.D.
Adjunct Clinical Professor of Pediatrics
University of California at San Francisco
Director of Medical Research
Children's Hospital Oakland Research Institute
51st and Grove Streets
Oakland, California 94609

Rita Maccarrio, Ph.D.
Department of Pediatrics
University of Pavia
Clinica Pediatrica
IRCCS Policlinico S. Matteo
P.le Golgi
27100 Pavia
ITALY

Bruno Marino, M.D.
Professor at Postgraduate School of Cardiology
Catholic University, Medical School
Consultant Pediatric Cardiologist
Bambino Gesù Hospital
Istituto di Ricovero e Cura a Carattere Scientifico
Piazza San'Onofrio, 4
00165 Rome
ITALY

Beverly A. Myers, Ph.D.
Clinical Assistant Professor
Brown University School of Medicine
Consultant in Child Psychiatry
Child Development Center
Rhode Island Hospital
593 Eddy Street
Providence, Rhode Island 02903

Peggy L. Pipes, M.P.H., R.D.
Lecturer, School of Nursing
Assistant Chief Nutritionist
Child Development Mental Retardation Center
CTU-CDMRC
Mail Drop IWJ-10
University of Washington
Seattle, Washington 98195

Jeanette K. Pueschel
Child Development Center
Rhode Island Hospital
593 Eddy Street
Providence, Rhode Island 02903

Siegfried M. Pueschel, M.D., Ph.D., M.P.H.
Professor of Pediatrics
Brown University School of Medicine
Director, Child Development Center
Rhode Island Hospital
593 Eddy Street
Providence, Rhode Island 02903

Adele D. Sadovnick, Ph.D.
Assistant Professor
Departments of Medical Genetics and Medicine
University of British Columbia
226–6174 University Boulevard
Vancouver, British Columbia V6T 1Z3
CANADA

James M. Scherbenske, M.D.
Chief, Department of Dermatology
Fort Evans Army Community Hospital
Fort Carson, Colorado 80913

Patricia S. Scola, M.D., M.P.H.
Clinical Assistant Professor
Brown University School of Medicine
Associate Physician
Department of Pediatrics
Child Development Center
Rhode Island Hospital
593 Eddy Street
Providence, Rhode Island 02903

Mark Scott, Ph.D.
Assistant Research Biochemist
Children's Hospital Oakland Research Institute
747 Fifty Second Street
Oakland, California 94609

Yigal Shvil, M.D.
Senior Lecturer in Pediatrics
The Hebrew University—Hadassah Medical School
Chief Pediatric Nephrologist
Department of Pediatrics
Hadassah University Hospital Kiryat Hadassah
P.O. Box 12000
91120 Jerusalem
ISRAEL

Patricia M. Solga, M.D.
Assistant Professor of Orthopaedics
Brown University School of Medicine
Rhode Island Hospital
593 Eddy Street
Providence, Rhode Island 02903

Horace C. Thuline, M.D.
Clinical Professor
Department of Pediatrics
School of Medicine
University of Washington
16353 129th Avenue, SE
Renton, Washington 98058

Alberto G. Ugazio, M.D.
Professor of Pediatrics
University of Brescia
Head, Department of Pediatrics
Clinica Pediatrica
Spedali Civili di Brescia
25100 Brescia
ITALY

Merete Vigild, D.D.S., Ph.D.
Associate Professor of Dentistry
Institute of Community Dentistry and Graduate
  Studies
The Royal Dental College
20 Norre Alle
2200 Copenhagen N
DENMARK

Preface

Since Down (1866) described the condition that today bears his name, a multitude of publications on this subject have permeated the medical literature. In 1980, Pueschel and Steinberg conducted an intensive literature search and compiled more than 6,000 articles relating to various aspects of Down syndrome. It is estimated that an even larger number of publications appeared in print during the 1980s. This enormous information explosion in recent years is in part a reflection of the progress that has been made in the field of Down syndrome. The knowledge that has accumulated necessitates a thorough discussion of the various biomedical concerns in a form that would be meaningful for professionals who are pursuing investigative work, as well as for those who are providing care for individuals with Down syndrome—and this is the main reason that this book was written.

The task of describing these advances succinctly and scholarly was accomplished because of the expertise of the contributors of this volume, a group of internationally renowned scientists and physicians. They are uniquely qualified to discuss the unforeseen progress that has been made in the biomedical arena pertaining to Down syndrome with a clarity, sensitivity, and the specific knowledge that is unmatched. It is of note that the authors of this volume have been actively involved in investigations and clinical work in the field of Down syndrome. They are foremost experts in their respective subspecialty; hence, they can provide insight into the various conditions and disorders prevailing in individuals with Down syndrome that would not be possible for the less involved professional.

Because of the increasing volume of articles on Down syndrome and, more importantly, because of the specific focus on biomedical concerns of this book, developmental, educational, behavioral, psychologic, social, and environmental circumstances are not discussed here. In addition, because of limited space, important aspects such as cytogenetic, epidemiologic, and etiologic issues have not been included. Also, the emerging field of molecular genetics as it relates to chromosome 21 is only briefly mentioned throughout the text.

The main objective of this book is to provide a basic description of various organ systems and their underlying pathology and also focus on specific issues such as phenotype, growth, and life expectancy, as well as management issues relating to Down syndrome. Although comprehensiveness was an important factor in the composition of most of the chapters, the primary objective in the selection of the various topics was to present students, clinicians, and other professionals in the field of developmental disabilities with up-to-date information that will permit optimal care provision for persons with Down syndrome. Essentially, this is the main theme of this book—for if we provide excellent care to individuals with Down syndrome based on the present state of knowledge, then these individuals will be able to enjoy life more fully and to function more effectively. If in good health, persons with Down syndrome will be able to participate to the best of their abilities in educational processes and vocational pursuits. With appropriate medical care, the quality of life of persons with Down syndrome can be significantly enhanced, and they can become productive and contributing members of society.

REFERENCES

Down, J.L. (1866). Observations on an ethnic classification of idiots. *London Hospital Clinical Lectures and Reports, 3,* 259–262.
Pueschel, S.M., & Steinberg, L. (1980). *Down syndrome: A comprehensive bibliography.* New York: Garland STPM Press.

Biomedical Concerns
in Persons with Down Syndrome

Phenotypic Characteristics

Siegfried M. Pueschel

Although there are suggestions in the literature that persons with Down syndrome have been sculpturally and pictorially represented in the past (Pueschel, 1990), no well-documented reports of individuals with Down syndrome were published prior to the 19th century. The first description of a child who presumably had Down syndrome was provided by Esquirol in 1838. Shortly thereafter, in 1846, Seguin described a child with features suggestive of Down syndrome, a condition he called "furfuraceous idiocy." In 1866, Duncan noted a girl "with a small round head, Chinese looking eyes, projecting a large tongue who only knew a few words." That same year, Down (1866) published a paper describing some of the characteristics of the syndrome that today bears his name:

> The hair is not black, as in the real Mongol, but of a brownish colour, straight and scanty. The face is flat and broad, and destitute of prominence. The cheeks are roundish, and extended laterally. The eyes are obliquely placed, and the internal canthi more than normally distant from one another. The palpebral fissure is very narrow . . . . The lips are large and thick with transverse fissures. The tongue is long, thick, and is much roughened. The nose is small . . . (p. 261)

Down deserves credit for describing some of the classical features of this condition, thus distinguishing these children from others with mental retardation, in particular, those with cretinism. Thus, Down's great contribution was his recognition of the physical characteristics and his description of the condition as a distinct and separate entity.

GENERAL CONSIDERATIONS

Since Down's (1866) description of some of the characteristics observed in persons with Down syndrome, a multitude of articles have appeared in the medical literature reporting numerous features associated with this syndrome (e.g., Clark, Cowell, McCracken, & Bennett, 1978; Coleman, 1978; Domino & Newman, 1965; Gustavson, 1964; Hall, 1964, 1966; Johnson & Barnett, 1961; Lee & Jackson, 1972; Levinson, Friedman, & Stamps, 1955; Öster, 1953; Richards, 1965; W. Schmid, Lee, & Smith, 1961; Singh, 1976; Strelling, 1976; Wahrman & Fried, 1970). Some of the characteristics observed in individuals with Down syndrome occur with a high frequency and thus are considered to be typical of this syndrome. Henceforth, some investigators have used certain cardinal signs for the development of diagnostic indices in the clinical identification of young children with Down syndrome (Preus, 1977). Professionals have emphasized the importance of recognizing the clinical features in children with Down syndrome for diagnostic purposes. Yet, such physical stigmata are not identified on a regular basis in every child with Down syndrome, and it is well known that none of the observed features in children with Down syndrome can be considered pathognomonic for this chromosome disorder.

Although the vast majority of individuals with Down syndrome can be diagnosed clinically, and the physician's diagnostic acumen is still of significance today, a chromosome analysis is necessary to determine the child's cytogenetic make-up. Hence, a chromosome study should be performed at once when the clinical diagnosis of Down syndrome has been entertained or if there is a suspicion of Down syndrome or other chromosome disorder in the child. Karyotyping not only serves as confirmation of the clinical impression, but also identifies the type of chromosome disorder (trisomy 21, translocation, mosaicism, or partial trisomy 21). Moreover, one will uncover those children with a resemblance of the Down syndrome phenotype who may have a karyotype of 48, XXXX, or 49, XXXXY. In addition, children with Down syndrome who have double aneuploidy or previously unidentified chromosome aberrations will also be detected.

Because physical features of any human being are to a large extent determined by his or her genome, the child with Down syndrome will have some physical similarity to the biological parents from whom he or she received the genes. He or she will also have common features with other children who have Down syndrome due to the presence of extra genetic material in the form of a supernumerary chromosome 21 in these children. Although the pathogenetic mechanisms leading to the observed phenotypic findings in Down syndrome are not known, it is the presence of three #21 chromosomes that is responsible for the altered development during embryogenesis and organogenesis. Presently, limited information is available about how this additional chromosome material interferes with normal developmental processes or how structural changes are produced in the embryo. Moreover, there is no explanation of why some children with Down syndrome have certain abnormal features and others who also have the extra #21 chromosome do not show the same characteristics. Some children will display nearly all of the features described in this chapter whereas others will exhibit only a few of them. There have been premature infants with Down syndrome who had only a few stigmata, whereas on other occasions the presence of most of the characteristics of Down syndrome leaves no doubt as to the diagnosis of this chromosome disorder.

It is of note that some investigators reported only such Down syndrome characteristics that are apparent on surface examination (Clark et al., 1978; Hall, 1966; Wahrman & Fried, 1970). Others described in more detail additional parameters, such as anthropologic findings, roentgenologic features, and various aspects of psychological and socioeducational functions (Lee & Jackson, 1972; Pueschel, 1984). Some investigators focused also on internal organ systems and reported cardiac, respiratory, gastrointestinal, hematologic, immunologic, and other abnormalities in individuals with Down syndrome (Pueschel, 1984). Frequently, observers studied specific features of Down syndrome according to their respective preference. Furthermore, the recording of Down syndrome characteristics often took place at various age periods. Some physicians studied individuals with Down syndrome during infancy, whereas others assessed them during later childhood or adolescence. A few reports on phenotypic delineation in Down syndrome included all age groups, whereas others provided no age range (Clark et al., 1978; Öster, 1953; Singh, 1976). Moreover, detailed postmortem anatomic dissection of persons with Down syndrome has provided information on an "internal phenotype" that, according to Bersu (1980), comprises variations in facial muscles, peripheral arteries, and first cervical and spinal accessory nerves.

It is well known that some physical features in persons with Down syndrome change over time. Certain characteristics, such as single palmar creases, overlapping helices, and brachycephaly, can be observed at any age. Others, however, such as epicanthal folds or the sometimes initially abundant neck tissue, will become less prominent as the child grows. A few stigmata, however, such as the fissured tongue or dental anomalies, may become apparent with increasing age.

It should be pointed out that many of the physical features noted in individuals with Down syndrome are also observed at various frequencies in children with 46 chromosomes. For example, 4%–5% of "normal" children have a single palmar crease, 6%–8% of "normal" infants display epicanthal folds, and 26%–43% of "normal" newborns have overlapping helices (Holmes,

1976; Ŏster, 1953). Clark et al. (1978) reported that small teeth, abnormally aligned teeth, furrowing of the tongue, slanting of palpebral fissures, flat occipital area, small ears, a flat nasal bridge, and strabismus, which were present in 53.7%–70.9% of persons with Down syndrome, also were noted in 25%–50% of persons who do not have Down syndrome. Although the latter data appear to be high estimates of normal variation, they emphasize the fact that almost none of the so-called Down syndrome stigmata are specific for this chromosome disorder, and they may occur in any human being.

With this in mind, it is important to make parents aware of the fact that children with Down syndrome are more similar to "normal" children than they are different. When physical features are discussed with the parents, it should be emphasized that many of the observed findings in Down syndrome will not cause any disability in the child. For example, the incurved little finger will not limit the function of the hand, nor will the slanting of the palpebral fissure interfere with the child's vision. Yet, other defects, such as severe congenital heart disease and duodenal atresia, are serious and require prompt medical attention. It is also important to reassure parents that although physical changes will take place during the process of development and maturation, the features will not become "worse" over time. The professional who is counseling parents in the diagnosis of Down syndrome should be aware of these issues and should relate them to the parents. The physician should also realize that the diagnosis of Down syndrome implies much more to the parents than the mere enumeration of various physical characteristics; it exerts a deep and far-reaching effect upon the individual parent and the entire family.

The following description of various physical features does not provide a complete and comprehensive account of all observed phenotypic stigmata of the person with Down syndrome. Rather, the focus is on characteristics that can be identified on routine physical examination. Table 1.1 charts the frequency of many of the characteristics seen in persons with Down syndrome. Also, it should be noted that some characteristics not discussed here are included in subsequent chapters of this book.

SPECIFIC PHENOTYPIC STIGMATA

Skull

The skull of the child with Down syndrome is usually small and the anterior-posterior diameter is shortened. According to Rett (1977), brachycephaly is found in 80% of children with Down syndrome. Yet, true microcephaly is rarely observed in Down syndrome. Benda (1969) reported that the head measurements in newborns with Down syndrome are within normal limits. However, Hall's studies (1964, 1966), as well as Cronk and Pueschel's investigations (1984), indicated that the mean head circumference of infants with Down syndrome is markedly below the mean head circumference of the "normal" child, but not in the microcephalic range.

In the newborn, the anterior fontanel is frequently wide open with a metopic suture sometimes extending to the forehead. The sagittal suture is often open, with a widening at the parietal area that is referred to as false or third fontanel. There is a delay in the closing of sutures and fontanels in children with Down syndrome. It is not uncommon for the anterior fontanel still to be open at the age of 2–3 years. Ŏster (1953) reported that the anterior fontanel was open in 25 of 77 children with Down syndrome at the age of 2–5 years.

In addition, children with Down syndrome reportedly have hypoplasia of their midfacial bones. Strelling (1976) pointed to the size and grouping of the midfacial features as a significant characteristic of the child with Down syndrome. He emphasized that the eyes, nose, and mouth are not only small, but are grouped more closely together at the center of the face. In quantitative studies of the face, Gerald and Silverman (1965) and Lowe (1949) noted that the interorbital distance is often reduced, the maxilla is underdeveloped, and the angle of the mandible may be somewhat obtuse. Benda (1969) reported abnormalities of the sphenoid bone, displacement of the cribriform plate, and changes

Table 1.1. Frequency of physical characteristics in persons with Down syndrome

Characteristic	Öster (1953)	Levinson, Friedman, and Stamps (1955)	Gustavson (1964)	Domino and Newman (1965)	Hall (1966)	Wahrman and Fried (1970)	Lee and Jackson (1972)	Singh (1976)	Clark, Cowell, McCracken, and Bennett (1978)	Pueschel (1984)
Skull										
brachycephaly	74	82	81	73			75	98	63	75
Eyes										
oblique palpebral fissures	75	88	86	75	80		85		70	98
epicanthal folds	28	50	55	67		76	79	76		57
Brushfield spots	70		70	58			35	59	55	75
Nose										
flat nasal bridge	59	62	62				87		57	83
Ears										
folded helix/dysplastic ear	49		28		62	78	43	91	56	34
Mouth										
open mouth	67	62	59	53			40			65
protruding tongue	49	32	38	45		63	38	89	50	58
furrowed tongue	59	44	44	80			22		80	
high arched palate	67	74	70	59			68	55		
narrow palate			76				68			
abnormal teeth	71	56	65				31		80	85
Neck										
short neck	39	50		71			70			
loose skin on neck nape					80	94	60	17	76	87
Cardiac										
congenital heart defects			19				25	55		39
Extremities										
short broad hands	69	74	75	66			61	55		38
transverse palmar crease	43	48	60	64	45	42	60	77	45	57
short fifth finger	57		74	61			51	77		51
incurved fifth finger	48	68	52	58	58		43	89	73	51
gap between first and second toes	97	44	87			67	64		82	96
Musculoskeletal										
hyperflexibility	47		85	77	77		60			92
muscular hypotonia	21		72	40	77	82	40	41		85

Note: All data are reported as percentages.

4

in the sella turcica. Roche, Roche, and Lewis (1972) carried out a cephalometric X-ray study of the cranial base in 131 children and adults with Down syndrome and found a reduction in cranial base length. Another significant observation related to the cranial bones is that the sinuses are underdeveloped (Benda, 1969).

Eyes

The eyes and features surrounding the eyes of persons with Down syndrome had already attracted interest in the 19th century (Down, 1866; Seguin, 1866). The palpebral fissures are usually obliquely placed, and epicanthal folds and a depressed nasal bridge are often present. Since these findings impressed Down as Asian features, he coined the terms "mongoloid" and "mongolism." During the same year when Down's paper was published, Seguin (1866, p. 11) also described the epicanthal folds in Down syndrome as "skin at the margin of the lid." Tredgold (1908) remarked that if Seguin's observation had received greater recognition, there would not have been general approval of the idea that the child with Down syndrome is related to the Mongolian race, and many contributions dealing with the racial retrogression theory would never have been written.

Epicanthal folds in children with Down syndrome are often found bilaterally and, on occasion, unilaterally. These inner canthal skin folds may be prominent at the time of birth. However, as the child grows they often fade, become less apparent, or sometimes disappear. Epicanthal folds have been reported to be present in 28%–80% of individuals with Down syndrome (Gustavson, 1964; Hall, 1964; Lee & Jackson, 1972; Levinson et al., 1955; Öster, 1953). Pueschel (1984) found that 57% of children with Down syndrome had epicanthal folds. Epicanthal folds are also occasionally seen in "normal" children (Holmes, 1976). It should be noted that the inner canthal folds in persons with Down syndrome are different in structure from the folds observed in Asian people. In most Asian individuals, the inner canthal fold continues with the pars orbitalis of the upper eyelid. The pars orbitalis overlaps the pars tarsalis with a skin fold, which turns medially and partially covers the caruncula

lacrimalis. The epicanthal fold of the child with Down syndrome, in contrast, starts at the upper eyelid, continues around the medial angle of the eye, and ends beneath in the skin of the sulcus infrapalpebralis. The inner canthal folds of the child with Down syndrome are thought to be due to the hypoplasia of the nasal bone (Benda, 1969). As the nasal bone develops during the first few years of life, the adjacent skin will be pulled medially and the epicanthal folds often will become less prominent.

The oblique placement of the palpebral fissures in individuals with Down syndrome is a common finding and was observed in 97% of young children with Down syndrome followed in Pueschel's (1984) longitudinal study. Other investigators (Gustavson, 1964; Hall, 1964; Öster, 1953) have also described the upward slant of palpebral fissures in persons with Down syndrome. In addition, the palpebral fissures are usually narrow (Benda, 1969). In contrast to the eye of the Asian person, the palpebral fissure in individuals with Down syndrome is said to be more almond shaped. In order to identify whether there is a significant obliquity of palpebral fissures, one should measure the angle produced by a line connecting the two medial canthi and the line connecting the medial and lateral canthi of each eye. If the lateral canthus is above the medial canthus, the obliquity is considered to be positive (Wahrman & Fried, 1970).

Various observers have interpreted the obliquity of the palpebral fissures in different ways. Whereas Benda (1969) suggested that the palpebral slant is due to the underlying abnormal bony structure, Lowe (1949) attributed the obliquity of the palpebral fissures to a soft tissue defect.

Both hypertelorism and hypotelorism (increased distance or closeness between the eyes, respectively) have been reported to be present in Down syndrome. The described variations in the intercanthal distance is primarily due to a lack of accurate measurements. Hypertelorism has been suggested because of the presence of a flat nasal bridge with marked epicanthal folds covering the inner canthi. Hypotelorism in Down syndrome had already been observed in the beginning of the century by Barr (1904) and was later reported by Brushfield (1924). Lowe (1949) reported that the distance between the inner canthi of persons with Down syndrome is approximately 1.5 cm less than in "normal" adults.

Ordinarily, measurements of interpupillary distance will identify the presence of hypertelorism or hypotelorism. Since, however, esotropia and exotropia have been observed with increased frequency in persons with Down syndrome, interpupillary measurements are only of value in those children without strabismus. As an accurate approach to recording the presence of hypertelorism or hypotelorism, measurements between both the outer and inner canthi as well as interpupillary distance should be obtained.

Brushfield spots had been observed by Down as fine white spots in the periphery of the iris. He brought them to the attention of Tredgold, who described this observation in 1908, long before Brushfield published his paper in 1924. These Brushfield spots are white-gray protuberant areas on the surface of the iris. According to Purtscher (1958), these spots consist of connective tissue that is localized within the anterior layer of the iris. Benda (1969) thought that the Brushfield spots were related to the thinning of the iris stroma as well as to abnormal pigment distribution.

In newborns with Down syndrome, Brushfield spots are not always identified. In a cohort of infants, Brushfield spots were observed in 75% (Pueschel, 1984). Other investigators reported that the presence of Brushfield spots in Down syndrome is between 30%–70% (Gustavson, 1964; Hall, 1964; Lee & Jackson, 1972; Öster, 1953). Singh (1976) found a higher percentage of Brushfield spots in whites, both females and males, than in a black study population. It has also been found that Brushfield spots are more often noted in children with a light blue-gray iris than in children with a dark brown pigmentation of the iris (Donaldson, 1961; Pueschel, 1984; Solomons, Zellweger, Jahnke, & Opitz, 1965). (For further discussion of ophthalmologic findings, see Catalano, chap. 6, this volume.)

Nose

The nose of the child with Down syndrome is characterized by its reduced size and depression of the nasal bridge. The nares are sometimes anteverted and the nostrils are narrow. Deviations of the nasal septum are common. The nasal bone is usually not ossified and is underdeveloped in the newborn. Pueschel (1984) noted that a hypoplastic nose was observed in 83% of newborns with Down syndrome. Other investigators (Clark et al., 1978; Domino & Newman, 1965; Gustavson, 1964; Hall, 1964; Lee & Jackson, 1972; Levinson et al., 1955; Öster, 1953; Wahrman & Fried, 1970) also described the flattening of the nasal bridge at a similar frequency, between 57.4%–86.7%. The hypoplastic nose, in addition to the underdevelopment of the already-mentioned midfacial region, makes the faces of young children with Down syndrome appear flat. This flat facial profile has been emphasized as one of the most frequently observed characteristics (Hall, 1964).

Ears

An abnormal structure and reduction in the size of the ear are common findings in persons with Down syndrome. Aase, Wilson, and Smith (1973) and Thelander and Pryor (1966) reported shortened ears. Lower and oblique implantation of the ears occurring unilaterally or bilaterally have been described in young children with Down syndrome (F. Schmid, 1976). Pueschel (1984) noted that an abnormal structure was observed in 28% and low implantation of ears was found in 16%. The most prominent finding is the overlapping or folding of the helix. This has been reported at a frequency between 28%–78% (Clark et al., 1978; Domino & Newman, 1965; Gustavson, 1964; Hall, 1964; Lee & Jackson, 1972; Levinson et al., 1955; Öster, 1953; Wahrman & Fried, 1970). It is of interest that this slightly broadened and downturned top of the helix has also been noted to occur at a high frequency in "normal" newborns (Holmes, 1976). In addition to the overfolding of the helix, other structural ear anomalies include a prominent antihelix, absent or attached earlobes, and projecting ears (F. Schmid, 1976). Narrow ear canals are very common and have been described by Wallis (1955). Structural aberrations of the middle ear and its ossicles have been reported by Balkany, Mischke, Downs, and Jafek (1979).

(For further discussion of audiologic/otolaryngologic findings, see Dahle & Baldwin, chap. 7, this volume.)

Lips

In the neonatal period, the lips of the infant with Down syndrome are not considered to be abnormal. As the child grows, the lips become more prominent, thickened, and fissured (Benda, 1969). This change with advancing age is probably related to a combination of factors, including the frequently open mouth, protrusion of tongue, and excessive moisture at the lips. During the cold season, the lips may become cracked and chapped. Butterworth, Leoni, Beeman, Wood, and Stern (1960) reported a frequent thickening and white appearance of the membranes of the lips, which later fissured with gradual enlargement. The corners of the mouth are usually turned downward; this was found to be present in 84% of children examined by Wahrman and Fried (1970).

Tongue

As previously mentioned, some persons with Down syndrome keep the mouth open and the tongue protruding. Singh (1976) reported that protrusion of the tongue appears more often in white males (37 out of 38) than in white females (28 out of 33). There is a significant difference in the frequency of tongue protrusion when white males (92%) are compared with black males (67%).

In an attempt to explain the tongue protrusion, it has been postulated that there is an absolute increase in the size of the tongue and that the underdeveloped maxilla, the narrow palate with broadened alveolar ridges, and/or the enlarged tonsils and adenoids cause the oral cavity to be small (Barnes, 1923; Jensen, Cleal, & Yips, 1973). In the newborn with Down syndrome, the tongue is usually smooth, has a normal texture, and does not show significant pathologic changes. However, as the child grows, papillary hypertrophy and fissuring of the tongue are observed. This fissuring and papillary hypertrophy are thought to be due to excessive sucking or chewing of the tongue. Papillary hypertrophy is often noted during the early preschool years, and fis-

suring of the tongue becomes more apparent in the later school years. Although Engler (1949) reported that all persons with Down syndrome over 5 years of age exhibit fissuring of the tongue, a number of children do have normal-appearing tongues (Pueschel, 1984).

Some observers have noted an abnormally large tongue in the person with Down syndrome. Öster (1953) found 57% of children with Down syndrome in his study had enlarged tongues. It is difficult, however, to measure or estimate the exact size of the tongue. Ardron, Harker, and Kemp (1972) assessed the size of the tongue by roentgenologic means. The 8 children in their study did not have a generalized enlargement of the tongue; yet, 5 children had some localized increase in tongue size near the lingual tonsil. The tongue of many children with Down syndrome may appear large because of the relatively small oral cavity. (For discussion of how a large and/or protruding tongue affects the oral health of persons with Down syndrome, see Vigild, chap. 8, this volume.)

Neck

The neck of the child with Down syndrome, especially the newborn, appears to be short and broad. There is sometimes abundant skin and subcutaneous tissue in the posterior neck area in the newborn. The base of the neck will stay broad; however, the increased tissue observed will become less apparent as the child grows older.

Usually, the neck is supple, and there is full range of motion. In those children who have symptomatic atlantoaxial dislocation, torticollis, head tilt, and limited range of motion in the neck area are common features (Pueschel, Scola, Perry, & Pezzullo, 1981; see also Pueschel & Solga, chap. 15, this volume).

Chest

The chest of the child with Down syndrome is usually normally shaped. The rib cage may appear somewhat shortened since some children have only 11 instead of the normal 12 ribs (Beber, 1965; Murray, Sylvester, & Gibson, 1966). An extensive study by Thuline and Islam (1966) found 12th rib anomalies in 26% of females and

15% of males with Down syndrome. Some individuals had complete absence of the 12th rib whereas others had a rudimentary 12th rib unilaterally or bilaterally.

Pectus excavatum has been observed in 18% and pectus carinatum was noted to be present in 11% of children with Down syndrome (Pueschel, 1984). Other investigators also found pectus excavatum in 12% (Levinson et al., 1955) and in 14% (Domino & Newman, 1965) of children with Down syndrome. Pectus carinatum was noted in 40% of children with Down syndrome by Levinson et al., (1955) and in 6% by Domino and Newman (1965). Öster (1953) reported that both pectus excavatum and pectus carinatum were present in 5% of his study population. It is of note that these deformities of the sternum ordinarily do not interfere with respiratory or cardiovascular functions (see Howenstine, chap. 10, this volume). Surgery is usually not indicated since it is only a minor cosmetic defect in the majority of cases.

Abdomen

The abdomen of young children with Down syndrome often appears distended and protuberant, which is thought to be due to the reduced muscle tone. In addition, diastasis recti is frequently observed in the young child with Down syndrome. Levinson et al. (1955) reported diastasis recti in 76% and Domino and Newman (1965) in 87% of children. Umbilical hernias are referred to less often in the literature. Levinson et al. and Domino and Newman reported a 4% and 6% frequency of umbilical hernias, respectively. Pueschel (1984) found a much higher prevalence of umbilical hernias: 89% of infants with Down syndrome had umbilical hernias measuring 2 mm–25 mm in diameter. Benda (1969) recorded umbilical hernias in 90% and Rett (1977) found umbilical hernias in 47% of his patients. This discrepancy among various observers is most likely due to the examination approach used. If one merely describes the hernias noted on super-ficial visual inspection, one will not uncover the majority of hernias, which require careful palpation. Although some umbilical hernias are of impressive size, no surgical intervention is usually needed since a gradual spontaneous involution is observed in the majority of cases (Pueschel, 1984).

Extremities

The extremities of persons with Down syndrome are often described as short, particularly in their distal portions (Benda, 1969). Rett (1977) found that the metacarpals and the phalanges are 10%–30% shorter in children with Down syndrome than in "normal" children. The hands and feet of children with Down syndrome have been described as broad and stubby.

Clinodactyly or brachyclinodactyly is seen in approximately half of the individuals with Down syndrome (Benda, 1969). Pueschel (1984) noted that brachyclinodactyly of the left hand was observed in 51%, and of the right hand in 50% of children with Down syndrome. Similar findings were reported by Roche, Seward, and Sutherland (1961), who found 55% of children to have clinodactyly, and Öster (1953), who noted that 48% of children had brachyclinodactyly.

Brachyclinodactyly is thought to be due to a hypoplastic, slightly wedge-shaped, small middle phalanx of the finger. Garn, Gall, and Nagy (1972) reported a hypoplastic middle phalanx (brachymesophalangia) in 21% of children with Down syndrome, while Roche (1961) found this skeletal abnormality slightly more often (25%). In situations where there is marked brachyclinodactyly, there is usually one crease (90%), instead of the typical two creases (Pueschel, 1984).

The single palmar transverse crease or the four-finger line at the midpalmar surface of the hand have attracted special attention as a diagnostic sign in Down syndrome. However, it should be noted that a single palmar crease is not present in every child with Down syndrome. Reports from the literature have indicated that 42%–64% of children with Down syndrome have a single transverse palmar crease (Clark et al., 1978; Domino & Newman, 1965; Gustavson, 1964; Hall, 1964; Lee & Jackson, 1972; Levinson et al., 1955; Öster, 1953; Wahrman & Fried, 1970). Benda (1969) noted that the single palmar crease occurs in "normal" persons primarily bilaterally, whereas in individuals with Down syndrome, a unilateral single palmar crease is found more often. It is known that in approximately 4%–5% of a "normal" population a single palmar crease is observed either unilaterally or bilaterally (Holmes, 1976).

Partial or complete syndactyly (webbing or fusion of fingers or toes) has also been reported at a higher frequency in children with Down syndrome. In Pueschel's (1984) study, 10.7% of children displayed partial or complete syndactyly at both hands and feet. Hanhart (1960) noted syndactyly between toes in 2.1% and Beckman, Gustavson, and Akesson (1962) observed syndactyly in 11.4% of the children.

Dignan (1973) reported infrequent occurrence of polydactyly in people with Down syndrome. Pueschel and O'Donnell (1974) reported 3 patients with partial adactyly, where the second, third, and fourth digits were absent from one hand only. Since publishing this report on unilateral partial adactyly in persons with Down syndrome, the authors have encountered 4 other persons with this hand malformation.

Short and stubby feet are as common as shortened hands. Short feet were noted in 33% of children with Down syndrome (Pueschel, 1984). A wide space between the first and second toes was recorded in 96% of the children (Pueschel, 1984); in addition, a plantar crease was often found between the first and second toes (94%). This finding was observed by Brushfield in 1924 and has been noted by many other investigators (Clark et al., 1978; Domino & Newman, 1965; Gustavson, 1964; Hall, 1964; Lee & Jackson, 1972; Levinson et al., 1955; Öster, 1953; Wahrman & Fried, 1970).

Benda (1969) mentioned that the third toe is frequently longer than the second toe and that these two toes may be grouped together in a fork-like position. Radial deviation of the third, fourth, and fifth toes, with unusual positioning, is also a common finding in children with Down syndrome. In addition, Hanhart (1960) noted a retroposition of the fourth toe in approximately 10% of his patients.

CONCLUSION

Although Down (1866) described some of the features of children with this chromosome disorder, the delineation of the phenotype took place primarily during the first half of the 20th century. Also, in subsequent decades investigators provided further details of specific characteristics of children with Down syndrome (Clark et al., 1978; Coleman, 1978; Domino & Newman, 1965; Gustavson, 1964; Hall, 1964, 1966; Johnson & Barnett, 1961; Lee & Jackson, 1972; Levinson et al., 1955; Öster, 1953; Pueschel, 1984; Richards, 1965; W. Schmid et al., 1961; Singh, 1976; Strelling, 1976; Wahrman & Fried, 1970).

Since the mid-1970s, however, there have been significant efforts that go beyond the descriptive phase and focus more on the pathogenesis of the observed dysmorphic features and on the search for gene loci at the long arm of chromosome 21 that are responsible for the phenotypic characteristics in trisomy 21. The phenotypic map of Down syndrome (see Figure 1.1) based on molecular analysis of specific duplications on the long arm of chromosome 21 is now emerging from several investigations (Korenberg et al., 1990; McCormick et al., 1988; Rahmani et al., 1989). In a recent international workshop on Genotype–Phenotype Correlations in Down syndrome, protocols were developed that will provide the basis for analyzing and comparing phenotypes and genotypes of individuals with various duplications at the long arm of chromosome 21 (Epstein et al., 1991).

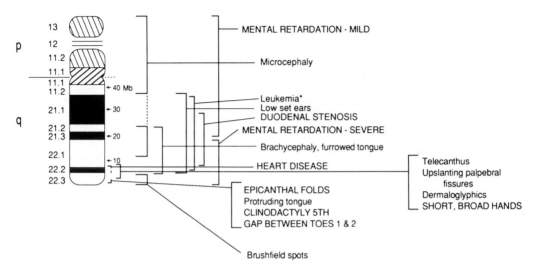

Figure 1.1.   Phenotypic map of Down syndrome: 1973–1989. From molecular mapping of the Down syndrome phenotype by J.R. Korenberg. In D. Patterson, & C.J. Epstein (Eds.), *Progress in clinical and biological research: Vol. 36. Molecular genetics of chromosome 21 and Down syndrome* (p. 109). Copyright © 1990 by John Wiley & Sons, Inc. Reprinted by permission of Wiley-Liss, a division of John Wiley & Sons, Inc.

REFERENCES

Aase, J.M., Wilson, A.C., & Smith, D.W. (1973). Small ears in Down's syndrome: A helpful diagnostic aid. *Journal of Pediatrics, 82,* 845–852.

Ardron, G.M., Harker, P., & Kemp, F.H. (1972). Tongue size in Down's syndrome. *Journal of Mental Deficiency Research, 16,* 160–166.

Balkany, T.J., Mischke, R., Downs, M.P., & Jafek, B.W. (1979). Ossicular abnormalities in Down's syndrome. *Otolaryngology and Head and Neck Surgery, 87,* 372–384.

Barnes, N.P. (1923). Mongolism—Importance of early recognition and treatment. *Annals of Clinical Medicine, 1,* 302–306.

Barr, M.W. (1904). *Mental defectives: Their history, treatment and training.* London: Rebman.

Beber, B.A. (1965). Absence of a rib in Down's syndrome. *Lancet, ii,* 289–290.

Beckman, L., Gustavson, K.H., & Akesson, H.O. (1962). Studies of some morphological traits in mental defectives. *Hereditas, 48,* 105–112.

Benda, C.E. (1969). *Down's syndrome: Mongolism and its management.* New York: Grune & Stratton.

Bersu, E.T. (1980). Anatomical analysis of the developmental effects of aneuploidy in man: The Down syndrome. *American Journal of Medical Genetics, 5,* 399–420.

Brushfield, T. (1924). Mongolism. *British Journal of Childhood Diseases, 21,* 241–244.

Butterworth, T., Leoni, E.P., Beeman, H., Wood, M.G., & Stern, L.P. (1960). Cheilitis of mongolism. *Journal of Investigative Dermatology, 35,* 347–352.

Clark, A.M., Cowell, H.R., McCracken, A.A., & Bennett, W.C.L. (1978). A survey of Down syndrome at the Hospital for the Mentally Retarded, Georgetown, Delaware. *Delaware Medical Journal, 50,* 13–23.

Coleman, M. (1978). Down's syndrome. *Pediatric Annals, 7,* 90–103.

Cronk, C.E., & Pueschel, S.M. (1984). Anthropometric studies. In S.M. Pueschel (Ed.), *A study of the young child with Down syndrome* (pp. 105–141). New York: Human Science Press.

Dignan, P. St. J. (1973). Polydactyly in Down's syndrome. *American Journal of Mental Deficiency, 77,* 486–489.

Domino, G., & Newman, D. (1965). Relationship of physical stigmata to intellectual subnormality in mongoloids. *American Journal of Mental Deficiency, 69,* 541–545.

Donaldson, D.C. (1961). The significance of spotting of the iris in mongoloids. *Archives of Ophthalmology, 65,* 26–28.

Down, J.L. (1866). Observations on an ethnic classification of idiots. *London Hospital. Clinical Lectures and Reports, 3,* 259–262.

Duncan, P.M. (1866). *A manual for the classification, training and education of the feeble-minded, imbecile and idiotic.* London: Longmans, Green & Co.

Engler, M. (1949). *Mongolism (peristatic amentia).* London: Wright.

Epstein, C.J., Korenberg, J.R., Annerén, G., Antonarakis, S.E., Aymé, S., Courchesne, E., Epstein,

L.B., Fowler, A., Groner, Y., Huret, J.L., Kemper, T.L., Lott, I.T., Lubin, B.H., Magenis, E., Opitz, J.M., Patterson, D., Priest, J.H., Pueschel, S.M., Rapaport, S.I., Sinet, P-M., Tanzi, R.E., & de la Cruz, F. (1991). Protocols to establish genotype-phenotype correlations in Down syndrome: Report of a workshop. *American Journal of Human Genetics, 49*, 207–235.

Esquirol, J.E.D. (1838). *Des maladies mentales considerees sous les rapports medical, hygienique et medico-legal* [Mental illness considered by the medical, health, and medical-legal reports]. Paris: Bailliere.

Garn, S.M., Gall, J.C., Jr., & Nagy, J.M. (1972). Brachymesophalangia-5 without cone-epiphysis mid-5 in Down's syndrome. *American Journal of Physical Anthropology, 36*, 253–255.

Gerald, B.E., & Silverman, F.C. (1965). Normal and abnormal interorbital distances with special reference to mongolism. *American Journal of Roentgenology, 95*, 154–161.

Gustavson, K.H. (1964). *Down's syndrome: A clinical and cytogenetical investigation.* Uppsala, Sweden: Almqvist and Wiksell.

Hall, B. (1964). *Mongolism in newborns—A clinical and cytogenetic study.* Lund: Berlingska Boktryckeriet.

Hall, B. (1966). Mongolism in newborn infants. An examination of the criteria for recognition and some speculations on the pathogenic activity of the chromosomal abnormality. *Clinical Pediatrics, 5*, 4–12.

Hanhart, E. (1960). 800 fälle von mongoloidismus in konstitutioneller betrachtung [Clinical features of 800 cases with mongolism]. *Archiv der Julius Klaus-Stiftung, Vererbungsforschung und Sozialanthropologische Rassenhygiene, 35*, 1–16.

Holmes, L.B. (1976). *The malformed newborn: Practical perspectives.* Boston: Massachusetts Developmental Disabilities Council.

Jensen, G.M., Cleal, J.F., & Yips, A.S.G. (1973). Dentoalveolar morphology and developmental changes in Down's syndrome (trisomy 21). *American Journal of Orthodontics, 64*, 607–611.

Johnson, C.D., & Barnett, C.D. (1961). Relationship of physical stigmata to intellectual status in mongoloids. *American Journal of Mental Deficiency, 66*, 435–437.

Korenberg, J.R. (1990). Molecular mapping of the Down syndrome phenotype. In D. Patterson, & C.J. Epstein (Eds.), *Progress in clinical and biological research: Vol. 360. Molecular genetics of chromosome 21 and Down syndrome* (p. 109). New York: Wiley-Liss.

Korenberg, J.R., Kawashima, H., Pulst, S.M., Ikeuchi, T., Ogasawara, N., Yamamoto, K., Schonberg, S.A., Kojis, T., Allen, L., Magenis, E., Ikawa, H., Taniguchi, N., & Epstein, C.J. (1990). Molecular definition of the region of chromosome 21 that causes the classical Down syndrome phenotype. *American Journal of Human Genetics, 47*, 236–246.

Lee, L., & Jackson, J. (1972). Diagnosis of Down's syndrome: Clinical vs. laboratory. *Clinical Pediatrics, 11*, 353–356.

Levinson, A., Friedman, A., & Stamps, F. (1955). Variability of mongolism. *Pediatrics, 16*, 43–49.

Lowe, R. (1949). Eyes in mongolism. *British Journal of Ophthalmology, 33*, 131–174.

McCormick, M.K., Schinzel, A., Peterson, M.B., Mikkelsen, M., Driscoll, D.J., Cantu, E.S., Stetten, G., Watkins, P.C., & Antonarakis, S.E. (1988). Molecular genetic characterization of the "Down syndrome region" of chromosome 21. *American Journal of Human Genetics, 43*, A90.

Murray, J.B., Sylvester, P.E., & Gibson, J. (1966). Rib absence in Down's syndrome. *Lancet, i*, 1375.

Öster, J. (1953). *Mongolism: A clinico-geneological investigation comprising 526 mongols living in Seeland and neighboring islands of Denmark.* Copenhagen: Danish Science Press.

Preus, M. (1977). A diagnostic index for Down syndrome. *Clincal Genetics, 12*, 47–55.

Pueschel, S.M. (1984). *A study of the young child with Down syndrome.* New York: Human Science Press.

Pueschel, S.M. (1990). *A parent's guide to Down syndrome: Toward a brighter future.* Baltimore: Paul H. Brookes Publishing Co.

Pueschel, S.M., & O'Donnell, P. (1974). Unilateral partial adactyly in Down's syndrome. *Pediatrics, 54*, 466–469.

Pueschel, S.M., Scola, F.H., Perry, C.D., & Pezzullo, J.C. (1981). Atlantoaxial subluxation in children with Down syndrome. *Pediatric Radiology, 10*, 129–132.

Purtscher, E. (1958). Knotenförmige verdichtungen im irisstroma bei mongolismus [Knot-like structures in the iris in mongolism]. *Von Graefes Archiv der Ophthalmologie, 160*, 200–203.

Rahmani, Z., Blouin, J.L., Creau-Goldberg, N., Watkins, P.C., Mattei, J.F., Poissonnier, M., Prieur, M., Chettough, A.N., Aurias, A., Sinet, P-M., & Delabar, J-M. (1989). Critical role of the D21S55 region on chromosome 21 in the pathogenesis of Down syndrome. *Proceedings of the National Academy of Sciences of the United States of America, 86*, 5958–5962.

Rett, A. (1977). *Mongolismus* [Mongolism]. Bern: Huber.

Richards, B.W. (1965). The diagnosis of Down syndrome. *Developmental Medicine and Child Neurology, 7*, 286–288.

Roche, A.F. (1961). Clinodactyly and brachymesophalangia of the fifth finger. *Acta Paediatrica, 50*, 387–389.

Roche, A.F., Roche, P.J., & Lewis, A.B. (1972). The cranial base in trisomy 21. *Journal of Mental Deficiency Research, 16*, 7–20.

Roche, A.F., Seward, F.S., & Sutherland, S. (1961). Nonmetrical observations on cranial roentgenograms in mongolism. *American Journal of Roentgenology, 84,* 659–662.

Schmid, F. (1976). *Das Mongolismus-Syndrom* [The mongolism syndrome]. Muensterdorf: Hansen and Hansen.

Schmid, W., Lee, C.H., & Smith, P.M. (1961). At the borderline of mongolism. *American Journal of Mental Deficiency, 64,* 449–455.

Seguin, E. (1846). *Le traitement moral, l'hygiene et l'education des idiots* [The moral treatment, hygiene and education of idiots]. Paris: Bailliere.

Seguin, E. (1866). *Idiocy and its treatment by the physiological method.* New York: Wood.

Singh, D.M. (1976). Down's syndrome: A study of clinical features. *Journal of the National Medical Association, 68,* 521–524.

Solomons, G., Zellweger, H., Jahnke, P.G., & Opitz, E. (1965). Four common eye signs in mongolism.

American Journal of Diseases of Children, 110, 46–50.

Strelling, M.K. (1976). Diagnosis of Down's syndrome at birth. *British Medical Journal, 2,* 1386–1389.

Thelander, H.E., & Pryor, H.B. (1966). Abnormal patterns of growth and development in mongolism: An anthropometric study. *Clinical Pediatrics, 5,* 493–498.

Thuline, H., & Islam, A.R. (1966). Absence of a rib in Down's syndrome. *Lancet, i,* 1156–1157.

Tredgold, R.F. (1908). *Mental deficiency (amentia).* London: Bailliere, Tindall, and Cox.

Wahrman, J., & Fried, K. (1970). The Jerusalem Prospective Newborn Survey of Mongols. *Annals of the New York Academy of Science, 171,* 341–360.

Wallis, H.R.E. (1955). The diagnosis of mongolism in infancy: Small auditory meatus. *British Medical Journal, 1,* 30–32.

CHAPTER
2

Dermatoglyphics

Horace C. Thuline

Dermatoglyphs describe the patterns and systems of lines formed by epidermal ridges. This strict definition has been broadened in clinical application to include the flexion creases and other secondary folds of the areas with ridged skin on the volar surfaces of the hands and feet (Holt, 1968). Dermatoglyphics refers to the study of dermatoglyphs and may be done directly from the skin or from prints or other reproductions made of the ridged skin.

The clinical use of ridged skin patterns of fingers, palms, and soles for the diagnosis of Down syndrome has given way to the more powerful methods of cytogenetic and molecular genetic analyses. However, it would not be appropriate to omit the subject of dermatoglyphics in a discussion of Down syndrome since it is of phenotypic importance.

TYPES OF RIDGE PATTERNS

Ridge patterns of the fingertips and toes are described as arch, loop, or whorl (Figure 2.1). The loop is further identified as to whether the open end of the pattern is directed toward the ulnar or radial side of the finger. Palm and sole patterns are described as to form (open fields, loops, and whorls), location on the palm or sole (thenar, hypothenar, interdigital area, hallucal), and exit direction of lines from palm or sole (ulnar, radial, tibial, fibular), as seen in Figures 2.2–2.5.

Essential to the definition of arch, loop, and whorl patterns is the triradius, which is the point where three ridge systems meet (Figure 2.1). Ideally, the angle between adjacent ridge systems in forming the triradius would be 120°, but angles from 90°–180° may be accepted in the same triradius. Two triradii are basic to the definition of a whorl, one triradius is required for a loop, and the arch has no true triradius. There are many variations on these basic themes, and the reader is referred to Penrose (1968) and Schaumann and Alter (1976) for more details.

The mainline is another characteristic described for ridge patterns. This is the ridge that originates in a triradius of the palm or sole, then courses across the palm or sole to exit at a border of the ridged skin surface, or reverses to form a loop. Mainlines are described as to transversality and whether they form loops.

Ridge count is also an element used to describe ridge patterns. This involves a count of the number of ridges crossed by a line drawn between the triradius and the core of a pattern (Figure 2.1). It gives a measure relating to ridge width and intensity of patterns.

HISTORICAL ASPECTS

Scientific interest in ridged skin was traced back to at least 1684 by Cummins and Midlo (1961). The anatomists of the 1700s described dermal ridges, but the accepted landmark report is that of Purkinje (1823/1940), who developed a systematic classification of fingerprint patterns. In the 1860s and 1870s, Europeans observed that fingerprints are unique and useful for identification of individuals. By the 1890s, systems of identification by fingerprinting were introduced; modern methods of analysis are based on this early work. Interests in ridged skin patterns as possible genetic and racial characteristics grew with the general interest in genetics that developed after 1900.

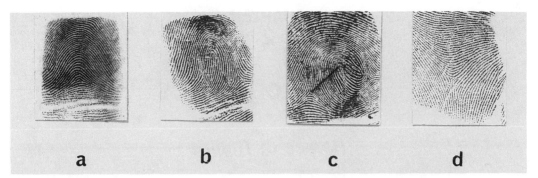

Figure 2.1. Fingertip dermatoglyph patterns. Illustrated are the three basic patterns seen in all patterned areas of ridged skin: (a) an arch, no triradius; (b) a loop, one triradius; and (c) a whorl, two triradii (the line drawn in the figure is used to determine a "ridge-count"). A triradius is illustrated in (d). In each case, the ulnar side of the print is on the left, the radial side on the right.

Efforts to quantitate dermatoglyphs for genetic studies began in the 1920s (Cummins & Midlo, 1926), and, by the late 1930s, ridge patterns had been characterized in terms of height, depth, ridge count, and angular measurements. Use of this quantitative approach for the study of Down syndrome resulted in independent confirmation of the characteristic patterns for Down syndrome by Cummins (1939) and Workman (1939). In summarizing the data up to 1943, Cummins and Midlo (1961) recorded the distinct features of dermatoglyphs in persons with Down syndrome as:

- Hypothenar patterns
- Central location of the palmar axial triradius
- Alteration in size and complexity of thenar/first interdigital patterns
- Increased frequency of second and third interdigital patterns with reduction in frequency of fourth interdigital patterns
- Transverse coursing of palmar mainlines
- Reduction in bimanual symmetry of ridge direction
- Increased proportion of ulnar loops with decrease in whorls on fingertips
- Shift for maximum frequency of radial loops

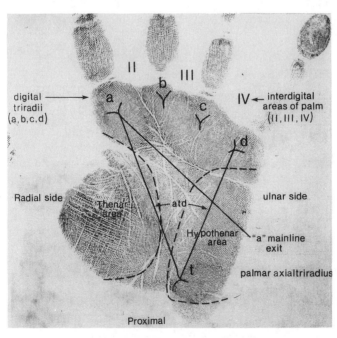

Figure 2.2. Normal palm (contact print of right hand) with significant features identified.

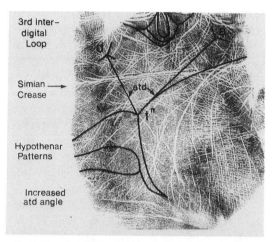

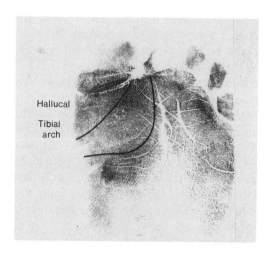

Figure 2.3. Tape-lifted print of right hand in person with Down syndrome showing four features commonly found: simian crease (four finger line), third interdigital area loop pattern, hypothenar area with patterning, and increased atd angle.

Figure 2.5. Tape-lifted print of left sole illustrating the common arch tibial pattern seen in the hallucal area in persons with Down syndrome.

from the second digit to the fourth and fifth digits
- Frequent presence of a single palmar crease

Cummins and Platou (1946) and Cummins, Talley, and Platou (1950) reported an 85% correlation of two dermatoglyphic features, transversality of distal palmar ridges and large hypothenar patterns, with the phenotype of Down

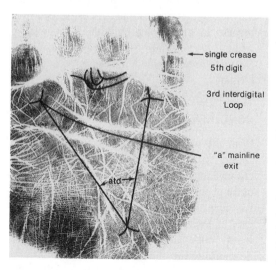

Figure 2.4. Tape-lifted print of left hand in person with Down syndrome showing presence of abnormal (single flexion crease in fifth digit, distal exit of "a" mainline, third interdigital area loop pattern) and normal (palmar crease and atd angle) dermatoglyphic features.

syndrome. This use of two items was a move toward the concept of an index.

DEVELOPMENT OF DERMATOGLYPHIC INDICES

Walker (1957a, 1957b, 1958) used dermatoglyphs as an "objective" method to diagnose Down syndrome. She developed the concept that, for given features, the observed frequency in control and Down syndrome populations constitutes a ratio. This ratio could be used as an index of the probability for a given individual to have or not to have Down syndrome. By using the observed frequencies for each of 8 items on both hands (16 in all) for 540 controls and 150 individuals with Down syndrome, she arrived at ratios of pattern frequencies in Down syndrome versus controls. To make these ratios easier to use, they were changed to their logarithms, which was called a probability for Down syndrome. Combining the probabilities for 16 variables gave a single score or index for an individual. This Walker index had a distribution for individuals with Down syndrome that did not overlap that of 70% of control individuals. Conversely, the distribution of the index for controls did not overlap that for persons with Down syndrome in 76%. Thus, the Walker index for Down syndrome would have a 70% probability of clearly confirming the diagnosis of Down syndrome, but in 30% of individuals the score would be in the control range and therefore inconclusive.

After cytogenetic verification of Down syndrome became common, Borgaonkar, Davis, Bolling, and Herr (1967, 1971) developed a scoring method based on the principles of predictive discrimination. They examined 15 dermatoglyphic features from each side of 106 individuals without Down syndrome (controls) and from 106 individuals with cytogenetically verified Down syndrome. The ratio for frequency of specific features found in the two populations studied was analyzed using likelihood ratio statistics to derive a sum of positive and negative logarithmic values, which they termed the "log odds score." This method of scoring dermatoglyphs achieved 96.6% correct discrimination for individuals between the two groups. This approach was refined further by combining the scores for given features from right and left sides into a single score for the feature examined. Analysis as done for the log odds score then produced 97.7% correct discrimination for the same original data. This was reported by Bolling, Borgaonkar, Herr, and Davis (1971), who called it the "Hopkins Combined Score." For more detailed information about these methods, the reader is referred to the original reports.

In Europe, Greyerz-Gloor, Auf der Maur, and Riedwyl (1969) reported a dermatoglyphic index based on 24 items. The nearly complete discrimination between individuals with Down syndrome and controls appears to be the result of virtually no overlap in the values for "atd" angles between their test and control populations. (An abnormal atd angle is illustrated in Figure 2.3.) This index has not been used for reports in the United States, probably because it appeared after cytogenetics had become widely available for diagnosis.

The easiest method for diagnostic use of dermatoglyphics for Down syndrome is the nomogram reported by Reed, Borgaonkar, Conneally, and Yu (1970). The use of stepwise regression analysis reduced the number of dermatoglyphic features analyzed from the 30 reported by Borgaonkar et al. (1971) to 14. Further evaluation by Reed, Christian, and Nance (1971) showed that only 4 of the 14 features were contributing the major portion of the discriminatory power in the analysis. Using patterns of these four locations (the right hallucal area, right and left index fingers, and right atd angle), a nomogram was constructed that gave an 80% confidence level for the diagnosis of Down syndrome. This is less accurate than the Hopkins Combined Score, but it is less complex to use. The nomogram has been produced by Indiana University School of Medicine as the "Down Syndrome Dermatogram."

A more elaborate method for distinguishing several chromosome disorders by means of discriminant functions derived from dermatoglyphs was reported by Penrose and Loesch (1971a, 1971b). This method has not been widely used.

The latest dermatoglyphic index for Down syndrome was published in a series of papers by Deckers (1974) and Deckers, Oorthuys, and Doesburg (1973a, 1973b). These authors also selected variables for discriminating capacity, as had Reed et al. (1970), and used four right–left pairs (eight variables in all) to construct their "Radboud" score.

Reed and Christian (1976) compared the Dermatogram score, Hopkins and composite score, the Radboud score, and the Walker index for 119 individuals with Down syndrome. Although they found that none of the indices were entirely precise in classifying individuals as with or without Down syndrome, the ease of use of the Dermatogram justified its use in the original format.

CONCLUSION

With the wide availability of cytogenetic procedures to assist the clinician in confirming the clinical diagnosis of Down syndrome, the importance of dermatoglyphics for diagnostic purposes has been minimized to a marked degree. However, in those situations where cytogenetic studies are not available, dermatoglyphics may still be useful to the clinician. If Down syndrome is suspected, the physician can determine whether there is a distally placed palmar axial triradius in either hand, whether there is a tibial arch pattern in the hallucal area of a sole, and whether all or most of the fingertip patterns are ulnar loops. With these positive dermatoglyphic findings, common for a majority of individuals with Down syndrome, the probability of the clinical diagnosis being correct will increase significantly.

REFERENCES

Bolling, D.R., Borgaonkar, D.S., Herr, H.M., & Davis, M. (1967). *Evaluation of dermal patterns in Down's syndrome by predictive discrimination.* Toronto: American Society of Human Genetics, Program and Abstracts.

Borgaonkar, D.S., Davis, M., Bolling, D.R., & Herr, H.M. (1967). *Evaluation of dermal patterns in Down's syndrome by predictive discrimination.* Toronto: American Society of Human Genetics, Program and Abstracts.

Borgaonkar, D.S., Davis, M., Bolling, D.R., & Herr, H.M. (1971). Evaluation of dermal patterns by predictive discrimination. I. Preliminary analysis based on frequencies of patterns. *Johns Hopkins Medical Journal, 28,* 141–152.

Cummins, H. (1939). Dermatoglyphic stigmata in mongoloid imbeciles. *Anatomy Records, 73,* 407–415.

Cummins, H., & Midlo, C. (1926). Palmar and plantar epidermal ridge configurations (dermatoglyphics) in European-Americans. *American Journal of Physiology and Anthropology, 9,* 471–502.

Cummins, H., & Midlo, C. (1961). *Finger prints, palms and soles: An introduction to dermatoglyphs.* New York: Dover.

Cummins, H., & Platou, R.V. (1946). Mongolism: Objective early sign. *Southern Medical Journal, 39,* 925.

Cummins, H., Talley, C., & Platou, R.V. (1950). Palmar dermatoglyphs in mongolism. *Pediatrics, 5,* 241–248.

Deckers, J.F.M. (1974). [Letter]. *Clinical Genetics, 6,* 237.

Deckers, J.F.M., Oorthuys, M.A., & Doesburg, W.H. (1973a). Dermatoglyphs in Down's syndrome: I. Evaluation of discriminating ability of pattern areas. *Clinical Genetics, 4,* 311–317.

Deckers, J.F.M., Oorthuys, M.A., & Doesburg, W.H. (1973b). Dermatoglyphs in Down's syndrome: III. Proposal of a simplified scoring method. *Clinical Genetics, 4,* 381–387.

Greyerz-Gloor, R.D.V., Auf der Maur, P., & Riedwyl, H. (1969). Beurteilung des diagnostichen Wertes der Finger—und Handleistenmerkmale von Mongoloiden unter Anwendung einer Diskrimineirungsanalyse [Assessment of diagnostic use of finger and hand dermatoglyphs of mongoloids by use of discriminant analysis]. *Humangenetik, 8,* 195–207.

Holt, S.B. (1968). *The genetics of dermal ridges.* Springfield, IL: Charles C Thomas.

Penrose, L.S. (1968). Memorandum on dermatoglyphic nomenclature. In *Birth Defects Original Article Series, IV*(3). New York: National Foundation–March of Dimes.

Penrose, L.S., & Loesch, D. (1971a). Dermatoglyphic patterns and clinical diagnosis by discriminant functions. *Annals of Human Genetics, 35,* 51–60.

Penrose, L.S., & Loesch, D. (1971b). Diagnosis with dermatoglyphic discriminants. *Journal of Mental Deficiency Research, 15,* 185–195.

Purkinje, J.E. (1823). Commentatio de examine physiologico organi visus et systematis cutanei [External physiological examination of the integumentary system]. Thesis, University Press of Breslau. (English translation [1940] by H. Cummins & R.W. Kennedy, *American Journal of Criminal Law and Criminology, 31,* 343–356.)

Reed, T.E., Borgaonkar, D.S., Conneally, P.M., & Yu, P. (1970). Dermatoglyphic nomogram for the diagnosis of Down's syndrome. *Journal of Pediatrics, 77,* 1024–1032.

Reed, T.E., & Christian, J.C. (1976). A comparison of the Dermatogram with other indices for the diagnosis of Down's syndrome. *Clinical Genetics, 10,* 139–144.

Reed, T.E., Christian, J.C., & Nance, W.E. (1971). Diagnosis of mongolism with a dermatoglyphic nomogram. *Southern Medical Journal, 64,* 70–72.

Schaumann, B., & Alter, M. (1976). *Dermatoglyphics in medical disorders.* New York: Springer Verlag.

Walker, N.F. (1957a). The use of dermal configurations in the diagnosis of mongolism. *Journal of Pediatrics, 50,* 19–26.

Walker, N.F. (1957b). Inkless method of finger, palm, and sole printing. *Journal of Pediatrics, 50,* 27–29.

Walker, N.F. (1958). The use of dermal configurations in the diagnosis of mongolism. *Pediatric Clinics of North America, 5,* 531–543.

Workman, G. (1939). *A study of the palmar dermatoglyphics of mongoloid idiots.* Unpublished thesis, University of Toronto.

CHAPTER 3

Growth

Christine E. Cronk and Göran Annerén

Growth is an important measure of health and developmental progress during the childhood years. In addition, size and body conformation throughout childhood and the adult years influence lifestyle choices, activity patterns, and health. This chapter reviews the characteristics of growth and size in individuals with Down syndrome, and considers some of the mechanisms that might be responsible for these abnormalities. The discussion of growth characteristics is presented by periods of development (prenatal through adolescence), with primary attention given to infancy growth. Special attention is given to issues of overweight. Each of the possible mechanisms or contributors to growth retardation is considered. Finally, recommendations for how to approach growth assessment are provided.

PRENATAL GROWTH

Until the broad clinical use of ultrasound, most data on prenatal growth in fetuses with Down syndrome came either from birth size in newborn infants of varying gestational ages or data on abortuses. Smith and McKeown (1956) found a difference of about 0.3 kg between the average weight of their Down syndrome sample ($n = 103$) and that of "normal" controls. This difference was due in part to differences in gestational age, but their data also suggested that values were significantly less than the mean, commencing at about 38 weeks of gestational age. These findings were corroborated in studies by Kučera and Dolezalova (1973) and Papp, Adam, and Szabo (1976).

Marmol, Scriggins, and Vollman (1969) found a 220 g difference, controlling for hospital, race, maternal age, and time of conception, in a cohort of infants with Down syndrome followed in the Perinatal Collaborative Project. Using this same data set, Ershow (1986) found a difference in birth size between black and white infants with Down syndrome. This difference disappeared after maternal cigarette consumption and maternal weight at delivery were controlled. As with "normal" newborns, infants with Down syndrome born to mothers smoking 10 or more cigarettes per day weighed about 345 g less and were 1 cm shorter than infants with mothers having low or no cigarette use. The deficit introduced by maternal cigarette use persisted throughout childhood to 7 years of age in this group of children.

Pueschel, Rothman, and Ogilby (1976) matched their sample with a control sample of siblings and found that the mean birth weight for infants with Down syndrome (3.07 kg) was significantly less (using a paired comparison) than that for their siblings (3.52 kg), even when adjusting for gestational age, birth order, and maternal age. These authors concluded that growth retardation was associated with the presence of the extra chromosome and was independent of other possibly confounding factors.

Few studies have directly evaluated birth length of a large sample of infants with Down syndrome, and comments from studies including small numbers of newborns have been contradictory. For example, Roche (1965) examined data from early studies of Brousseau and Brainerd (1928), Benda (1946), and Öster (1953) and suggested that birth length was well below the normal range. However, the total number of infants in the combined samples was less than 30, and some infants from the Öster sample were stillborn. Using data from the same sample evaluated in Pueschel et al. (1976), Cronk and Pueschel (1984) found that average birth lengths reported in hospital birth records were slightly, though significantly, less than those for a "normal" control group (48.9 cm for infants with Down syndrome versus 50 cm for "normal" infants). However, when infants with Down syndrome having a gestational age of less than 38 weeks were excluded from the analysis, there was no difference in birth length.

Ultrasound studies have provided data on longitudinal growth of fetuses with Down syndrome who reach birth. Kurjak and Kirkinen (1982) evaluated 8 fetuses with trisomy 21 using serial cephalometry and measurements of abdomen and head-to-abdomen ratio from 16 through 38 weeks of gestation. They found normal biparietal diameters in all of the fetuses, but slightly reduced body dimensions. It is noteworthy that the typical brachycephalic conformation of the skull in individuals with Down syndrome, if manifest prenatally, would lead to normal findings for biparietal diameter. Ultrasound studies have suggested that fetal femur length is slightly shortened compared to reference values, though values are within 2 SD of the norm (Benacerraf, Gelman, & Frigoletto, 1987).

In a study of radiographically or directly measured long bones (femur, tibia, fibula, ulna, radius, and humerus) of a sample of abortuses with Down syndrome, Fitzsimmons and colleagues (1989) found that most values were within 2 SD of the control mean, but with a tendency for all values to cluster at the low end of the normal distribution. This finding was statistically significant by sign test and was more marked for upper than for lower extremities. The authors concluded that there is growth retardation of the long bones that is subtle and more marked in the upper extremities. Because of small sample sizes at various gestational ages, they were unable to detect the time of onset of reduced long bone growth.

In summary, it appears that prenatal growth of fetuses with Down syndrome is slightly reduced compared to normal. Birth weight is slightly less

than normal even when gestational age, parity, maternal age, and genetic determinants of size are controlled. The weight difference of newborns with Down syndrome probably arises during the third trimester of pregnancy when fat accumulation accounts for the greatest percentage of weight gain. Linear growth during fetal life also appears to be slightly reduced. Age of onset of the linear growth deficit is uncertain.

POSTNATAL GROWTH

Postnatal shortness of stature has been a clearly identified associate of Down syndrome from the earliest studies. The nature of the postnatal growth deficit in infancy and childhood was not well understood until the 1970s and 1980s, when longitudinal data on home-reared children became available. Indeed, adequate longitudinal data for childhood and adolescence are still lacking.

Early Studies of Growth Over the Life Cycle

Studies of growth and size of individuals with Down syndrome agree that by adulthood, stature is reduced by an average of about two standard deviations (i.e., is less than 5th percentile) (Benda, 1939, 1946; Dutton, 1958; Gustavson, 1964; Öster, 1953; Rarick & Seefeldt, 1974; Roche, 1965). The earliest studies of institutionalized individuals have suggestd that the largest growth deficits occur in the first years of life. Benda (1939) maintained that growth was lower than normal in the first 5 years but normal from about 8 years onward. Dutton (1958) estimated the curve of growth for boys with Down syndrome 6–18 years by computing the percentage of average adult stature achieved at each age. He concluded that progress of growth during the entire period he studied was similar to that for "normal" boys, thus partially supporting Benda's (1939) assertion. Gustavson (1964) and Roche (1965) evaluated the average number of standard deviations below the mean for various age groups of individuals with Down syndrome. In general, these data indicated deficits of nearly 2 SD (less than 5th percentile) by 2 years of age, with varying deficits of up to 4 SD between 2 years and adulthood. Roche (1965) found no difference in the degree of deficit between the sexes in his sample. In addition, there was a greater range of variation in size for the Down syndrome sample than for his "normal" controls.

Roche (1965) and Rarick and Seefeldt (1974) also analyzed serial records focusing on the period of 10–18 years of age. Roche (1965) found that most (36 of 41) of his sample experienced an adolescent growth spurt (i.e., growth velocity of greater than 5 cm/year). Rarick and Seefeldt found that their sample was already more than 2 *SD* below the mean at 10 years, with few individuals within the normal range of variation. This group had greater variability than "normal" adolescents in size. Their growth velocity during the period of observation differed only slightly from normal (about 0.5 cm/yr less).

Growth During Infancy

The longitudinal study of infants with Down syndrome carried out at the Children's Hospital of Boston, 1970–1976, forms the basis for most of the following statements on infancy and early childhood growth (Cronk, 1978; Cronk & Pueschel, 1984; Pueschel, 1984). The sample consisted of about 100 home-reared infants followed from birth to age 3 years (some until age 7 years), at 3- and then 6-month intervals until 3 years and

then yearly thereafter. (References are also made to other studies.)

Recumbent Length/Height

Figures 3.1 and 3.2 present the curve of growth for height for the sample of children followed at Children's Hospital of Boston from birth to 3 years compared with mean values for the National Center for Health Statistics sample (Hamill, Johnson, Reed, Roche, & Moore, 1979). At birth, length and weight were slightly, though statistically significantly, different from "normal" infants (≤ 1 cm in each sex). From birth to 3 years, there was a progressive decline in average recumbent length relative to "normal" controls. At 3 months, the absolute difference between the Down syndrome and "normal" mean was about 2 cm (-0.9 *SD* or at about the 15th percentile). By 3 years, the absolute difference in the means was about 3.5 cm (-2.5 *SD* or at about the 1st percentile). Variability (i.e., total range of variation from smallest to largest individuals) was broader in the children with Down syndrome, as can be seen from the slightly larger *SD* bars on Figures 3.1 and 3.2 for the children with Down syndrome. In this respect, boys with Down syndrome were more variable than "normal" boys throughout the age range

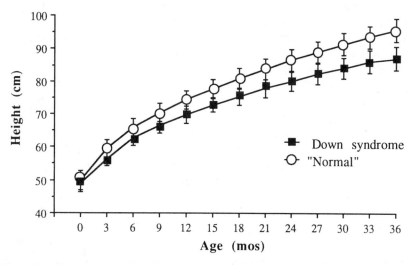

Figure 3.1.   Mean height (recumbent length) (cm) birth to 36 months for girls from the Children's Hospital of Boston sample (Cronk, 1978) compared with age- and sex-specific mean (±*SD*) from National Center for Health Statistics (Hamill, Johnson, Reed, Roche, & Moore, 1979).

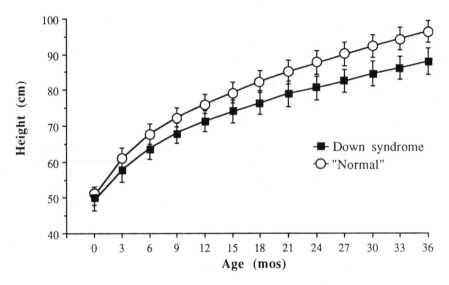

Figure 3.2.   Mean height (recumbent length) (cm) birth to 36 months for boys from the Children's Hospital of Boston sample (Cronk, 1978) compared with age- and sex-specific mean (±SD) from National Center for Health Statistics (Hamill, Johnson, Reed, Roche, & Moore, 1979).

birth to 36 months, whereas girls with Down syndrome had variability similar to "normal" girls beginning at about 9 months of age.

As these data indicate, growth rate for length in children during all 6-month intervals from birth to 36 months was reduced by about 1 *SD* (around the 10th – 25th percentile). For the full 36 months, the average child with Down syndrome grew 38.2 cm (*SD* 4.05 cm, range 28.2–47.5 cm), whereas the average "normal" child grew 46 cm during this same period.

Individual children manifested deficient growth in different ways. About 70% had deficient growth in all intervals from birth to 36 months of age, and these children were always outside the range of normal size by the end of infancy. About 30% showed intermittent normal growth velocity punctuated with periods of deficient growth relative to "normal" children. Only about 10% had growth velocity within the normal range throughout this period, and these children were often between the 3rd–50th percentile for "normal" children at 3 years. It should be noted that growth deficiency in length was often so marked that periods of "no growth" (i.e., growth undetectable because it is within measurement error for recumbent length or height) lasting 3–6 months were not uncommon. Cronk and Reed (1981) speculated that the stop-and-go quality of growth

in these children might be evidence of poor canalization of growth and a possible destabilizing effect of the extra chromosome 21. However, recent studies (Cronk, Stallings, Spender, Ross, & Widdoes, 1989; Hermanussen, Geiger-Benoit, Burmeister, & Sippell, 1988; Lampl & Emde, 1983) have shown that "normal" children also grow sporadically over the short term (i.e., 1 week to 1 month). It is therefore alternatively possible that growth in Down syndrome is simply a slower (and also ultimately deficient) process as has been suggested by Cicchetti and Sroufe (1976) for cognitive and emotional development in these children.

Weight

Mean values for weight from birth to 36 months for boys and girls with Down syndrome from the Children's Hospital of Boston sample compared with the National Center for Health Statistics reference data are shown in Figures 3.3 and 3.4, respectively. These values and those for weight velocity mirrored those for length. Absolute differences between Down syndrome and control data at 3 months were a little less than 1 kg (−1 *SD* or about the 10th percentile). By 3 years, the difference was 3 kg in each sex (− 2 *SD* or less than the 3rd percentile). Velocity of weight gain was deficient for all intervals between 6–18

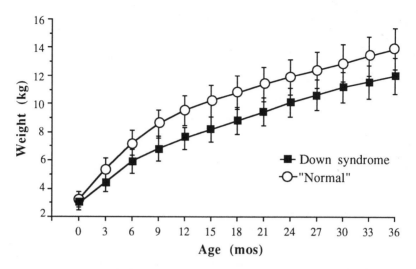

Figure 3.3. Mean weight (kg) birth to 36 months for girls from the Children's Hospital of Boston sample (Cronk, 1978) compared with age- and sex-specific mean (±*SD*) from National Center for Health Statistics (Hamill, Johnson, Reed, Roche, & Moore, 1979).

months when weight gain was 22% less than expected for "normal" children. Between 18–36 months, velocity was not different from average. (Issues relating to the relationship of weight and length are discussed in the section "Overweight in Children with Down Syndrome.")

Head Circumference and Other Dimensions

Figures 3.5 and 3.6 show mean values ±*SD* for head circumference for the Children's Hospital of Boston sample, birth to 3 years for each sex, compared with the National Center for Health Statistics data. Growth in head circumference is also deficient for children with Down syndrome during infancy. At 3 months, average head circumference for infants with Down syndrome (about 38 cm) is already about 1.5 cm less than "normal" controls. By 36 months, the difference is slightly greater than 3 cm (46 cm for Down syndrome versus 50 cm for controls). When head circumference was plotted against length, however, values were within the normal range, suggesting that head circumference deficit is primarily a reflection of small body size rather than

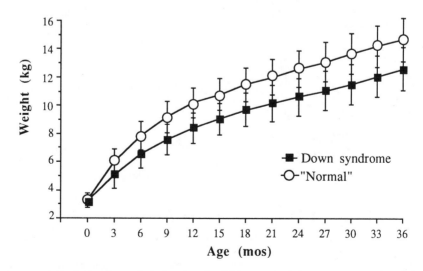

Figure 3.4. Mean weight (kg) birth to 36 months for boys from the Children's Hospital of Boston sample (Cronk, 1978) compared with age- and sex-specific mean (±*SD*) from National Center for Health Statistics (Hamill, Johnson, Reed, Roche, & Moore, 1979).

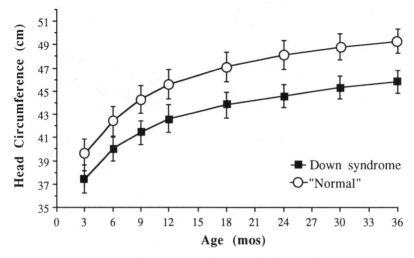

Figure 3.5.   Mean head circumference (cm) birth to 36 months for girls from the Children's Hospital of Boston sample (Cronk & Pueschel, 1984) compared with age- and sex-specific mean (±SD) from National Center for Health Statistics (Hamill, Johnson, Reed, Roche, & Moore, 1979).

an abnormally small brain size. Indeed, the primary deficit in head size is in head length. Head length reflects growth at the cranial base, which grows under the same controls as the postcranial body, whereas growth in head breadth is more closely related to brain size and growth. The differential deficiency in growth of head length leads to the characteristic brachycephalic head shape.

The best study of the external head dimensions was reported by Roche and co-workers (1961). They evaluated about 150 individuals with Down syndrome, ranging from birth to adulthood. They found that both head breadth (the largest lateral diameter of the head) and head length (measured from nasion to the largest length across the occiput) were not different from "normal" control values from birth to age 1 year. Beginning between 6 months and 1 year, mean values for each dimension were significantly less than those for "normal" infants. For head breadth, the deficit was about 1 *SD*, whereas

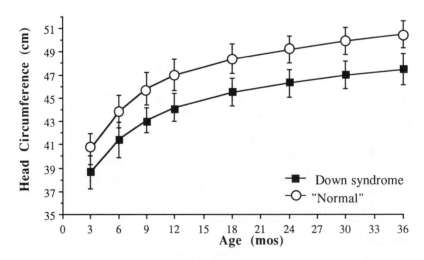

Figure 3.6.   Mean head circumference (cm) birth to 36 months for boys from the Children's Hospital of Boston sample (Cronk & Pueschel, 1984) compared with age- and sex-specific mean (±SD) from National Center for Health Statistics (Hamill, Johnson, Reed, Roche, & Moore, 1979).

for head length it was as much as 3 *SD*, suggesting that growth was much more markedly reduced at cranial base than in elements contributing to the growth of head breadth.

Factors Affecting Growth in Infancy

For the Children's Hospital sample, a number of factors with potential influence on infancy growth were evaluated, including gestational age at birth, presence of significant congenital heart disease, and genetic endowment for body size.

Gestational Age At birth and at 3 months, average length and weight for infants born before 38 weeks of gestational age (range 31–38, $n = 22$) were significantly smaller than children with gestational age $\geq$ 38 weeks. The difference disappeared by 6 months of age, thus indicating that, as in "normal" prematurely born infants, preterm infants with Down syndrome have faster growth velocity in very early infancy than their full-term age peers.

Cardiac Disease As with otherwise "normal" infants with congenital heart disease, children who have Down syndrome and a significant cardiac defect grow and gain weight more slowly during infancy. In the Children's Hospital of Boston sample, the absolute size differences between children with moderate and severe congenital heart disease and those with mild or no congenital heart disease increased from less than 1 cm near birth to around 2.5 cm by 3 years of age. Growth velocity differences were small but consistent (0.3–0.6 cm per 6 months) until about 30 months of age, after which velocity in both groups was similar. Average weight of children with significant congenital heart disease was also lower than children with mild or no cardiac problems, though weight velocity in the two groups did not differ consistently across the age interval. Ershow (1986) also observed an effect from cardiac disease in the Perinatal Collaborative Project sample of children with Down syndrome. Deficits in these children were restricted to weight. However, she evaluated differences between children with any heart defect and those without disease.

It should be noted that effects of surgical correction on growth were not evaluated in the Chil-

dren's Hospital of Boston data, nor have they been reported elsewhere. This and developmental amelioration of the defect may account for the lack of differences at older ages between children with and without significant congenital cardiac disease.

Genetic Endowment for Size A small group of parents and siblings from the Children's Hospital of Boston sample were measured, and standard scores for their heights were compared with height at age 3 years for children with Down syndrome. Correlations were low and statistically not significant for parent size. A statistically significant but modest association was apparent with sibling height ($r = 0.40$, $p < 0.05$, $n = 34$). This supports the contention that genetic endowment for size is weakly manifest in growth of children with Down syndrome, and perhaps (as with "normal" children) should be considered in growth assessment.

Growth After Infancy

Whereas there are adequate cross-sectional data on growth during childhood and adolescence, no study has been carried out carefully following a series of children at frequent intervals to allow generalizations about growth velocity after infancy. Figures 3.7 and 3.8 summarize available data on cumulative height from ages 4 to 18 years for four different data sets, along with values from the National Center for Health Statistics data (Hamill et al., 1979). The means for "normal" children and children with Down syndrome appear to be similar until about 11 or 12 years of age for girls, and 15 or 16 years of age in boys. After these ages, the distance between the "normal" and Down syndrome curves is larger.

Growth During Childhood

Using mixed longitudinal data on institutionalized children, Roche (1965) found stature to be reduced by 2–4 *SD* below the mean for all ages 3–10 years. This reduction did not differ from *SD* values computed for stature/recumbent length for children 1–3 years of age. Roche's (1965) data agreed with data from the studies of Brousseau and Brainerd (1928), Benda (1946), Öster (1953), and Gustavson (1964).

Ikeda, Higurashi, Hirayama, and Ishikawa

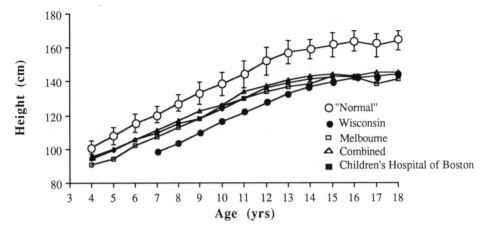

Figure 3.7. Height (cm) for 4–18 years for four samples of girls with Down syndrome: Children's Hospital of Boston (Cronk, unpublished observation); Wisconsin (Rarick & Seefeldt, 1974); Combined (Cronk et al., 1988); Melbourne (Roche, 1965); and "Normal" (National Center for Health Statistics; Hamill, Johnson, Reed, Roche, & Moore, 1979).

(1977) followed a small group of Japanese home-reared children with Down syndrome from infancy to 4 years. Figure 3.9 shows standard scores for the means in each sex for this sample. A decline in scores is evident until about 30 months, after which values are similar (about 3 SD below the control group mean) through 48 months of age. In this sample, growth velocities were intermittently deficient (though always similar to "normal" children) prior to 36 months of age. Six-month velocities for intervals after 36 months were usually lower than normal. These findings are somewhat in agreement with those of Roche (1965) and earlier works. However, the pattern of early childhood growth

velocities suggests that some children in this sample were still growing deficiently after 4 years of age.

Ershow's (1986) data from the Perinatal Collaborative Project study included height and weight at 7 years for 12 girls and 19 boys. Reduction below the National Center for Health Statistics mean was between 2–3 SD for height and around 0.5 SD for weight for this small group. At 12 months (the closest earlier measurement), these children had mean values reduced by about 1.5 SD (similar to the reduction observed in the Children's Hospital of Boston sample). Longitudinal data collected by Rarick and Seefeldt (1974) included a small number of institutional-

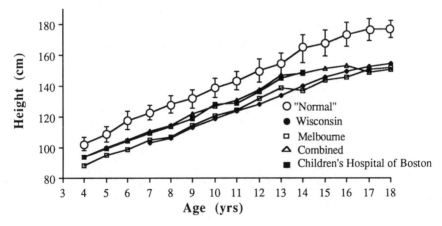

Figure 3.8. Height (cm) for 4–18 years for four samples of boys with Down syndrome: Children's Hospital of Boston (Cronk, unpublished observation); Wisconsin (Rarick & Seefeldt, 1974); Combined (Cronk et al., 1988); Melbourne (Roche, 1965); and "Normal" (National Center for Health Statistics; Hamill, Johnson, Reed, Roche, & Moore, 1979).

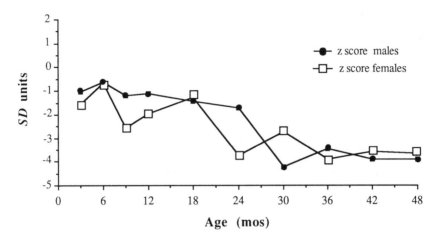

Figure 3.9. Mean z scores for height for children 3–48 months (Ikeda, Higurashi, Hirayama, & Ishikawa, 1977).

ized children ages 7–10 years. At 7 years, the stature of these children was reduced by 3–4 *SD* and did not appear to change across this 3-year age interval. These data, taken in concert with other infancy and childhood growth data just discussed, suggest maintenance of a similar level of growth retardation from the end of infancy through mid-childhood.

Using mixed longitudinal data gathered from three East Coast centers, Cronk et al. (1988) found that from 2 to about 11.5 years, girls with Down syndrome were around 2 *SD* below the National Center for Health Statistics mean with minor fluctuations (-1.51 to -2.49 *SD*) depending upon the age. For the same period, boys were also about 2 *SD* reduced below the National Center for Health Statistics mean, with a tendency for values to fall between -2 and -3 *SD* (-2.3 to -3 *SD*). Reductions for weight were substantially less, ranging from -1.2 to 0 *SD* (i.e., average weight equal to that for "normal" children). It is notable that children included in this data set showed more normal growth than did institutionalized children included in the samples of Roche (1965), Rarick and Seefeldt (1974), and earlier studies cited. Pseudovelocities (i.e., rate of gain computed by subtracting an earlier from a later mean value) showed that in each sex, velocity was between the 3rd and 25th percentile for males, and between the 3rd and 50th percentile in females for height growth. For weight in each sex, pseudovelocities were

usually the 25th – 50th percentile with excursions at some ages up to the 75th percentile.

A subset of children from the Children's Hospital of Boston study were followed intermittently during childhood. Sample sizes ranged from 43 seen at 4 years to only 6 seen at 10 years of age. Figure 3.10 shows mean 6-month velocity from birth through 10 years for the Children's Hospital of Boston sample and for reference data from the Fels Institute study (Baumgartner, Roche, & Himes, 1986). Error bars show the standard deviation for this reference group. For both the Down syndrome and the reference samples, mean values for the two sexes are combined. From this graph, it is clear that velocity of growth is less than normal at least until 8 years of age. These findings are in agreement with the pseudovelocities extracted from the Cronk et al. (1988) study and reinforce the observation that growth through at least mid-childhood is slow in children with Down syndrome. This is corroborated by the observation of Rarick, Wainer, Thissen, and Seefeldt (1975) that the prepubertal component of growth curves fitted using the double logistic function contributed importantly to the difference between the final height of children with Down syndrome in their sample as compared with "normal" controls.

Growth During Adolescence

As with childhood values, means for both sexes are reduced by 2–4 *SD* below the normal mean

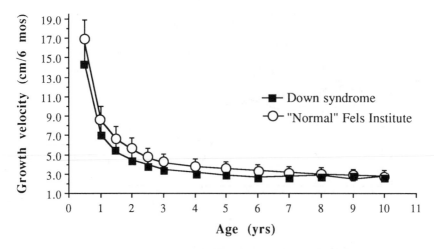

Figure 3.10.   Mean growth velocity (cm/6 months) birth to 10 years for children from the Children's Hospital of Boston sample (Cronk, 1978) contrasted with mean ±SD for the Fels Institute sample (Baumgartner, Roche, & Himes, 1986).

throughout the adolescent years in all of the samples plotted on Figures 3.7 and 3.8. The means are similar for males and females for the whole period. In each sex, values for the two institutionalized samples (Rarick & Seefeldt, 1974; Roche, 1965) are significantly lower than the Children's Hospital of Boston sample. This difference amounts to between 7–12 cm in males throughout this period. At the end of adolescence, however, means for all of the Down syndrome samples appear to converge at a similar level between −3.5 and −4 SD below the normal mean. It is possible that home-reared children have a nutritional and/or emotional advantage throughout the childhood growing period, such that an individual's final height is achieved earlier. Pseudovelocities for the various samples suggest that growth rate is generally in the lower percentiles (25th–50th percentile) for normal in each sex.

Roche (1965) found that 90% of the group of children he followed through adolescence experienced an adolescent growth spurt (annual height increment ≥4 cm). Maximum increments ranged from 5 cm to about 13 cm per year, which is similar to normal, and these spurts occurred at roughly similar age ranges to those of "normal" adolescents. Cessation in height growth for Roche's (1965) sample occurred significantly earlier than in "normal" adolescents (15.5 years,

range 13.9–18 years in boys; 14.3 years, range 12.1–16 years in girls). Bone ages at the time of growth cessation were not fully mature.

Rarick and Seefeldt (1974) were able to demonstrate less growth in the period 10–18 years using an ANOVA with "normal" control data. They found that growth of boys with Down syndrome was significantly lower than "normal" adolescents during this age interval, whereas growth during this period in girls with Down syndrome was not different from "normal" girls in their control sample. When they subdivided the full period into two shorter ones (10–14 years and 14–18 years), they found that in later puberty, girls with Down syndrome actually had significantly greater growth than "normal" girls, suggesting the occurrence of a later pubertal growth spurt in girls. Further analyses suggested that continued late growth was in the upper segment (as measured by sitting height). There was, however, not a parallel finding for boys.

Maximum annual height velocity was 7.83 cm for boys with Down syndrome (compared with 9.14 cm for "normal" boys), and 6.61 for girls (compared with 7.83 cm for "normal" girls). The age of maximum growth was similar in adolescents with Down syndrome (11.8 years for girls and 13.79 years for boys) and "normal" adolescents (12 years for girls and 14 years for boys). However, analyses using double logistic curves fitted to the Down syndrome and control data indicated that, on average, the growth spurt for both boys and girls with Down syndrome occurred 1 year later than for "normal" adolescents (Rarick et al., 1975). Using data on body water determined from deuterium oxide dilution, Culley, Chilko, and Coburn (1974) determined that boys with Down syndrome begin their adolescent growth spurts at a shorter average height than "normal" boys.

Secondary Sex Characteristics

There are little data on timing of maturation and appearance of secondary sex characteristics in children with Down syndrome. Roche (1965) found the mean menarcheal age of girls in his sample (13 years) to be slightly later than "normal" girls. Rundle (1970) found that menarcheal age and breast and pubic hair stages were slightly delayed in girls with Down syndrome. Pueschel (1987) reported that the average age of menarche was 12½ years, that menstrual periods occurred at normal intervals (average 27 days), and were of normal duration (4 days). Moreover, physiological symptoms (headache, mood swings, abdominal bloating) similar to those in "normal" girls occurred in two thirds of the sample.

Secondary sex characteristics in males with Down syndrome were found to be similar to those in "normal" males in Pueschel, Orson, Boylan, and Pezzullo (1985). However, development of axillary and facial hair (particularly hair on the upper lip) was delayed compared to normal. Testicular volume and penile length did not differ from "normal" controls. These investigators also found that changes of hormone levels including follicle-stimulating hormone, luteinizing hormone, and testosterone during the adolescent period were similar to those of "normal" adolescents (see also Pueschel & Blaymore Bier, chap. 22, this volume).

OVERWEIGHT IN CHILDREN WITH DOWN SYNDROME

Although clinical and observational evidence for overweight in children with Down syndrome had been available for some time, only unsystematic

documentation of its occurrence in these children was available until the 1980s. Brousseau and Brainerd (1928) and Benda (1939) noted a lack of uniformity in weight/height relationships and a tendency to be overweight for height.

Data on three samples, two institutionalized (the Melbourne sample originally reported by Roche, 1965; and the Wisconsin sample originally reported by Rarick & Seefeldt, 1974) and one home-reared sample (the Children's Hospital of Boston sample) were analyzed for evidence of overweight (Chumlea & Cronk, 1982). Sex- and age-specific medians for body mass index (weight ÷ height^2), a convenient and valid measure of overweight (Roche, Siervogel, Chumlea, & Webb, 1981), in these three samples were compared to those for a sample of "normal" children. Beginning at about 2 years of age, children with Down syndrome in all three groups had greater median values than the control group. These values were equivalent to between the 75th and 90th percentile values for normal at some ages between 2–12 years. After 12 years, median values for the two institutionalized samples were not different from those for the controls. However, clearly at these ages the timing of the adolescent growth spurt and the expected increase in total body fatness accompanying puberty probably obscures the continued propensity for overweight in these children.

Using the same data sets, Cronk, Chumlea, and Roche (1985) also compared weight for 5-cm height intervals by sex to control data, as shown in Figures 3.11 and 3.12. Values were clearly above those for "normal" children beginning at about the 100-cm interval for height (around 4–6 years of age). Values remained above the normal mean for all the remaining intervals. There was evidence that institutionalized children have a greater propensity for overweight than those who are home reared.

Cronk and Howard (1977) evaluated data from the first 36 months of life for the Children's Hospital of Boston sample for age of onset of overweight in specific children using three indices of overweight (weight ÷ height^2, weight ÷ height^3, and weight for height relationship). About 30% of the 90 children in this sample were ≥1 SD

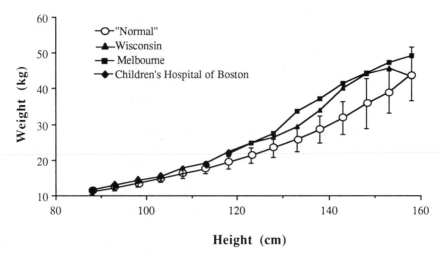

Figure 3.11. Mean weight (kg) for height (cm) for three samples of girls with Down syndrome: Children's Hospital of Boston (Cronk, Chumlea, & Roche, 1985); Wisconsin (Rarick & Seefeldt, 1974); Melbourne (Roche, 1965); and "Normal" (National Center for Health Statistics; Hamill, Johnson, Reed, Roche, & Moore, 1979).

above the normal mean for at least one of these indices sometime in the first 3 years of life. The mean age of onset of overweight was 20 months, and the largest percentage of these children became overweight in the 2nd year of life.

The etiology of overweight in children with Down syndrome has not been adequately investigated. Studies assessing nutrient intake are inconclusive with regard to this issue. Culley,

Goyal, Jolly, and Mertz (1965) analyzed intakes of 23 institutionalized children 5–12 years of age with trisomy 21. Only three children had "stocky" builds (relative weight >110%) and each child consumed adequate calories per centimeter of body stature, although the total caloric intake was less than normal for age. Calvert, Vivian, and Calvert (1976) reported the dietary intakes of 40 home-reared children with trisomy

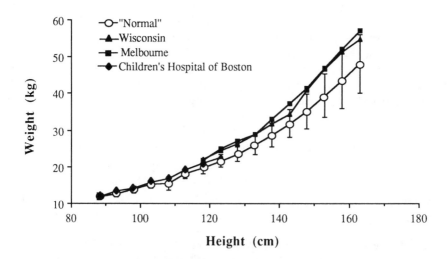

Figure 3.12. Mean weight (kg) for height (cm) for three samples of boys with Down syndrome: Children's Hospital of Boston (Cronk, Chumlea, & Roche, 1985); Wisconsin (Rarick & Seefeldt, 1974); Melbourne (Roche, 1965); and "Normal" (National Center for Health Statistics; Hamill, Johnson, Reed, Roche, & Moore, 1979).

21 between 1–12 years old. The caloric intake of more than 50% of these children was less than normal, and fewer than 25% exceeded recommended daily caloric intake by more than 50%. Calvert et al. did not state how the recommended intake was assessed (i.e., by age, cm of body stature, or kg of body weight) or the relationship of the anthropometric data to the dietary data. In a third study by Madsen (1979), 26 home-reared children with trisomy 21 between 3.4–26.5 months of age had three 3-day food diaries. No differences in kcal per cm of body height or kg of body weight were evident between this sample and control data. The relationships between caloric intake and ponderal index were not analyzed.

Several other factors causing overweight in "normal" individuals may play a part in its etiology in children with Down syndrome. The hypotonia characteristic of the syndrome is often associated with decreased activity. Delay in achievement of motor milestones typical in these children may also contribute to limitation of activity during infancy. Finally, limitation of gross motor performance may decrease activity during childhood and adolescence when "normal" children participate in active play and organized sports.

Using multiple regression analysis, Cronk and Howard (1977) evaluated associates of obesity measures in the Children's Hospital of Boston sample. About 25% of the variation in ponderal index at 3 years was explained by a combination of muscle tone, age of walking, and growth velocity. Children with poor muscle tone, late walking age, and slower growth velocity tended to have higher ponderal indices, and were probably overweight.

Overweight also may be related to poorly synchronized body composition development that is, in turn, secondary to the presence of the additional chromosome. The average pace of growth in infancy differs for height and weight, with deficiencies in height velocity outpacing those for weight velocity within the first 2 years of life. Finally, the range of endocrine and metabolic abnormalities characteristic of the syndrome may contribute to the presence of overweight (Cronk & Chumlea, 1985).

GROWTH OF BODY SEGMENTS

A small number of studies have evaluated growth of lateral and segmental dimensions of children with Down syndrome allowing assessment of proportionality of growth. Both Rundle (1970) and Thelander and Pryor (1966) evaluated the relative retardation of sitting height and height, and found greater deficiency in lower body growth than in upper body growth. Rarick, Rapaport, and Seefeldt (1966) studied tibial length in persons with Down syndrome ages 7–18 years, and found mean values were 4 years below normal at the beginning of this period.

The best studies demonstrating disproportionality of growth are those of Ikeda et al. (1977) and Rarick and Seefeldt (1974). Ikeda et al. found that the upper limb length/stature and lower limb length/stature ratios of children with Down syndrome were significantly different at most ages from 3–48 months, indicating disproportionately short limbs. In contrast, the intermembral index (upper limb/lower limb) was similar to that of "normal" children. Rarick and Seefeldt found the ratio of sitting height to height to be significantly different from normal in their sample of 7–18 year olds, demonstrating the relatively shorter leg lengths of these children at all ages. Sex differences and age changes in the ratio of sitting height to height were not, however, different from normal in this group.

SKELETAL MATURATION

Maturation as measured by bone age using hand and wrist radiographs is a useful index of biologic age. Using the Greulich and Pyle (1959) standards, children from the Children's Hospital of Boston sample had a bone age of about 17 ± 6 months at 24 months, whereas at 36 months the average bone age was 28 ± 7 months. These values are about 1 and 2 *SD* below the mean, respectively. The variability for bone ages of children with Down syndrome was similar to that for "normal" children. When analyzed categorically, about 75% had retarded, 9% had advanced, and 16% had normal bone ages at 24 or 36 months. Most children who had bone age evaluations at both ages showed enhanced skeletal retardation at the later assessment. In general, findings from other studies of skeletal maturation in children with Down syndrome are in accordance with these findings.

After infancy, Roche (1967) observed that skeletal maturation levels rose with relation to normal from about 4 through about 10 years of age. During this time, children with Down syndrome have bone age delays of 1.5–2 years (about −1 SD below the normal mean). After 10 years, he found the average values to remain similar through the end of the growing period. Observations of Rarick et al. (1966) indicated that mean skeletal age levels increased through middle childhood, with average skeletal age levels retarded by 3 years from 7–9 years of age, but only by 1 year for children 12–14 years old. They also observed marked variability among children, with 67% of boys and 72% of girls more than 2 SD below the normal mean for age.

ETIOLOGY OF POOR GROWTH IN DOWN SYNDROME

A large number of potential factors may cause poor growth and slowed development in children with Down syndrome. Some factors are known, such as abnormalities of the growth hormone/insulin-like growth factor system (Annerén, Gustavson, Sara, & Tuvemo, 1990), hypothyroidism (Pueschel & Pezzullo, 1985) and celiac disease (Similä & Kokkonen, 1990). It is also probable that genes mapped within the Down syndrome–specific segment of chromosome 21 and coding for growth-regulating factors are responsible for the growth retardation. These genes might also underlie the developmental delay in individuals with Down syndrome. At present, however, no known genes for growth factors or receptors of growth-regulating systems are mapped on chromosome 21.

Growth Retardation— A Gene Dosage Effect?

The distal segment of the long arm of chromosome 21 is responsible for the Down syndrome phenotype (Hagemeijer & Smit, 1977; Neibuhr, 1974). This Down syndrome–specific segment contains the genes, which in triplicate constitute gene-dosage effects that give rise to the features of Down syndrome. In spite of the fact that no growth-regulating genes have yet been mapped on chromosome 21, gene coding for growth-regulating proteins may play a part in the growth retardation observed in individuals with Down syndrome. In addition, overproduction of certain proteins encoded by otherwise normal genes on the Down syndrome–specific segment may distort the delicate balance of biochemical pathways essential to proper development and function of the organs affected in Down syndrome (Epstein, 1986). The resulting destabilization of developmental processes may disrupt the integrity of the growth process, which depends upon the coordination of many different underlying developmental processes (Barden, 1983; Cronk & Reed, 1981; Shapiro, 1975).

Growth Hormone in Down Syndrome

The onset of the greatest growth deficiency for children with Down syndrome is at 6 months, the age at which growth comes under the regulation of growth hormone. Serum levels of growth hormone have been reported to be normal in children with Down syndrome (Milunsky, Lowy, Rubenstein, & Wright, 1968; Ruvalcaba, Thuline, & Kelley, 1972). Torrado and Castells (1991) and Castells, Torrado, and Gelato (1991) recently reported poor response of serum growth hormone to dopamine and clonidine, and decreased physiological growth hormone secretion in 5 children with Down syndrome. They suggested that hypothalamic dysfunction may underlie growth retardation. Annerén, Sara, Hall, and Tuvemo (1986) found normal growth hormone secretion during sleep and after arginine-insulin-loading tests. An evaluation of 24-hour serum secretion of growth hormone in children with Down syndrome showed a pattern of few but normal peaks, typical in "normal," healthy children with short stature. This suggests that a partial hypothalamic dysfunction and delayed maturation of the hypothalamus might underlie growth retardation in children with Down syndrome.

Insulin-Like Growth Factors

Abnormal serum patterns of insulin-like growth factors have been found in persons with Down syndrome. The receptor levels for insulin-like growth factors and insulin (Sara et al., 1984) as well as serum levels of insulin-like growth factor-II (Annerén, Enberg, & Sara, 1984) are normal in Down syndrome. From 2 years of age, persons with Down syndrome demonstrate a serum deficit in insulin-like growth factor-I, which fails to increase during childhood and adolescence (Sara, Gustavson, Annerén, Hall, & Wetterberg, 1983). A radioreceptor assay for insulin-like growth factor-I and -II revealed scarcely any activity in the fetal circulation (Sara, Hall, Rodeck, & Wetterberg, 1981). By contrast, such hormone levels are elevated throughout postnatal life (Sara et al., 1983).

Persons with Down syndrome appear to have a selective deficiency of insulin-like growth factor-I. The elevated serum levels of radioreceptor assay insulin-like growth factor found postnatally in persons with Down syndrome could be explained by the presence of a variant form of fetal insulin-like growth factor-I in the circulation long after birth. There may be a delayed maturation of the insulin-like growth factor system in Down syndrome, with an incomplete switching from production of the fetal form of insulin-like growth factor-I to the growth hormone–regulated insulin-like growth factor-I (Annerén et al., 1990). This might be explained by a hypothalamic dysfunction and thereby a partial growth hormone deficiency (see also Pueschel & Blaymore Bier, chap. 22, this volume).

It has been shown that healthy children with short stature respond to human growth hormone therapy with increased growth velocity and increased serum levels of insulin-like growth factor-I (Hayek & Peake, 1981; Rudman et al., 1981). It was therefore of interest to study the effect of human growth hormone treatment on children with Down syndrome. Five short children with Down syndrome, with normal endogenous production of growth hormone and thyroid hormones, were treated with human growth hormone for 6 months (Annerén et al., 1986). The serum levels of both insulin-like growth factor-I and insulin-like growth factor-II increased to normal and the growth velocity increased from a mean of 2.5 cm per 6 months before human growth hormone treatment to 4.8 cm per 6 months during the human growth hormone treatment period in all 5 children. Skeletal maturation did not accelerate as a result of the treatment.

An ongoing study was initiated in 1989 to evaluate whether human growth hormone therapy of young children with Down syndrome can result in normalization of body growth and improve mental development (Annerén, 1991). From the age of 6–9 months, 16 children with Down syndrome have been treated for a period of 3 years with standard doses of human growth hormone. No results concerning mental development have yet been obtained. Preliminary results after 2 years of human growth hormone treatment reveal normal growth velocity in all 16 children compared to healthy, "normal" children.

In conclusion, growth retardation, retarded skeletal maturation, and serum insulin-like growth factor-I deficit in individuals with Down syndrome could be explained by a partial deficit of growth hormone on the basis of a hypothalamic dysfunction or delay in maturation of the growth hormone/insulin-like growth factor system. Children with Down syndrome are thought to respond to human growth hormone therapy (see also Pueschel & Blaymore Bier, chap. 22, this volume).

GROWTH ASSESSMENT OF CHILDREN WITH DOWN SYNDROME

Assessment of growth in children with Down syndrome requires careful anthropometric measurement, thorough recording of relevant medical history and intercurrent information, and the use of growth charts for "normal" children and those specific to children with Down syndrome.

Anthropometric Measurements

The reader is referred to Lohman, Roche, and Martorell (1988) for description and illustration of appropriate measurement technique. Recumbent length should be used for children less than 3 years of age and should be taken on a measuring table with a fixed headpiece and movable footpiece. Standing height should be taken with equipment that is fixed to the wall with a movable headpiece. The sliding bar available on most beam balance scales is inappropriate and inaccurate. Head measurements should be taken with plastic, fiber glass, or metal tape. All measurements should be repeated at least once and the average of the replicates used.

Normal Growth Charts

The National Center for Health Statistics growth charts are preferred (Hamill et al., 1979) for height, weight, head circumference, and height-for-weight. Detailed information for computing standard scores can be obtained from Frisancho (1990). Measurements should always be plotted on normal growth charts or assessed using standard scores so that the child's status relative to normal is known. This is particularly important where obesity and failure to thrive are of concern, because reference data for children with Down syndrome were developed from small, nonrandom samples. Thus, values at outlying percentiles may indeed represent pathologic states.

Charts for Children with Down Syndrome

Charts for height and weight for children 1–36 months, and 2–18 years are available from Castle Mead Publications (12 Little Mundells, Welwyn Garden City, Herts AL7 1EW, England). Values for weight-for-length can be obtained from Cronk, Chumlea, and Roche (1985). Charts for head circumference are available from Palmer et al. (1992).

Medical and Background History

There are several possible mechanisms underlying the growth retardation in Down syndrome, some of which are easy to treat (e.g., hypothyroidism and celiac disease). For this reason, it is important to exclude these disorders in every child with Down syndrome, especially when growth retardation is present. Neonatal screening for congenital hypothyroidism, as well as yearly investigations of thyroid-stimulating hormone and thyroxine levels is recommended

(Pueschel & Pezzullo, 1985). For the same reason, serum levels of gliadin antibodies should be assayed if there are signs of decreased growth velocity and/or gastrointestinal problems, such as diarrhea or constipation.

It is important to note the presence of heart or other major organ disease. Children with significant major medical problems will not grow well. Frequent lower respiratory tract infections as well as other serious infectious illnesses may affect growth in children with Down syndrome as they do in all children. Finally, it is important to note parental size, even though the relationship between size of family members and children with Down syndrome is weaker than that usually observed in the general population. It should be assumed that children with taller parents have a greater genetic potential for larger size.

CONCLUSION

Growth in children with Down syndrome differs from normal growth beginning prenatally. Beginning during the second or third trimester of fetal life, length and weight of fetuses with Down syndrome are slightly less than normal. During infancy, deficits in length, weight, and head circumference gain are most marked, being reduced by as much as 25% from normal growth rates. By the age of 3 years, children with Down syndrome are on average smaller than 90% of "normal" children. Growth during mid-childhood is closer to normal growth, with only small deficits in growth rate. At adolescence, young persons with Down syndrome tend to have smaller pubertal growth spurts than normal. Most adolescents with Down syndrome have normal development of secondary sex characteristics. Average final height for adults with Down syndrome is reduced by 2 SD from the mean for "normal" adults. Weight gain during late infancy and during childhood and adolescence is often excessive relative to gains in height during development. As a consequence, individuals with Down syndrome are often overweight.

The etiology of growth retardation in individuals with Down syndrome is multifactorial. It is partially due to the multiple abnormalities in endocrine and metabolic systems that are in turn related to the presence of the extra genetic material. Insulin-like growth factors are specifically known to be abnormal.

Clinical assessment of growth in children with Down syndrome should include accurate, carefully taken measurements that are then plotted both on growth charts for children with Down syndrome and growth charts for "normal" children. Careful medical history and intercurrent illness assessment is essential to evaluate whether growth failure beyond that usually associated with Down syndrome is present.

Despite encouraging preliminary work, treatment of growth retardation in children with Down syndrome with human growth hormone is not generally recommended at this time. Before treatment with this potent hormone can be recommended for children with Down syndrome, careful investigation must be made of the long-term effects and possible side effects.

REFERENCES

Annerén, G. (1991). Unpublished raw data. Uppsala, Sweden.

Annerén, G., Enberg, G., & Sara, V.R. (1984). The presence of normal levels of serum immunoreactive insulin-like growth factor 2 (IGF-2) in patients with Down's syndrome. *Uppsala Journal of Medical Sciences, 89,* 274–278.

Annerén, G., Gustavson, K-H., Sara, V.R., & Tuvemo, T. (1990). Growth retardation in Down syndrome in relation to insulin-like growth factors and growth hormone. *American Journal of Medical Genetics Supplement, 7,* 59–62.

Annerén, G., Sara, V.R., Hall, K., & Tuvemo, T. (1986). Growth and somatomedin responses to growth hormone in children with Down's syndrome. *Archives of Disease in Childhood, 61,* 48–52.

Barden, H. (1983). Growth and development of selected hard tissues in Down syndrome: A review. *Human Biology, 55,* 539–576.

Baumgartner, R.N., Roche, A.F., & Himes, J.H. (1986). Incremental growth tables: Supplementary to previously published charts. *American Journal of Clinical Nutrition, 43,* 711–722.

Benacerraf, B.R., Gelman, R., & Frigoletto, F.D. (1987). Sonographic identification of second trimester fetuses with Down's syndrome. *New England Journal of Medicine, 317,* 1371–1376.

Benda, C.E. (1939). Studies in mongolism: Growth and physical development. *Archives of Neurological Psychiatry, 41,* 83–95.

Benda, C.E. (1946). *Mongolism and cretinism.* New York: Grune & Stratton.

Brousseau, K., & Brainerd, H.G. (1928). *Mongolism.* Baltimore: Williams & Wilkins.

Calvert, S.D., Vivian, V.M., & Calvert, G.P. (1976). Dietary adequacy, feeding practices and eating and behavior of children with Down's syndrome. *Journal of the American Dietetic Association, 69,* 152–156.

Cartlidge, P.H.T., & Curnock, D.A. (1986). Specific malabsorption of vitamin B12 in Down's syndrome. *Archives of Disease in Childhood, 61,* 514–515.

Castells, T., Torrado, C., & Gelato, M.C. (1991). Growth hormone (GH) responses to GH-releasing hormone (GH-RH) suggest hypothalamic dysfunction as a cause for growth retardation in Down syndrome (DS) [Abstract]. *Pediatric Research, 29,* 75A.

Chumlea, W.C., & Cronk, C.E. (1982). Overweight among children with trisomy 21. *Journal of Mental Deficiency Research, 25,* 275–279.

Cicchetti, D., & Sroufe, L.A. (1976). The relationship between affective and cognitive development in Down's syndrome infants. *Child Development, 47,* 920–926.

Cronk, C.E. (1978). Growth of children with Down's syndrome: Birth to age 3 years. *Pediatrics, 61,* 564–568.

Cronk, C.E., & Chumlea, W.C. (1985). Obesity in trisomy 21. *Trisomy 21, 1,* 19–26.

Cronk, C.E., Chumlea, W.C., & Roche, A.F. (1985). Assessment of overweight in children with trisomy 21. *American Journal of Mental Deficiency, 89,* 433–436.

Cronk, C.E., Crocker, A.C., Pueschel, S.M., Shea, A.M., Zackai, E., Pickens, G., & Reed, R.B. (1988). Growth charts for children with Down syndrome: 1 month to 18 years of age. *Pediatrics, 81,* 102–110.

Cronk, C.E., & Howard, R.B. (1977, April). *Excess weight for length relations in Down syndrome children.* Paper presented at the 46th annual meeting of the American Association of Physical Anthropologists, Seattle.

Cronk, C.E., & Pueschel, S.M. (1984). Anthropometric studies. In S.M. Pueschel (Ed.), *The young child with Down syndrome* (pp. 105–142). New York: Human Science Press.

Cronk, C.E., & Reed, R.B. (1981). Canalization of growth in Down syndrome. *Human Biology, 53,* 383–398.

Cronk, C.E., Stallings, V.A., Spender, Q.W., Ross, J.L., & Widdoes, H.D. (1989). Measurement of short term growth with the knee height measuring device. *American Journal of Human Biology, 1,* 421–428.

Culley, W., Chilko, J., & Coburn, S. (1974). Body water content of boys with Down's syndrome. *Journal of Mental Deficiency Research, 18,* 25–29.

Culley, W.J., Goyal, K., Jolly, D.H., & Mertz, E.T. (1965). Calorie intake of children with Down's syndrome (mongolism). *Journal of Pediatrics, 66,* 772–775.

Dutton, G. (1958). The physical development of mongols. *Archives of Disease in Childhood, 34,* 46–50.

Epstein, C.J. (1986). *The consequences of chromosome unbalance: Principles, mechanisms and models.* New York: Cambridge University Press.

Ershow, A.G. (1986). Growth in black and white children with Down syndrome. *American Journal of Mental Deficiency, 90,* 507–512.

Fitzsimmons, J., Droste, S., Shepard, T.H., Pascoe-Mason, J., Chinn, A., & Mack, L.A. (1989). Longbone growth in fetuses with Down syndrome. *American Journal of Obstetrics and Gynecology, 161,* 1174–1177.

Frisancho, A.R. (1990). *Anthropometric standards for the assessment of growth and nutritional status.* Ann Arbor: University of Michigan Press.

Greulich, W.W., & Pyle, I. (1959). *Radiographic atlas of skeletal development of the hand and wrist.* Stanford, CA: Stanford University Press.

Gustavson, K.H. (1964). *Down's syndrome: A clinical and cytogenetical investigation.* Uppsala, Sweden: Alonquist & Wiksell.

Hagemeijer, A., & Smit, E.M.E. (1977). Further evidence that trisomy of band 21q22 is essential for Down's syndrome. *Human Genetics, 38,* 15–23.

Hamill, P.V., Johnson, C.L., Reed, R.B., Roche, A.F., & Moore, W.M. (1979). Physical growth: National Center for Health Statistics percentiles. *American Journal of Clinical Nutrition, 32,* 607–629.

Hayek, A., & Peake, G.T. (1981). Growth and somatomedin-C responses to growth hormone in dwarfed children. *Pediatrics, 99,* 868–871.

Hermanussen, M., Geiger-Benoit, K., Burmeister, J., & Sippell, W.G. (1988). Periodical changes of short term growth velocity ("mini growth spurts") in human growth. *Annals of Human Biology, 15,* 103–110.

Ikeda, Y., Higurashi, M., Hirayama, M., & Ishikawa, N. (1977). A longitudinal study on the growth of stature, lower limb, and upper limb length in Japanese children with Down's syndrome. *Journal of Mental Deficiency Research, 21,* 139–151.

Kučera, J., & Dolezalova, V. (1973). Prenatal development of malformed fetuses at 28–42 weeks of gestational age. *Biologia Neonatorum, 22,* 319–324.

Kurjak, A., & Kirkinen, P. (1982). Ultrasonic growth pattern of fetuses with chromosomal aberrations. *Acta Obstetrica Gynecologica Scandinavica, 61,* 223–225.

Lampl, M., & Emde, R.N. (1983). Episodic growth in infancy: A preliminary report on length, head circumference, and behavior. In K.W. Fischer (Ed.), *Levels and transitions in children's development: New directions for child development* (No. 21, pp. 21–36.) New York: Jossey-Bass.

Lohman, T.G., Roche, A.F., & Martorell, R. (Eds.). (1987). *Anthropometric standardization reference manual.* Champaign, IL: Human Kinetics Books.

Madsen, A.L. (1979). *Height, weight and nutritional intake of young children with Down's syndrome.* Doctoral dissertation, University of Massachusetts, Amherst.

Marmol, J.G., Scriggins, A.L., & Vollman, R.F. (1969). Mothers of mongoloid infants in the Collaborative Project. *American Journal of Obstetrics and Gynecology, 104,* 533–543.

Milunsky, A., Lowy, C., Rubenstein, A.H., & Wright, A.D. (1968). Carbohydrate tolerance, growth hormone and insulin levels in mongolism. *Developmental Medicine and Child Neurology, 10,* 25–31.

Neibuhr, E. (1974). Down syndrome: The possibility of a pathogenetic segment on chromosome 21. *Human Genetics, 21,* 99–100.

Öster, J. (1953). *Mongolism.* Copenhagen: Danish Science Press.

Palmer, C.G.S., Cronk, C.E., Pueschel, S.M., Wisniewski, K.E., Laxova, R., Crocker, A.C., & Pauli, R.M. (1992). Head circumference of children with Down syndrome (0–36 months). *American Journal of Medical Genetics, 42,* 61–67.

Papp, Z., Adam, S., & Szabo, Z. (1976). Prenatal growth in Down's syndrome. *Orvosi Hetilap, 117,* 277–282.

Philipps, A.F., Persson, B., Hall, K., Lake, M., Skottner, A., Sanengen, T., & Sara, V.R. (1988). The effects of biosynthetic insulin-like growth factor-I supplementation on somatic growth, maturation and erythropoiesis on neonatal rats. *Pediatric Research, 23,* 298–305.

Pueschel, S.M. (1984). The study population. In S.M. Pueschel (Ed.), *The young child with Down syndrome* (pp. 39–58). New York: Human Science Press.

Pueschel, S.M. (1987). Health concerns of persons with Down syndrome. In S.M. Pueschel, C. Tingey, J.E. Rynders, A.C. Crocker, & D.M. Crutcher (Eds.), *New perspectives on Down syndrome* (pp. 113–133). Baltimore: Paul H. Brookes Publishing Co.

Pueschel, S.M., Orson, J.M., Boylan, J.M., & Pezzullo, J.C. (1985). Adolescent development in males with Down syndrome. *American Journal of Diseases of Children, 139,* 236–238.

Pueschel, S.M., & Pezzullo, J.C. (1985). Thyroid dysfunction in Down syndrome. *American Journal of Diseases of Children, 139,* 636–639.

Pueschel, S.M., Rothman, K.J., & Ogilby, J.D. (1976). Birth weight of children with Down's syndrome. *American Journal of Mental Deficiency, 80,* 442–445.

Rarick, G.L., Rapaport, I.F., & Seefeldt, V. (1966). Long bone growth in Down's syndrome. *American Journal of Diseases of Children, 112,* 566–571.

Rarick, G.L., & Seefeldt, V. (1974). Observations from longitudinal data on growth in stature and sitting height of children with Down's syndrome. *Journal of Mental Deficiency Research, 18,* 63–78.

Rarick, G.L., Wainer, H., Thissen, D., & Seefeldt, V. (1975). A double logistic comparison of growth patterns of normal children and children with Down's syndrome. *Annals of Human Biology, 2,* 339–346.

Roche, A.F. (1965). The stature of mongols. *Journal of Mental Deficiency Research, 9,* 131–145.

Roche, A.F. (1967). Skeletal maturation and elongation in Down's disease (mongolism). *Eugenics Reviews, 59,* 11–21.

Roche, A.F., Seward, F.S., & Sunderland, S. (1961). Growth changes in the mongoloid head. *Acta Paediatrica Uppsala, 50,* 133–142.

Roche, A.F., Siervogel, R.M., Chumlea, W.C., & Webb, P. (1981). Grading of body fatness from limited anthropometric data. *American Journal of Clinical Nutrition, 34,* 2831–2838.

Rudman, D., Kutner, M.H., Blackston, R.D., Cushman, R.A., Bain, R.P., & Patterson, J.H. (1981). Children with normal-variant short stature: Treatment with human growth hormone for six months. *New England Journal of Medicine, 305,* 123–131.

Rundle S. (1970). Anthropometry: A ten-year survey of growth and sexual maturation. In B.W. Richards (Ed.), *Mental subnormality: Modern trends in research* (pp. 68–118). London: Pitman Medical and Scientific Publishing.

Ruvalcaba, R.H.A., Thuline, H.C., & Kelley, V.C. (1972). Plasma growth hormone in patients with chromosomal anomalies. *Archives of Disease in Childhood, 47,* 307–309.

Sara, V.R., Gustavson, K-H., Annerén, G., Hall, K., & Wetterberg, L. (1983). Somatomedins in Down's syndrome. *Biological Psychiatry, 18,* 803–811.

Sara, V.R., Hall, K., Rodeck, C.H., & Wetterberg, L. (1981). Human embryonic somatomedin. *Proceedings of the National Academy of Sciences of the United States of America, 78,* 3175–3179.

Sara, V.R., Sjogren, B., Annerén, G., Gustavson, K-H., Forsman, A., Hall, K., Wahlstrom, J., & Wetterberg, L. (1984). The presence of normal receptors for somatomedin and insulin in fetuses with Down's syndrome. *Biological Psychiatry, 19,* 591–597.

Shapiro, B. (1975). Amplified developmental instability in Down's syndrome. *Annals of Human Genetics, London, 38,* 429–437.

Similä, S., & Kokkonen, J. (1990). Coexistence of celiac disease and Down syndrome. *American Journal on Mental Retardation, 95,* 120–122.

Smith, A., & McKeown, T. (1956). Prenatal growth of mongoloids. *Archives of Disease in Childhood, 30,* 448–456.

Tanner, J.M. (1978). *Foetus to man.* Cambridge, MA: Harvard University Press.

Thelander, H.E., & Pryor, D. (1966). Abnormal growth patterns and development in mongolism. *Clinical Pediatrics, 5,* 493–499.

Torrado, C., & Castells, S. (1991). Decreased physiologic growth hormone (GH) secretion in Down syndrome (DS) children suggests hypothalamic dysfunction as the cause for growth retardation [Abstract]. *Pediatric Research, 29,* 86A.

CHAPTER
4

Nutritional Aspects

Peggy L. Pipes

Children and adults with Down syndrome have been stereotyped as hypotonic, obese individuals who have respiratory infections in childhood and experience early symptoms of aging and dementia in adulthood. Also, many individuals with Down syndrome present with symptoms of deficiency of certain nutrients (e.g., dry scaly skin, follicular hyperkeratosis indicative of vitamin A deficiency). As a result of these perceptions and the hypothesis of a few researchers that the chromosome anomaly may cause altered absorption and/or metabolism of some nutrients, a number of studies in the 1970s and 1980s investigated the absorption of fat-soluble vitamin A, the effect of supplemental zinc on the immune system, the possible effect of vitamin E and selenium on premature aging and Alzheimer disease, and approaches to the prevention of and intervention for obesity in persons with Down syndrome. Results of these studies have not always been in agreement. There have been limitations in the methodology. The studies of adults living in institutions have assumed that because food that provided an appropriate nutrient intake was available it was consumed. There have been no well-designed nutritional status studies of individuals with Down syndrome living in the community or in institutions. Studies of energy and nutrient intake and problems in achieving an adequate intake have focused on children. Biochemical studies have not been included.

It is clear from clinical reports and studies of children that some individuals with Down syndrome have conditions that require nutrition therapy and/or that can be prevented by anticipatory nutrition guidance. For example, there is a high incidence of cardiac anomalies among infants with Down syndrome. Constipation secondary to hypotonia is not uncommon and obesity, which is reported in up to 50% of children with Down syndrome by age 5 years, is a risk factor for all individuals with Down syndrome. In addition, psychosocial aspects of parent–child interactions coupled with the developmental delay may result in inappropriate nutrient intake in some infants and children. Most of the strategies for the management of nutrition and feeding problems have been accumulated from the clinical experience of nutritionists who provide services to persons with developmental disabilities.

STUDIES OF NUTRIENTS

Studies in institutions have found serum protein and amino acid levels to be both depressed and within the normal range, fasting blood sugar levels to be normal (Rundle, Atkins, & Clothier, 1973; Sutnick et al., 1974), but glucose tolerance curves flatter than expected, often with a double-hump curve suggesting delayed absorption. Cholesterol levels have been found to be both normal and elevated (Stern & Lewis, 1957). Both low and normal serum calcium have been reported (Sobel, Strazzulla, & Burton, 1958; Wachowicz & Kedziora, 1974). Depressed iron:copper ratios have also been noted (Sobel et al., 1958).

Malabsorption of some vitamins has been suggested. Matin, Sylvester, Edwards, and Dickerson (1981) found biochemical evidence of thiamine, niacin, and ascorbic acid deficiency in a study of 18 individuals in an institutionalized population, including 12 persons with Down syndrome, in spite of a supplement of 50 mg of ascorbic acid per day. They suggested an increased requirement or malabsorption. Low concentrations of calcium and copper were found in individuals with Down syndrome in the same institution compared to noninstitutionalized control individuals, without Down syndrome. Hair trace metals of institutionalized individuals studied were all significantly less than those noninstitutionalized controls (Barlow, Sylvester, & Dickerson, 1981).

A number of researchers have suspected that malabsorption of vitamin A might be a problem. Impaired dark adaptation was reported by Griffiths and Behrmian (1967) in individuals with Down syndrome compared to controls without Down syndrome. Palmer (1978) found that children supplemented with 1,000 IU/kg per month had improved absorptive capacity, increased vitamin A levels, and a reduction in infections. Pueschel et al. (1990) investigated vitamin A absorption in 40 individuals with Down syndrome 6–28 years of age who lived at home. Vitamin A absorption curves paralleled those of "normal" controls at 3 hours. However, at 6 hours after administration of vitamin A, there had been a greater decline in the serum vitamin A levels of individuals with Down syndrome than those of controls. Utilization of this nutrient between 3–6 hours remains a matter of speculation. Storm (1990) also noted normal vitamin A levels in 44 individuals with Down syndrome. However, 14 of these clients had high serum levels of beta-carotene, indicating hypercarotenemia. No dietary or medical reason for the carotenemia could be identified.

NUTRIENTS AND IMMUNE FUNCTION

The effect of nutrient supplements on the incidence of upper respiratory infection and the immune system has also been investigated. Low plasma and erythrocyte zinc have been found in some individuals with Down syndrome (Milunsky, Hackley, & Hasted, 1970). However, a number of studies have found normal plasma levels of zinc. Bjorksten et al. (1980) prescribed zinc supplements of 600 mg (135 mg elemental zinc) for 12 individuals with Down syndrome whose serum zinc levels were significantly below con-

trols. This normalized serum zinc concentrations and immune function in the supplemented individuals.

Francheschi et al. (1988) supplemented 18 individuals with Down syndrome with 1 mg zinc per kg of body weight per day for 2 months, then 10 months later repeated the supplemental dose. These individuals had zinc plasma levels that were higher than age-matched controls after the trial periods. A dramatic increase in serum thymic factor and a decrease in serum thymic inhibitory molecules were noted. A reduction in recurrent respiratory, auditory, and skin infections was observed in 13 of the 18 individuals. After 10 months, all immunologic parameters had returned to presupplementation values. As previously noted, Palmer (1978) found that children supplemented with 1,000 IU/kg/month of water-soluble vitamin A had a reduced incidence of infections and reductions in serum IgG.

NUTRIENTS AND AGING

There have also been investigations as to whether nutrients with antioxidant properties might be one factor in the early aging and dementia that sometimes occurs in individuals with Down syndrome. Some investigators have wondered if supplementation with selenium could protect against oxygen radicals that might cause damage by lipid peroxidation, especially in the brain. Neve, Sinet, Molle, and Nicole (1983) found low plasma selenium in 29 outpatients with Down syndrome. Erythrocyte selenium was identical in the control group; however, the activity of glutathione peroxidase was significantly increased above normal values in the group with Down syndrome as compared to controls. A study in Sweden (Annerén, Gebre-Medhin, & Gustavson, 1989) found that after supplementation with 10 mg per kg of body weight per day of selenium-rich yeast tablets for 6 months, the concentration of selenium in the plasma and erythrocytes increased. There was a significant decrease in glutathione peroxidase activity in erythrocytes.

Another group questioned if a gene coding for superoxide dismutase located on chromosome 21 might result in increased activity of the enzyme and play a role in the early aging and dementia often found in persons with Down syndrome (Jackson, Holland, Williams, & Dickerson, 1988). They investigated plasma levels of vitamin E in 24 individuals with Down syndrome over 30 years of age. Mean serum vitamin E values were less in the plasma of individuals with dementia compared to those of a nondementia group. However, all but two of the plasma vitamin E levels were within the normal range.

Storm (1990) wondered if the hypercarotenemia he found was an adaptation to increased amounts of unstable oxygen radicals formed in the metabolism of people with Down syndrome. Antioxidants such as beta-carotene, which scavenge the hydroxyl radicals, aid in protection against oxidative damage to body cells.

The practical significance of these studies and speculations remains unknown. If dietary analysis or clinical assessment is cause for concern, biochemical parameters should be investigated. Therapy should be individualized. Clinical experiences of the author have indicated that low blood levels of zinc and vitamin A in preschool children with Down syndrome have resulted from inadequate dietary intake.

MEGAVITAMIN THERAPY

Claims that megadoses of vitamins would increase the intelligence of individuals with Down syndrome have been made for a number of years. The evidence supporting these claims, however, has been unconvincing and not much attention has been focused on this therapy.

For example, in 1981, Harrell, Capp, and Davis reported gains in IQ when megavitamins were given to 16 children with developmental delays. The children who experienced the greatest gains had Down syndrome. To test this hypothesis, replication of the Harrell study was undertaken in a number of clinical settings using a double-blind control design (Bennett, McClelland, Kriegsman, Andrus, & Sells, 1983; Ellis & Tomporowski, 1983; Smith, Spiker, Peterson, Cicchetti, & Justin, 1983; Weathers, 1983). In no instance did the megavitamin therapy result in an increase in intelligence, motor performance,

or communicative abilities, or change the appearance of the children or adults studied. Unfortunately, some professionals continue to offer false hope to parents by promising changes with this therapy. (For further discussion of megavitamin therapy, see Pueschel, chap. 24, this volume.)

PHYSICAL GROWTH AND ENERGY NEEDS

Individuals with Down syndrome are growth retarded compared to the general population. The growth deficiency begins prenatally and continues until children are between 3–5 years of age (Cronk, 1978). Mean heights are reduced by 2 SD from the average by 5 years of age. By the onset of their pubescent growth spurt, which begins 6 months to 1 year later than in the average child, they are 3–5 cm shorter in stature than their age peers.

Basal metabolic rates of individuals with Down syndrome are not different from those of the average person when corrections are made for surface area and lean body mass (Schapiro & Rapoport, 1989). However, because children with Down syndrome have a smaller body mass and a slower rate of growth than do "normal" children, they require fewer total calories and nutrients that function in energy metabolism, such as thiamine and riboflavin. Culley, Goyle, Jolly, and Mertz (1965) noted that 5- to 11-year-old institutionalized well-nourished males with Down syndrome who were shorter and heavier than their age peers consumed 16.1 ± 0.8 and females 14.3 ± 1.1 kcal/cm/day. This was comparable to their age peers who were not overweight. Obese teenagers with Down syndrome have been found to consume 12–13 kcal/cm/day, between the 10th and 50th percentile of energy intake of "normal" children (Held & Mahan, 1978). Recommendations for energy intake should be individually determined for persons with Down syndrome.

Chumlea and Cronk (1981), using weight/height to determine overweight, suggest overweight as a characteristic of children with Down syndrome ages 2–3 years to adolescence. Others have made reference to the tendency of persons with Down syndrome to be obese, suggesting this as not inevitable but probably constitutional (Culley et al., 1965; Pipes & Holm, 1980). Regardless of its etiology, the hazards of obesity make prevention and intervention important (Chumlea & Cronk, 1981). (For further discussion of growth, see Cronk & Annerén, chap. 3, this volume.)

NUTRITION AND FEEDING PROBLEMS

Young Children

Feeding difficulties and concern about the adequacy of nutrient intake occur most frequently during the preschool years; however, such problems have been noted in children with Down syndrome at all ages. Problems in older children often appear to be multiple and more severe.

In a study of 40 children with Down syndrome, ages 1–12 years, Calvert, Vivian, and Calvert (1976) found that approximately half consumed foods providing less calcium, iron, vitamin A, and thiamine than the U.S. Recommended Dietary Allowances (RDAs). Another study of 47 children with Down syndrome, ages 6 months to 6½ years, noted that 16% had low intakes of calcium, 14% had low intakes of iron, and 10% had low intakes of vitamin D and ascorbic acid (Pipes & Holm, 1980).

Feeding problems (Figure 4.1) were also identified, including refusing to chew textured food when the child is developmentally ready to do so, resulting from lack of attention to the critical stage of development in relation to the addition of food with texture (Pipes & Holm, 1980). This results in the child's acceptance of a limited variety of foods, usually starchier and easier to masticate food items. Social-emotional situations have also been noted to result in problems that compromise feeding, children's nutrient intakes, and/or developmental progress in feeding behavior. Throwing food and utensils and refusing to progress in feeding behavior were often believed to result from such factors (Pipes & Holm, 1980).

It has been the author's experience that early individual or group intervention has proven effective in providing or remediating the above problems. Effective programs utilize an inter-disciplinary approach including a nutritionist, and occupational or physical therapist, and a behaviorist. Counseling and therapy focuses on developmental readiness for the transition to appropriate textures of foods, the use of food to support developmental progress, parental feelings about and interaction with their children, physical growth, maintenance of normal weight for height, and foods that supply appropriate nutrients. Individual counseling is provided for parents of children when dietary assessment indicates an inadequate or excessive intake of any nutrient.

Monitoring rates of weight gain and energy intake permits identification of potential problems of excessive weight gain and initiation of individual counseling regarding foods that support an appropriate energy intake. The long-term effectiveness of such a program was demonstrated at the Child Development and Mental Retardation Center; Seattle, Washington. On follow-up 7 years later, only 1 of 16 was obese. No inadequacies of nutrient intake were found. All 16 individuals continued to consume a variety of textured table foods in a socially acceptable manner (Pipes & Holm, 1980).

School-Age Children

Little definitive evidence has been collected on the nutrition and feeding problems of school-age and adolescent children with Down syndrome. However, unresolved conflicts about food and feeding may become severe. It is also at this age that obesity may become evident. Successful intervention strategies include the child, parents, teachers, and others in the food environment. Education of children in the school-age years should include approaches to teaching them to make wise food choices.

Many school-age children with Down syndrome lack the cognitive ability to understand nutritional needs. However, they are able to classify and understand relationships between groups. They must begin with something concrete in thinking and are unable to think of possibilities they cannot see. Food and food groups are appropriate concrete topics to use as opposed to "nutrient," which is abstract. Photographs of real food and people are necessary. Creativity

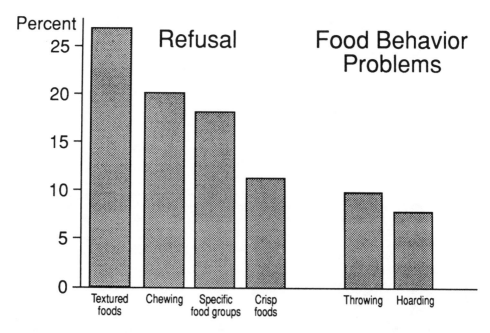

Figure 4.1.   Percentage of 49 children with Down syndrome with food refusals and food-related problems. (From Pipes, P.L., & Holm, V.H. [1980]. Feeding children with Down's syndrome. *Journal of the American Dietetic Association, 77,* 277; Copyright The American Dietetic Association; reprinted by permission.)

is needed to prevent boredom and enhance learning.

Parents' and school staff's attitudes, examples, and positive experiences with nutritious food can influence the children to make wise food choices. A strong force in forming good food habits is the food served at home and at school.

A 6-week demonstration weight control project for 6 children with developmental delay including 4 with Down syndrome conducted at a special education school in Kirkland, Washington, indicated that weight loss and changes in food patterns are possible if parents and teachers are included in the program (Held & Mahan, 1978). Classes were conducted weekly (Table 4.1). The goal of the session was to develop an awareness between the relationship of food, activity, and growth among obese children with developmental disabilities. Objectives of the classes were:

1. To help children with developmental disabilities learn to weigh and measure themselves
2. To teach children with developmental dis-

abilities how to prepare low-calorie snacks and beverages, emphasizing portion sizes
3. To help children with developmental disabilities increase physical activity and improve motor coordination
4. To teach children with developmental disabilities about "good" and "bad" snacks

Parent sessions focused on:

1. Children's lessons and encouraging them to reinforce children's lessons at home
2. Parent learning activities
3. Parental expressions of concern and sharing of successes and failures in attempts to control their children's rates of weight gain

Four children lost 0.25–0.9 kg during the 6 weeks of classes. The weight of 2 females increased an average of 0.27 kg. Energy intakes of those who reported food intakes were reduced from 12.0–13.5 kcal/cm of height to 7.0–8.0 kcal/cm of height.

Older Children and Adults

The transition from natural homes or foster homes to community group homes and/or inde-

Table 4.1. Effectiveness of weight control class

Age of client	Kg loss or gain[a]	Kcal/cm prior[b]	Kcal/cm after[c]
Males			
15, 9	−0.68	12.1	NA[d]
15, 2	−0.57	12.0	8.0
12, 5	−0.23	12.0	7.0
10, 11	−0.9	13.5	8.0
Females			
15, 2	+0.11	11.7	NA
10, 5	+0.27	NA	NA

From Held, M., & Mahan, K. (1978). *Nutrition education for obese developmentally delayed adolescents.* Unpublished nutrition fellowship project, University of Washington, Child Development and Mental Retardation Center, Seattle; reprinted with permission.

Note: All ages are years, months (e.g., 15, 9 = 15 years, 9 months).

[a]4 weeks of nutrition education.

[b]6-day food intake record.

[c]24-hour recall.

[d]information not reported.

pendent living may create another challenge if individuals involved are to have an adequate nutrient intake and maintain an appropriate weight for height. Menus in group homes usually reflect houseparents' food likes and attitudes. Residents of these facilities have limited food choices. The staff of sheltered workshops are often not supportive of programs to enhance nutrient or control energy intakes. In addition, money earned by residents in these facilities is often spent for food with high energy but low nutrient density. The finding that many individuals living in institutions have low blood levels of several vitamins compared to individuals living in the community may well result from dietary inadequacies because food served does not necessarily indicate food consumed.

Programs to correct obesity are difficult. A program of food denial has a tendency to encourage behaviors such as stuffing, sneaking, or hoarding food. This may result in greater food intake and improper eating habits. Individuals appear to respond better to programs that focus on activities rather than those that deny food.

A behavioral approach to weight loss has been documented as the most successful program in the general population. This program has been used with some modifications for both adolescents and adults with developmental delays. Such an obesity treatment program was conducted with 4 persons with severe retardation, including 1 with Down syndrome, living in a group home in Seattle, Washington (Warren, 1982). Plans for exercise were individualized based on fitness testing. A program of exercise was instituted for all 4, including a program of walking for 3 individuals.

Data collected on the eating habits record of individuals were used to plan a behavioral approach. All of the individuals initially took very large portions. When appropriate-size portions were taken, they were rewarded with a token. Second portions were not requested when they were no longer offered. Tokens were given to all 4 individuals for participation in each exercise, to be exchanged later for a trip to a concert. Eating time ranged from 8.7–20.0 minutes. Snacks were limited to one per day. Three of the 4 lost 0.23–0.45 kg per week.

Individuals with Down syndrome for whom independent living is planned must be educated not only in food selection but in food preparation skills as well. Unfortunately, no follow-up data are available on whether such individuals actually put this nutrition education into practice. Individual observations indicate that many convenience and already-prepared foods are used. An abundance of sweet foods of high caloric density are consumed and little support is given the individuals in selecting an adequate diet.

Thus, there continue to be many unknowns about the nutrient needs of individuals with Down syndrome and how to achieve an appropriate food and nutrient intake.

CONCLUSION

The nutrition problems and intervention strategies discussed in this chapter are by no means specific to individuals with Down syndrome. They are not uncommon in any population of individuals with developmental delays. Nutrition therapy should be individualized based on dietary, clinical (including anthropometric data), and laboratory assessment (when indicated). An assessment of feeding behavior including an oral-motor assessment and an assessment of the individual's interaction with others in the food environment may also be indicated. An interdisciplinary approach has been found to be effective.

Obesity can be prevented or corrected. Megavitamin therapy is *not* indicated. Studies of blood levels of nutrients should be accompanied by dietary intake data. Future investigations on the effect of nutrients with antioxidant properties are likely. Such studies may provide insight into aging not only in individuals with Down syndrome but in "normal" adults as well.

REFERENCES

Anneren, G., Gebre-Medhin, M., & Gustavson, K.H. (1989). Increased plasma and erythrocyte selenium concentrations but decreased glutathione peroxidase activity after selenium supplementation in children with Down syndrome. *Acta Paediatrica Scandinavia, 78*, 789–884.

Barlow, P.J., Sylvester, P.F., & Dickerson, J.W.T. (1981). Hair trace metal levels in Down's syndrome patients. *Journal of Mental Deficiency Research, 25*, 161–168.

Bennett, F.C., McClelland, S., Kriegsman, E.A., Andrus, L.B., & Sells, C.J. (1983). Vitamin and mineral supplements in Down's syndrome. *Pediatrics, 72*, 707–713.

Bjorksten, B., Back, O., Gustavson, K.H., Hallmans, G., Hagglof, B., & Tarnvik, A. (1980). Zinc and immune function in Down's syndrome. *Acta Paediatrica Scandinavica, 69*, 183–189.

Calvert, S.D., Vivian, V.M., & Calvert, G.P. (1976). Dietary adequacy, feeding practices, and eating behavior of children with Down's syndrome. *Journal of the American Dietetic Association, 69*, 152–156.

Chumlea, W.C., & Cronk, C.E. (1981). Overweight among children with trisomy 21. *Journal of Mental Deficiency Research, 25*, 275–280.

Cronk, C.E. (1978). Growth of children with Down's syndrome. *Pediatrics, 61*, 564–568.

Culley, W.J., Goyle, K., Jolly, D.H., & Mertz, E.T. (1965). Calorie intake of children with Down's syndrome. *Journal of Pediatrics, 66*, 772–775.

Ellis, N.R., & Tomporowski, R.D. (1983). Vitamin/mineral supplements and intelligence of institutionalized mentally retarded adults. *American Journal of Mental Deficiency, 88*, 211–214.

Francheschi, C., Chiricolo, M., Licastro, F., Zannotti, M.M., Mocchegini, E., & Fabris, N. (1988). Oral zinc supplementation in Down's syndrome: Restoration of thymic endocrine activity and some immune defects. *Journal of Mental Deficiency Research, 32*, 169–181.

Griffiths, A.W., & Behrmian, J. (1967). Dark adaptation in mongols. *Journal of Mental Deficiency Research, 11*, 23–30.

Harrell, R.J., Capp, R.H., & Davis, D.R. (1981). Can nutritional supplements help mentally retarded children? *Proceedings of the National Academy of Sciences of the United States of America, 78*, 574–578.

Held, M., & Mahan, K. (1978). *Nutrition education for obese children with Down's syndrome.* Unpublished nutrition fellowship project, University of Washington, Child Development and Mental Retardation Center, Seattle.

Jackson, C.V.E., Holland, A.J., Williams, C.A., & Dickerson, J.W.T. (1988). Vitamin E and Alzheimer's disease in subjects with Down's syndrome. *Journal of Mental Deficiency Research, 32*, 479–484.

Matin, M.A., Sylvester, P.E., Edwards, D., & Dickerson, J.W.T. (1981). Vitamin and zinc status in Down's syndrome. *Journal of Mental Deficiency Research, 25*, 121–126.

Milunsky, A., Hackley, B.M., & Hasted, J.A. (1970). Plasma erythrocyte and leucocyte zinc levels in Down's syndrome. *Journal of Mental Deficiency Research, 14*, 99–105.

Neve, J., Sinet, P.M., Molle, L., & Nicole, A. (1983). Selenium, zinc, and copper in Down's syndrome (trisomy 21): Blood levels and relations with glutathione peroxidase and superoxidase dismutase. *Clinica Chimica Acta, 133*, 209–213.

Palmer, S. (1978). Influence of vitamin A nurture on the immune response: Findings in children with Down's syndrome. *International Journal of Vitamin and Nutrition Research, 48*, 189–216.

Pipes, P., & Holm, V.A. (1980). Food and children with Down's syndrome. *Journal of the American Dietetic Association, 77*, 277–281.

Pueschel, S.M., Hillemeier, C., Caldwell, M., Senft, K., Mers, C., & Pezzullo, J.C. (1990). Vitamin A gastrointestinal absorption in persons with Down's syndrome. *Journal of Mental Deficiency Research, 34*, 269–275.

Rundle, A.T., Atkins, J., & Clothier, B. (1973). Serum proteins in Down's syndrome. *Developmental Medicine and Child Neurology, 15*, 736–747.

Schapiro, M.B., & Rapoport, S.I. (1989). Basal metabolic rate in healthy Down's syndrome adults. *Journal of Mental Deficiency Research, 33*, 211–219.

Smith, G.F., Spiker, D., Peterson, C., Cicchetti, D., & Justin, P. (1983). Failure of mineral and vitamin supplementation in Down's syndrome. *Lancet, ii,* 41.

Sobel, A.E., Strazzulla, M., & Burton, S. (1958). Vitamin A absorption and other blood composition studies in mongolism. *American Journal of Mental Deficiency, 62*, 642–656.

Stern, J., & Lewis, W.P. (1957). The serum cholesterol level in children with mongolism and other mentally retarded subnormal persons. *Journal of Mental Deficiency Research, 1*, 96–106.

Storm, W. (1990). Hypercarotenemia in children with Down's syndrome. *Journal of Mental Deficiency Research, 34*, 283–286.

Sutnick, A.I., London, W.T., Gerstley, B.J., Coyne, V.E., Blumberg, B.S., & Lustbader, E.D. (1974). Glucose tolerance in Down's syndrome. *Research Communications in Chemical Pathology and Pharmacology, 8*, 471–480.

Wachowicz, B., & Kedziora, J. (1974). Lower values of iron in blood of children with Down's syndrome. *Endokrynology Poland, 25*, 1–9.

Warren, L. (1982). *Development and implementation of an obesity treatment model for developmentally delayed clients.* Unpublished master's thesis, University of Washington, Seattle.

Weathers, C. (1983). Effect of nutritional supplementation on I.Q. and certain other variables associated with Down's syndrome. *American Journal of Mental Deficiency, 88*, 214–217.

CHAPTER
5

Life Expectancy

Adele D. Sadovnick and Patricia A. Baird

Life expectancy for persons with Down syndrome has increased dramatically since the early work of Record and Smith (1955). From 1942–1952, they reported that less than 50% of infants survived the 1st year; by age 5, only about 40% were still alive. In contrast recent studies (Baird & Sadovnick, 1987, 1989; McGrother & Marshall, 1990) found that over 80% of children with Down syndrome are still alive by age 5 and approximately 44% survive to age 60 (Baird & Sadovnick, 1988b). This improved survival probably reflects more effective treatment of the most common causes of death such as respiratory infection and congenital heart disease (Baird & Sadovnick, 1988a; McGrother & Marshall, 1990; Thase, 1981) as well as changing attitudes toward the neonatal care of such infants ("Declining mortality," 1990).

Comparison of maternal age–specific rates for Down syndrome over time has resulted in varying findings—increasing rates for older mothers in some regions (Evans, Hunter, & Hamerton, 1978; Hook & Cross, 1981; Mikkelsen, Fischer, Hanson, Pilgaard, & Nielsen, 1983), increasing rates for younger mothers in others (Leisti et al., 1985), and no change in yet others (Baird & Sadovnick, 1988c; Evers-Kieboom, Vlietinck, & Van Den Berghe, 1985). Although on an individual basis the risk of having a child with Down syndrome is greater for older mothers, the majority of births in children with Down syndrome are to younger mothers because of the relatively greater fertility for this group. With improved mortality rates, the number of surviving children and adults with Down

syndrome is increasing, especially in regions where the birth incidence for Down syndrome increases or remains the same over time. The same net effect can also be expected even if the incidence of births to older women is decreasing (due to increased utilization of prenatal diagnosis and subsequent termination of pregnancy), because of the fact that the majority of Down syndrome births are to younger women. Thus, it remains important for physicians and other health professionals to have accurate data on life expectancy for counseling families with respect to prognosis and long-term planning. In addition, such data are critical to those planning for the care, education, employment, and integration into the community of these individuals.

LIFE EXPECTANCY

British Columbia Population-Based Study on Life Expectancy in Persons with Down Syndrome to Age 68

British Columbia provided an excellent opportunity to examine life expectancy in people with Down syndrome because of the existence of the population-based Health Surveillance Registry that, for over 30 years, was designed to serve the entire province. Using these data, it was possible to examine life expectancy for persons with Down syndrome up to age 68 (Baird & Sadovnick, 1987, 1988b).

The Health Surveillance Registry was established in 1952. Ascertainment of each individual on the Health Surveillance Registry's caseload

This research was funded by the Scottish Rite Charitable Foundation of Canada and the Medical Research Council of Canada, Grant No. MA-9279.

may be made from over 60 different sources. All public health units register known persons with disabilities in their catchment areas. Other registering sources include physicians' notices of birth, hospital discharge diagnoses for children under age 7, institutions for persons with mental retardation, private physicians, genetics units, and provincial cytogenetics laboratories. In addition, the province provides a pension from age 18 to all persons with disabilities, and recipients are routinely registered with the Health Surveillance Registry. Thus, because of these multiple sources of ascertainment, there are several opportunities to register both institutionalized individuals and those living in the community. To avoid duplicate entry of cases, new registrations are compared with an alphabetic index of names before inclusion and are also linked with the provincial birth registration numbers to reduce further the likelihood of duplicate entry. Registration of births of children with Down syndrome for the period 1952 – 1981 is believed to be relatively complete.

The Health Surveillance Registry uses the World Health Organization's (WHO, 1977) *International Classification of Diseases Diagnostic Codes* (9th edition; *ICD-9*) to classify disabilities. Data on disabilities coded prior to January, 1979, when *ICD-9* codes were adopted, were converted to *ICD-9* prior to this study.

Life Expectancy to Age 30

Study Cohort All individuals with Down syndrome born in British Columbia from 1952 to 1981 inclusive, identified at year end 1982 as having Down syndrome (*ICD-9* code 758.0), were enrolled in the study. Chromosomal diagnoses confirmed Down syndrome for 459 cases. Clinical data on the remaining cases were reviewed by the medical consultant to the Health Surveillance Registry (the co-author of this chapter, P.A. Baird) and any clinically unclear cases were excluded. It was impossible to exclude the small number of children with translocation Down syndrome.

The final study cohort numbered 1,341 (703 males, 638 females) out of 1,066,508 consecutive live births in British Columbia. Of these,

388 (176 males, 212 females) had congenital heart disease, which had come to the attention of the Health Surveillance Registry by their requiring services for this at one of the registering sources (e.g., hospitals).

For comparison with the Down syndrome data, British Columbia–born individuals (1952–1981 inclusive) classified as having moderate mental retardation (*ICD-9* code 318.0, IQ 35–49) and having neither congenital heart disease nor Down syndrome were identified from the caseload of the Health Surveillance Registry at year end 1982. This comparison group was selected because the majority (41.5%) of individuals with Down syndrome on the Health Surveillance Registry's caseload for whom IQ levels were available fell within this range (Baird & Sadovnick, 1987). For the study period, there were a total of 579 births in British Columbia with moderate mental retardation but with neither congenital heart disease nor Down syndrome.

Life tables for the general population of British Columbia were obtained from Statistics Canada (1981).

Life Table Analyses Health Surveillance Registry data are continuously updated with respect to deaths from the provincial death lists. Information on deaths of British Columbia–born individuals with Down syndrome occurring elsewhere in Canada was obtained through Statistics Canada using a service available for research purposes (Smith & Newcombe, 1982). Although it was estimated at the time of the study that 0.3% of the British Columbia population were leaving Canada annually (Statistics Canada, 1981), the number of persons with Down syndrome emigrating was considerably less. It was thus estimated that very few deaths were missed during this study.

Life table analyses were conducted using standard actuarial methods (Lee, 1981). Survival for the various groups was compared using the z test. Differences in sample proportions were compared using the $2 \times K$ contingency χ^2 test with K-1 degrees of freedom. All differences were considered significant at the 5% level.

Survival to Age 30 Overall, 72% of the total Down syndrome cohort survived to age 30 (see Table 5.1), compared with 97% of the general population of British Columbia.

Of individuals with Down syndrome without congenital heart disease, 79% were still alive by age 30 (see Table 5.2). The highest probability of death (9%) was during the 1st year of life. There were no significant differences between males and females. Survival to age 30 for the Down syndrome group without congenital heart disease was significantly poorer compared with survival for the general population ($z = 12.6$; $p < 0.01$) and the moderately mentally retarded population, of which 92% were still alive at age 30 ($z = 6.05$; $p < 0.01$).

In contrast to the data for persons with Down syndrome not having congenital heart disease, fewer than 50% of persons with Down syndrome with congenital heart disease survived to age 30 (see Table 5.2). For this group, the highest probability of death (24%) was also during the 1st year. As for individuals with Down syndrome without congenital heart disease, life expectancy did not differ significantly according to sex. As seen in Table 5.2, survival was significantly poorer across all ages if congenital heart disease was present.

The data were examined separately for each decade of the study (1952–1961, 1962–1971, 1972–1981). No significant differences were observed from decade to decade for either the Down syndrome group as a whole or for those with or without congenital heart disease.

Life Expectancy from Age 31 to Age 68

Study Cohort Using Health Surveillance Registry data, the study group was extended to include live births in British Columbia from 1908–1951 inclusive. For this period, only those individuals who came to the attention of the Health Surveillance Registry after its inception in 1952 could be identified. It was thus necessary to estimate the number of live births of children with Down syndrome from 1908–1951, based on maternal-age–specific incidence rates for Down syndrome in British Columbia (Trimble & Baird, 1978), and from maternal-age–specific fertility rate data obtained from Statistics Canada (1981).

Table 5.1. Life expectancy for persons with Down syndrome to age 68

Age (years)	% survival at start of age interval
0	100.00
1	87.83
2	83.92
3	82.20
4	81.44
5	81.05
6	80.24
7	79.82
8	79.31
9	79.04
10	78.40
11	78.21
12	77.82
13	77.61
14	77.30
15	76.64
16	76.29
17	76.16
18	76.03
19	75.48
20	75.34
21	75.18
22	75.01
23	74.08
24	74.08
25	73.61
26	73.61
27	72.62
28	72.62
29	72.12
30	72.12
31	72.12
32	72.12
33	72.12
34	71.83
35	71.83
36	71.48
37	71.48
38	70.67
39	69.78
40	69.78
41	69.25
42	69.25
43	68.61
44	67.89
45	67.89
46	65.47
47	65.47
48	62.74
49	62.74
50	60.68
51	60.68
52	59.53
53	56.91
54	55.49
55	53.90

(continued)

Table 5.1. *(continued)*

Age (years)	% survival at start of age interval
56	53.90
57	51.94
58	49.68
59	47.14
60	44.44
61	38.71
62	29.03
63	29.03
64	29.03
65	24.88
66	20.36
67	13.57
68	13.57

Adapted from Baird and Sadovnick (1989).

It was estimated that there should have been 1,010 live births of children with Down syndrome in the province during this period if single-year maternal-age–specific rates for Down syndrome remained constant over time as appears to be the case in British Columbia (Baird & Sadovnick, 1988c). As previously discussed, few individuals with Down syndrome are believed to have been lost to follow-up in the cohort born after 1952. The population born before 1952 was even less mobile; therefore, outmigration is not believed to represent a major source of inaccuracy in the survival estimates from ages 33 to 68 (Baird & Sadovnick, 1988b).

Life Table Analyses In order to extend the earlier life table beyond age 30, it was important to verify that survival in adulthood for individuals with Down syndrome born prior to 1952 did not differ significantly from that for the group born after 1952. The study on life expectancy for adults with Down syndrome was done after the earlier study (Baird & Sadovnick, 1987); thus, it was possible to extend the life table for the Down syndrome group born after 1952 from ages 30 to 32. Survival from ages 20–32 was then compared for individuals with Down syndrome born before and after 1952 using the Mantel-Haenszel statistic and the χ^2 goodness-of-fit (Elandt-Johnson & Johnson, 1980). The life table from the earlier study to age 30 (Baird & Sadovnick, 1987) was extended into the 7th decade with data from individuals with Down syndrome born prior to 1952 according to the method outlined by Lawless (1982).

The earlier study (Baird & Sadovnick, 1987) showed that the probability of death was greatest for all persons with Down syndrome (with and without congenital heart defect) in early childhood. By about age 20, a "plateau" appeared to be reached. As part of the extension of that study, the authors wished to identify the age at which survival no longer followed this plateau (Baird & Sadovnick, 1988b). To evaluate this, the data were analyzed by comparing the average hazard function (Larsson & Sjogren, 1954) over different age ranges.

Life Expectancy After Age 30 For the two Down syndrome groups (born before and after 1952), life expectancy from age 20 to 32 did not differ significantly ($z = 0.674, p = 0.50$; $\chi^2 = 18.68, df = 13, p > 0.10$). Thus it was appropriate to extend the life table by use of observed data for the Down syndrome group born prior to 1952.

Table 5.2. Life expectancy to age 30 for persons with Down syndrome with and without congenital heart disease

Age interval	% survival to end of age interval		Comparison of survival rates (z-test[a])
	Without congenital heart disease	With congenital heart disease	
0	90.66	76.29	6.10
5	86.57	60.59	9.43
10	84.65	57.03	9.62
15	83.05	54.34	9.58
20	80.49	49.91	8.72
25	80.49	49.91	8.72
30	79.17	49.91	8.09

Adapted from Baird and Sadovnick (1987).
[a]All values highly significant at $p < 0.001$.

As seen in Table 5.1, 14% of the population with Down syndrome were still alive at age 68, compared with 78% of the general British Columbia population (Baird & Sadovnick, 1988b). Analyses with the hazard function showed that the previously observed survival plateau continued until the early 40s with a fairly abrupt end after age 44 ($t = 2.90$, $df = 47$, $p < 0.01$).

Life Expectancy for Males and Females with Down Syndrome   Life expectancy was not observed to differ significantly according to sex at any age (Mantel-Haenszel statistic z = 1.69; $p = 0.09$).

Discussion of Life Expectancy in Persons with Down Syndrome

Data spanning the long period needed for life expectancy estimates are difficult to obtain and thus most reports on this topic for Down syndrome have focused on survival to age 10. Even with this limitation, population-based data are not easy to obtain. For example, Masaki et al. (1981) looked at Down syndrome survival to age 10 in Japan. Their data actually appear to be based on two separate studies, one for an institutionalized population (Kabuto, 1979 cited in Masaki et al., 1981) and one carried out at a different time on cases in the community (Masaki et al., 1981) using different methods of case ascertainment. These combined data give a life expectancy to age 10 of 46.6% (Masaki et al., 1981). McGrother and Marshall (1990) reported survival rates for persons with Down syndrome with and without congenital heart defect for the Leicestershire birth cohort (1976–1985). Survival to age 10 for those without congenital heart defect approached 90% and that for the group with congenital heart defect was approximately 45%, indicating improved survival to age 10 for both groups compared with earlier work.

The British Columbia data are important as they represent an overall view of mortality in persons with Down syndrome as the Health Surveillance Registry caseload includes both institutionalized individuals and those living in the community. The data should be relevant to regions such as North America and Europe where there is fairly universal financial access to a modern medical care system. However, care

must be taken in extrapolating these data to those parts of the world where marked differences in medical care exist as these differences and differences in standards of living may well affect survival.

To assess whether Down syndrome (apart from complications related to the existence of congenital heart defect) results in greater mortality, life expectancy for persons with Down syndrome without congenital heart defect was compared with that for a comparative mentally retarded population having neither congenital heart defect nor Down syndrome. The data indicate that life expectancy for the Down syndrome group without congenital heart defect is still significantly lower than that for the mentally retarded comparison group, suggesting that there appears to be an effect on life expectancy related to Down syndrome that is separate from the effect of either congenital heart defect or moderate mental retardation (Baird & Sadovnick, 1987).

Richards and Siddiqui (1980), using an institutionalized population, compared survival for individuals with Down syndrome with that for persons with mental retardation from other causes and found no differences in survival until after age 40. However, data from institutionalized populations are subject to many biases and do not necessarily reflect the situation for the overall Down syndrome population. Balakrishnan and Wolfe (1976) and Thase (1981) used pooled data from various geographic regions, rather than institutions, to compare survival for persons with Down syndrome, persons with other types of mental retardation, and the general population.

The findings from these two studies were similar to those for British Columbia, with survival for both persons with Down syndrome and those with other causes of mental retardation being poorer than that for the general population (Baird & Sadovnick, 1987). However, in contrast to the authors' data, neither study reported differences in survival between persons with Down syndrome and the groups with other causes of mental retardation until age 30. Their data, based on populations from the same geographic region, ascertained from the same source (Health Surveillance Registry), and matched for both the level of mental retardation and the absence of congenital heart defect, indicate that differences in survival occur as early as the 1st year of life.

The British Columbia data showed that survival into the 7th decade for persons with Down syndrome is much improved over earlier estimates. Gallagher and Lowry (1975) extrapolated that about 50% of British Columbia–born persons with Down syndrome would be alive at age 30, in contrast to the authors' findings of more than 70% (see Table 5.1) (Baird & Sadovnick, 1987). Down syndrome survival still remains far poorer than that for the general population. As seen in Table 5.1, about 44% and 14% of individuals with Down syndrome are still alive at ages 60 and 68, respectively, compared with 86% and 78% of the general population (Baird & Sadovnick, 1988b).

The results of work by Forssman and Åkesson (1965, 1967) on a limited institutionalized population are congruent with the findings for British Columbia. They reported that mortality between the ages of 5–40, the age period more or less corresponding to the authors' "plateau," was only 3%–7% higher than that for the general population; after age 40, the survival rate dropped sharply compared with that for the general population and from age 50, the mortality rate for persons with Down syndrome was 30% higher than that for the general population. However, it must be noted that they did not follow a full population cohort as was done in the British Columbia study, but an institutionalized subgroup. Their analyses did not allow for live withdrawals (see Baird & Sadovnick [1989] for a complete life table for the British Columbia data showing live withdrawals) and so proper life tables could not be provided.

The British Columbia data indicate better survival for adults with Down syndrome than estimated by other work in Denmark (Dupont, Vaeth, & Videbech, 1986) and Western Australia (Malone, 1988). The Danish study followed their group for 8.5 years and predicted that about 9% and 5% would be alive at age 50 and 70 years, respectively. The Western Australia study predicted that about 42% and 7% of the study group would be alive at ages 40–49 and 60–69 respectively. There were, however, several methodological differences between the studies (Baird & Sadovnick, 1988b).

Dementia of the Alzheimer type has a high incidence in the Down syndrome population from ages 40–50 onward (Dalton & Crapper-McLachlan, 1986; Evenhuis, 1990; Thase, 1982). The impact of improved survival for individuals with Down syndrome into the 4th, 5th, 6th, and 7th decades in light of the apparent increased risk for dementia of the Alzheimer type in the older Down syndrome population must be taken seriously by those involved in long-term planning for the aging Down syndrome population (Steffelaar & Evenhuis, 1989). As more individuals with Down syndrome are being integrated into the community, family members, health professionals, and planners may be lulled into a false complacency about the long-range ability of these individuals to cope in society.

CAUSE OF DEATH IN PERSONS WITH DOWN SYNDROME

As discussed in the section on life expectancy, British Columbia data indicate that although survival has improved for Down syndrome, this is still considerably lower than survival for the general population and a "matched" group with mental retardation from other causes. The data suggest that Down syndrome itself may have an effect on survival in addition to the expected complications directly related to congenital heart defect and moderate mental retardation.

British Columbia Population-Based Study on Causes of Death to Age 30 in Persons with Down Syndrome

The existence of the Health Surveillance Registry provided an excellent opportunity to compare the underlying cause of death for the Down syndrome cohort, born 1952–1981, with the age-matched general population of British Columbia (Baird & Sadovnick, 1988a). The Health Surveillance Registry caseload allowed identification of the total population with Down syndrome "at risk" for dying over the entire study period, enabling the data to be analyzed with rates rather than proportional mortality ratios used by others (Scholl, Stein, & Hansen, 1982). Proportional mortality ratios have drawbacks in that an excessive proportional mortality ratio may be obtained either because the risk of death from a specific cause is increased or because the risks associated with other causes are decreased. Most previous studies have also focused on institutionalized persons and, unlike the British Columbia study, were not population based with virtually complete ascertainment.

Available data on the general population were such that the study could only be conducted using underlying cause of death information as recorded in vital statistics death data. Although it is recognized that these data have flaws, as long as the limitations of the information are borne in mind, they are still of value for epidemiologic research (Comstock & Markush, 1986; Seely, 1987).

Methodology

Underlying Cause of Death Data for Persons with Down Syndrome and the General Population In British Columbia, as is standard elsewhere, underlying cause of death is categorized according to International Classification of Disease categories (all Health Surveillance Registry data were coded to *ICD-9* at the time of the study). Underlying cause of death is defined by *ICD-9* as "(a) the disease or injury which initiated the train of morbid events leading directly to death, or (b) the circumstances of the accident or violence which produced the fatal injury" (WHO, 1977, p. 763).

To allow comparison with the data for the general population, underlying cause of death data for the Down syndrome group were used exactly as given on the death certificates with the following necessary exceptions: 1) in calculating rates for the general population of British Columbia, both numerators and denominators were adjusted to subtract the Down syndrome cohort; and 2) the underlying cause of death data for the Down syndrome group were adjusted to omit cases where Down syndrome was given as the underlying cause of death since, by definition, *all* individuals in the study cohort had Down syndrome. This approach was also taken by Scholl et al. (1982).

Study Group At the time of the study, 324 of the original Down syndrome cohort identified through the Health Surveillance Registry (*vide infra*) had died. The underlying cause of death could be determined for 259 (79.9%) of these. For nine persons (2.8%), the underlying cause of death was given as "unknown" on the death certificate. In the remaining 56 persons (17.3%), the underlying cause of death was given as Down syndrome and it was impossible to obtain other information to help delineate the actual underlying cause of death.

Data Analyses Underlying cause of death data for the Down syndrome cohort and the age-matched general population of British Columbia were compared as rates (number in a particular category per total risk group × 1,000) rather than as raw numbers (see Tables 1–4 in Baird & Sadovnick [1988a] for detailed age-specific rates/underlying cause of death categories for the general population and Down syndrome group). The ability to compare such data by rates (i.e., knowing the "at-risk" group) is an important difference between the British Columbia study and others. For each underlying cause of death category, differences in rates were compared using the z test and relative risks were calculated with 95% confidence intervals (Armitage, 1971).

Results

Table 5.3 lists the relative risk data for the Down syndrome cohort compared with the age-matched general population of British Columbia for age groups <1, 1–9, 10–19, and 20–29 according to underlying cause of death categories. Although life expectancy data show that the greatest absolute likelihood of dying in persons with Down syndrome occurs during the 1st year of life, the age group with the greatest relative risk of dying (17.3) is actually 1–9 years. In order, the three underlying cause of death categories with the highest relative risk in persons with Down syndrome are congenital anomalies, circulatory system, and respiratory system. The data in Table 5.3 show that individuals with Down syndrome do not die more often from perinatal complications and accidents compared with the age-matched general population. The distribution of the Down syndrome cohort into the underlying

Table 5.3. Age-specific relative risks (per 1,000) for cause of death in Down syndrome compared with the age-matched general population of British Columbia

Underlying cause of death	Relative risk[a] for Down syndrome at age			
	<1	1–9	10–19	20–29
Infections	17.1 (8.8,33.2)	23.9 (11.8,48.3)	21.0 (2.9,152.1)	.0 (.0,341.7)
Neoplasia	0.0 (.0,67.6)	7.4 (3.3,16.5)	6.2 (1.5,24.8)	4.9 (.7,35.0)
Endocrine	6.7 (1.1,48.0)	4.2 (1.1,17.0)	20.8 (2.9,150.5)	.0 (.0,333.6)
Blood diseases	15.0 (2.1,108.6)	25.3 (3.5,184.6)	65.8 (8.8,493.1)	.0 (.0,1647.3)
Mental diseases	35.2 (4.8,261.2)	49.1 (6.6,367.5)	.0 (.0,352.6)	.0 (.0,303.2)
Nervous system	5.3 (1.7,16.5)	8.0 (2.6,24.9)	.0 (.0,63.8)	.0 (.0,131.0)
Circulatory system	60.5 (24.3,150.3)	73.6 (29.6,183.4)	27.1 (6.7,110.2)	10.0 (1.4,71.7)
Respiratory system	4.3 (2.6,6.9)	25.7 (16.6,39.8)	68.2 (29.2,155.8)	53.1 (12.9,218.9)
Digestive system	7.3 (3.2,16.3)	8.6 (2.1,34.5)	32.4 (4.4,236.3)	.0 (.0,181.6)
Genitourinary system	0.0 (.0,158.8)	16.2 (2.2,117.0)	.0 (.0,336.8)	102.2 (13.4,780.2)
Congenital anomalies	13.5 (10.4,17.6)	76.9 (56.6,104.5)	113.6 (59.2,218.1)	112.2 (40.3,312.2)
Perinatal	1.2 (.8,2.0)	.0 (.0,2770.4)	.0 (.0,10988.1)	.0 (.0,5597.7)
Ill-defined conditions	5.0 (1.6,15.5)	59.7 (14.3,249.5)	158.2 (19.7,1272.1)	.0 (.0,355.7)
Accidents	0.8 (.1,6.0)	1.3 (0.5,3.5)	.0 (.0,2.2)	.0 (.0,2.9)
Unknown or "Down syndrome"	—	—	—	—
Total	6.2 (5.2,7.3)	17.3 (14.3,20.9)	6.0 (4.1,8.9)	3.8 (2.2,6.7)

Adapted from Baird and Sadovnick (1988c).

[a]95% confidence intervals given; numbers in parentheses are (upper, lower) bounds of the true value (Armitage, 1971).

cause of death categories did not differ significantly according to sex ($\chi^2 = 14.8$, $df = 15$, $p > 0.10$).

Causes of Death in Persons with Down Syndrome

Respiratory tract infections have long been recognized as a major cause of death in persons with Down syndrome (Brothers & Jago, 1954; Cant, Gibson, & West, 1987), although a recent study by McGrother and Marshall (1990) found that the proportion of deaths from this cause decreased from 39% (1944–1955) to 5% (1976–1985). British Columbia data (Baird & Sadovnick, 1988a), comparing relative risks rather than percentages, found that deaths from respiratory tract infections occurred significantly more often in the Down syndrome group compared with the general population.

It is now well established that leukemia occurs more often in persons with Down syndrome compared with the age-matched general population (Baird & Sadovnick, 1988a; Brewster & Cannon, 1930; Fong & Brodeur, 1987; McGrother & Marshall, 1990). Although many theories have been postulated to explain this association, no specific mechanism has yet been shown (Fong & Brodeur, 1987). (See Lubin, Kahn, & Scott, chap. 21, this volume, for further discussion.)

Across all ages, congenital anomalies are a major cause of death for individuals with Down syndrome (Baird & Sadovnick, 1988a; Deaton, 1973; Fabia & Drollette, 1970; McGrother & Marshall, 1990; Öster, Mikkelsen, & Nielsen, 1975; Scholl et al., 1982) The major congenital anomaly category responsible for death in persons with Down syndrome is congenital heart defect. The British Columbia study (Baird & Sadovnick, 1988a) found that 4 out of 5 persons with Down syndrome dying from congenital anomalies had congenital heart disease. For the period 1976–1985, McGrother and Marshall

(1990) reported that up to 70% of deaths in their Down syndrome series were due to congenital heart defect. Congenital anomalies of the gastrointestinal tract have been noted as the next most common cause of death in this category and British Columbia data found that 15 out of 16 deaths due to this cause occurred within the 1st year of life (Baird & Sadovnick, 1988a).

Nonmalignant intestinal obstructions also have been reported as an important cause of death in both persons with Down syndrome and those with mental retardation from other causes (Baird & Sadovnick, 1988a; Carter & Jancar, 1984; Roy & Simon, 1987).

CONCLUSION

While overall life expectancy has improved for individuals with Down syndrome, this group still has a greater risk of dying compared with the age-matched general population, and compared with individuals with similar levels of mental retardation due to other causes. This is true for individuals with Down syndrome, both those having and not having congenital heart defects, suggesting that Down syndrome itself may have an additional effect on mortality over those directly associated with congential heart defects and mental retardation.

A recent population-based study on cause of death in British Columbia (Baird & Sadovnick, 1988a) found that under age 1, a child with Down syndrome is six times more likely to die compared with a child not having Down syndrome. For ages 1–9, the individual with Down syndrome is about 17 times more likely to die than others, and for ages 10–19 and 20–29, 6 times and 4 times more likely to die, respectively. These are very substantial differences in overall death rates.

The observed improved survival over time for persons with Down syndrome is expected to result in a larger population of such individuals in all geographic areas, even those where the incidence of births of children with Down syndrome to older mothers is decreasing because of increased utilization of prenatal diagnosis and subsequent termination of pregnancy. Also, since most persons with Down syndrome live in the community, and as congenital heart defects are now often diagnosed early and treated effectively (both medically and surgically), and since infections and nutritional disorders are attended to appropriately, life expectancy for individuals with Down syndrome will most likely improve even more with time. The implications of this improved survival into the 4th, 5th, 6th, and 7th decades must be seriously considered by health care planners, in view of the now quite consistent observation that adults with Down syndrome over age 40 appear to be at an increased risk for dementia of the Alzheimer type.

REFERENCES

Armitage, P. (1971). *Statistical methods in medical research*. Oxford: Blackwell Scientific.

Baird, P.A., & Sadovnick, A.D. (1987). Life expectancy in Down syndrome. *Journal of Pediatrics, 110*, 849–854.

Baird, P.A., & Sadovnick, A.D. (1988a). Causes of death to age 30 in Down syndrome. *American Journal of Human Genetics, 43*, 239–248.

Baird, P.A., & Sadovnick, A.D. (1988b). Life expectancy in Down syndrome adults. *Lancet, ii*, 1354–1356.

Baird, P.A., & Sadovnick, A.D. (1988c). Maternal age–specific rates for Down syndrome. *American Journal of Medical Genetics, 29*, 917–927.

Baird, P.A., & Sadovnick, A.D. (1989). Life tables for Down syndrome. *Human Genetics, 82*, 291–292.

Balakrishnan, T.R., & Wolfe, L.C. (1976). Life expectancy of mentally retarded persons in Canadian institutions. *American Journal of Mental Deficiency, 80*, 650–658.

Brewster, H.F., & Cannon, H.E. (1930). Acute lymphatic leukemia: Report of case in eleventh month mongolian idiot. *New Orleans Medical and Surgical Journal, 82*, 872–873.

Brothers, C.R.D., & Jago, G.C. (1954). Report on the longevity and causes of death in mongoloidism in the state of Victoria. *Journal of Mental Sciences (British Journal of Psychiatry), 100*, 580–582.

Cant, A.J., Gibson, P.J., & West, R.J. (1987). Bacterial tracheitis in Down's syndrome. *Archives of Disease in Childhood, 62*, 962–963.

Carter, G., & Jancar, J. (1984). Sudden deaths in the mentally handicapped. *Psychological Medicine, 14*, 691–695.

Comstock, G.W., & Markush, R.E. (1986). Comments on problems in death certification. *American Journal of Epidemiology, 124,* 180–181.

Dalton, A.J., & Crapper-McLachlan, D.R. (1986). Clinical expression of Alzheimer's disease in Down's syndrome. *Psychiatric Clinics of North America, 9,* 659–670.

Deaton, J.G. (1973). The mortalilty rate and causes of death among institutionalized mongols in Texas. *Journal of Mental Deficiency Research, 17,* 117–122.

Declining mortality from Down syndrome—No cause for complacency [Editorial]. (1990). *Lancet, i,* 888–889.

Dupont, A., Vaeth, M., & Videbech, P. (1986). Mortality and life expectancy of Down's syndrome in Denmark. *Journal of Mental Deficiency Research, 30,* 111–120.

Elandt-Johnson, R.C., & Johnson, N.L. (1980). *Survival models and data analysis.* New York: John Wiley & Sons.

Evans, J.A., Hunter, A.G., & Hamerton, J.L. (1978). Down syndrome and recent demographic trends in Manitoba. *Journal of Medical Genetics, 15,* 43–47.

Evenhuis, H.M. (1990). The natural history of dementia in Down's syndrome. *Archives of Neurology, 47,* 263–267.

Evers-Kieboom, G., Vlietinck, R., & Van Den Berghe, H. (1985). The relative risk for standard 21 trisomy has not increased in young mothers in Belgium, 1960–1978. *Clinical Genetics, 27,* 33–44.

Fabia, J., & Drollette, M. (1970). Life tables up to age 10 for mongols with and without congenital heart disease. *Journal of Mental Deficiency Research, 19,* 157–163.

Fong, C.-T., & Brodeur, G.M. (1987). Down's syndrome and leukemia: Epidemiology, genetics, cytogenetics and mechanisms of leukemogenesis. *Cancer Genetics and Cytogenetics, 28,* 55–76.

Forssman, H., & Åkesson, H.O. (1965). Mortality in patients with Down syndrome. *Journal of Mental Deficiency Research, 9,* 146–149.

Forssman, H., & Åkesson, H.O. (1967). Note on mortality in patients with Down syndrome. *Journal of Mental Deficiency Research, 11,* 106–107.

Gallagher, R.P., & Lowry, R.B. (1975). Longevity in Down's syndrome in British Columbia. *Journal of Mental Deficiency Research, 19,* 157–163.

Hook, E.B., & Cross, P.K. (1981). Temporal increase in the rate of Down syndrome livebirths to older mothers in New York State. *Journal of Medical Genetics, 18,* 29–30.

Larsson, T., & Sjögren, T. (1954). A methodological, psychiatric, and statistical study of a Swedish rural population. *Acta Psychiatrica et Neurologic Scandinavica Supplement, 89,* 40–54.

Lawless, J.F. (1982). *Statistical models and methods for lifetime data.* New York: John Wiley & Sons.

Lee, E.T. (1981). *Statistical methods for survival data analyses.* Belmont, CA: Lifetime Learning Publications.

Leisti, J., Vahtola, L., Linna, S.-L., Herva, R., Koskela, S-L., & Vitali, M. (1985). The incidence of Down syndrome in northern Finland with special reference to maternal age. *Clinical Genetics, 27,* 252–257.

Malone, Q. (1988). Mortality and survival of the Down's syndrome population in Western Australia. *Journal of Mental Deficiency Research, 32,* 59–65.

Masaki, M., Higurashi, M., Iijima, K., Ishikawa, N., Tanaka, F., Fujii, T., Kuroki, Y., Matsui, I., Iinumi, K., Matsuo, N., Takeshita, K., & Hashimoto, S. (1981). Mortality and survival for Down syndrome in Japan. *American Journal of Human Genetics, 33,* 629–639.

McGrother, C.W., & Marshall, B. (1990). Recent trends in incidence, morbidity and survival in Down syndrome. *Journal of Mental Deficiency Research, 34,* 49–57.

Mikkelsen, M., Fischer, G., Hanson, J., Pilgaard, B., & Nielsen, J. (1983). The impact of legal termination of pregnancy and of prenatal diagnosis on the birth prevalence of Down syndrome in Denmark. *Annals of Human Genetics, 47,* 123–131.

Öster, J., Mikkelsen, M., & Nielsen, A. (1975). Mortality and life-table in Down's syndrome. *Acta Paedicatrica Scandinavica, 64,* 322–326.

Record, R.G., & Smith, A. (1955). Incidence, mortality, and sex distribution of mongoloid defectives. *British Journal of Preventive and Social Medicine, 9,* 10–15.

Richards, B.W., & Siddiqui, A.Q. (1980). Age and mortality trends in residents of an institution for the mentally handicapped. *Journal of Mental Deficiency Research, 24,* 99–105.

Roy, A., & Simon, G.B. (1987). Intestinal obstruction as a cause of death in the mentally handicapped. *Journal of Mental Deficiency Research, 31,* 193–197.

Scholl, T., Stein, Z., & Hansen, H. (1982). Leukemia and other cancers, anomalies, and infections as causes of death in Down's syndrome: A 10-year retrospective survey in the United States during 1976. *Developmental Medicine and Child Neurology, 24,* 817–829.

Seely, S. (1987). Errors in mortality statistics. *Lancet, i,* 220–221.

Smith, M.E., & Newcombe, H.B. (1982). Use of the Canadian mortality data base for epidemiological follow-up. *Canadian Journal of Public Health, 73,* 39–46.

Statistics Canada. (1981). *International and interprovincial migration in Canada* (Catalogue 91-208, annual publication, 1961–1981). Ottawa: Author.

Steffelaar, J.W., & Evenhuis, H.M. (1989). Life expectancy, Down syndrome, and dementia. *Lancet, i,* 492–493.

Thase, M.E. (1982). Longevity and mortality in Down's syndrome. *Journal of Mental Deficiency Research, 26,* 177–192.

Trimble, B.K., & Baird, P.A. (1978). Maternal age and Down syndrome: Age-specific incidence rates by single year intervals. *American Journal of Medical Genetics, 2,* 1–5.

World Health Organization. (1977). *World Health Organization International Classification of Diseases Diagnostic Codes (ICD)* (9th ed.). Geneva: Author.

CHAPTER
6

Ophthalmologic Concerns

Robert A. Catalano

Ocular and orbital abnormalities are common in persons with Down syndrome. With the exception of the vitreous, structural abnormalities have been documented in every ocular tissue. Prior to the advent of karyotyping, ocular findings were of great importance in diagnosing the syndrome. Despite this propensity to involve the eye, a specific phenotypic ocular expression of Down syndrome does not exist. No ocular finding is pathognomonic, as similar anomalies occur in otherwise "normal" individuals or in persons with other mental or physical disabilities (Ginsberg, Ballard, Buchind, & Kinkler, 1980). Furthermore, no individual exhibits every noted abnormality; there do not even exist subcategories of individuals with concordant constellations of findings.

Ginsberg, Bofinger, and Roush (1977) characterized the ocular findings of Down syndrome as consisting of a variety of nonspecific hyperplasias, hypoplasias, tissue defects, hamartomas, and heterotopias. The nature of these anomalies suggests that the eye is affected late in its embryologic development. In discussing these manifestations, emphasis is placed on those findings that appear in more than 10% of individuals (Table 6.1). Isolated reports of associated anomalies are so noted.

EXTERNAL OCULAR FINDINGS

External ocular features are prominent among the ocular findings of Down syndrome. The facies of individuals with Down syndrome includes a narrowed interpupillary distance (Brushfield, 1924; Kerwood, Lang-Brown, & Penrose, 1954; Lowe, 1949), upward and outward slanting palpebral fissures, and epicanthus. (These external ocular features are discussed in detail in Pueschel, chap. 1, this volume.) Additional external findings include an increased prevalence of blepharitis (inflammation of the eyelids) and congenital eversion of the upper eyelids.

Blepharitis has been reported in 2%–47% of individuals with Down syndrome (Cullen & Butler, 1963; Eissler & Longenecker, 1962; Shapiro & France, 1985; Solomons, Zellweger, Jahnke, & Opitz, 1965). Periodic examination, in a 10-year study, noted that 17 of 30 individuals with Down syndrome had at least one documented occurrence of blepharitis (Gaynon & Schimeck, 1977). Daily scrubbing of the eyelid margins with cotton swabs dipped in baby shampoo can reduce the prevalence of blepharitis (Catalano, 1990).

Seven of the 20 reported cases of congenital eversion of the upper eyelids, occurring in the absence of other major ocular abnormalities, have been reported in infants with Down syndrome (Bleeker-Wagemakers, Delleman, & Van Walbeek, 1976; Gilbert, Smith, Barlow, & Mohr, 1973; Johnson & McGowan, 1969; Stern, Campbell, & Faulkner, 1973; Sutterle & Gottesleben, 1967; Young, 1954). A postulated pathogenic mechanism relates to a constitutional weakness and flaccidity of the eyelid (Erb, 1909; Sutterle & Gottesleben, 1967). Obstruction of venous outflow from prominent epicanthal folds, resulting in palpebral conjunctival edema and

Supported in part by an unrestricted grant from Research to Prevent Blindness, Inc. Modified in part, with permission, from: Catalano, R.A. (1990). Down syndrome. *Survey of Ophthalmology, 34*, 385–398.

Table 6.1. Major ocular features of Down syndrome

Features	Cullen (1963)	Eissler and Longenecker (1962)	Gaynon and Schimeck (1977)	Jaeger (1980)	Lowe (1949)	Shapiro and France (1985)	Skeller and Öster (1951)
Epicanthus	100	38	53	17	—	—	21
Upward oblique slant of palpebral fissure	100	43	73	83	—	89	41
Brushfield spots	38	—	50	59	90	81	86
Strabismus	32	44	33	41	33	43	30
Cataract	15	12	16	55	86	13	43
Keratoconus	5	—	—	3	—	15	6
Myopia	6	—	13	20	37	27	"few"
Nystagmus	4	15	20	11	13	9	18
Blepharitis	2	6	56	13	15	47	67

Note: All data are reported as percentages.

eversion of the eyelids, has also been surmised (Stillerman, Emanuel, & Padoor, 1966; Young, 1954). Although conservative treatment to protect the eye from desiccation is usually advocated for congenital eyelid eversion (Mazhar, 1955; Ostriker & Lasky, 1954; Smith & Berg, 1976), surgical intervention was needed in 5 of the 7 affected infants with Down syndrome (Gilbert et al., 1973; Johnson & McGowan, 1969; Sutterle & Gottesleben, 1967; Young, 1954).

KERATOCONUS

Keratoconus (conical cornea) is one of the most recently described ocular findings in Down syndrome. Rados first noted the association in 1948. Since then, various authors have reported the prevalence of keratoconus to be between 5.5%–8.0% (Cullen & Butler, 1963; Missiroli & Vanni, 1970; Pierse & Eustace, 1971; Skeller & Öster, 1951; Walsh, 1981). In 1956, Hofmann first described acute keratoconus, or hydrops, in 2 persons with Down syndrome (Figure 6.1). Subsequently, isolated individuals were reported in European medical journals (Applemans, Micheiels, Nelis, & Massa, 1961; Heinmuller, 1959; Leffertstra, 1959; Woillez & Dansaut, 1960). It is now recognized that hydrops occurs much more frequently as a complication of keratoconus in individuals with Down syndrome (Applemans et al., 1961; Kenyon & Kidwell, 1976; Krachmer, Feder, & Berlin, 1984; Pierse

& Eustace, 1971; Pouliquen, 1987; Slusher, Laibson, & Mulberger, 1968). In one report, acute keratoconus was cited as the second most common cause of blindness in persons with Down syndrome (Cullen, 1963). The most common cause is a complication from cataract surgery.

The increased prevalence of both keratoconus (Pierse & Eustace, 1971) and acute keratoconus (Krachmer et al., 1984; Slusher et al., 1968) may be due to eye rubbing. In turn, chronic blepharitis has been postulated to result in eye rubbing (Shapiro & France, 1985).

Rarely reported corneal findings include congenital corneal opacities, which may be related to thyrotoxicosis (Dark & Kirkham, 1968; Schirb, 1968), and an irregular thickening of the corneal stroma (Ginsberg et al., 1980). The reported association of megalocornea to Down syndrome likely represents a chance occurrence (Rogers & Poloiteno, 1964).

INFANTILE GLAUCOMA

Primary infantile (congenital) glaucoma has been described in only 12 infants with Down syndrome (Bardelli, Hadjistilianou, & Frezzotti, 1985; Catalano, 1990; Francois, Berser, & Saraux, 1975; Traboulsi et al., 1988). Signs and symptoms of infantile glaucoma include increased intraocular pressure, optic nerve cupping, corneal edema (cloudiness), corneal enlargement, tearing, blepharospasm, and photophobia

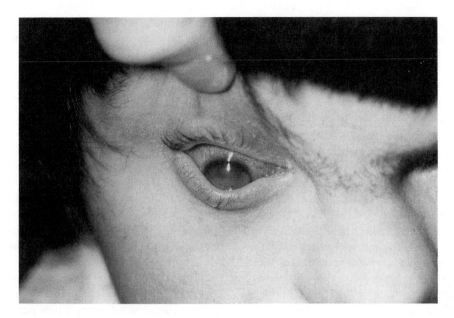

Figure 6.1. Acute keratoconus (hydrops) in a child with Down syndrome.

(Figure 6.2). This rarely reported association of infantile glaucoma with Down syndrome suggests a chance occurrence. The combination of infantile glaucoma, severe myopia, and cataracts in infants with Down syndrome, however, portends a poor visual outcome (Traboulsi et al., 1988).

IRIS ANOMALIES

Anomalies of the iris are common in individuals with Down syndrome (Ginsberg et al., 1977). An increased prevalence of iris spots or speckles, lighter colored irides, peripheral stromal iris hypoplasia, hypoplasia of the iris sphincter, and

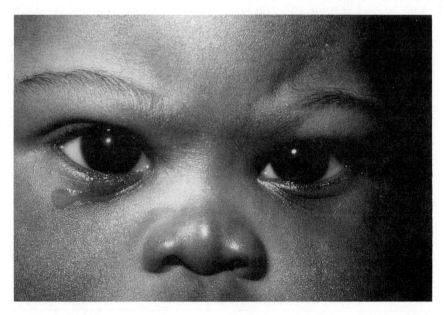

Figure 6.2. Primary infantile glaucoma in a child with Down syndrome. (From Catalano, R.A. [1990]. Down syndrome. *Survey of Ophthalmology, 34,* 392; reprinted with permission.)

iridoschisis have all been described (Beach, 1878; Cullen & Butler, 1963; Eissler & Longenecker, 1962; Gaynon & Schimeck, 1977; Ginsberg et al., 1977, Jaeger, 1980; Lowe, 1949; Shapiro & France, 1985; Skeller & Oster, 1951). None of these findings, however, is diagnostic for Down syndrome.

Speckling of the iris was first described by Wolfflin in 1902. He noted that 10% of all "normal" individuals had 10–20 whitish to light yellow, peripheral, pinpoint- to pinhead-size iris nodules. In 1924, Brushfield associated these nodules with Down syndrome. It is now well recognized that they occur in 38%–90% of persons with Down syndrome. They are more common in individuals with blue and hazel irides. Wallis (1951) suggested that they disappear in blue-eyed infants whose irises subsequently turn brown. They are not believed to be related to age, IQ, or sex (Donaldson, 1961; Jaeger, 1980). R.D.B. Williams (1981), in an excellent review of the subject, tabulated the differences between Brushfield spots and Wolfflin nodules (Table 6.2). Using his criteria, he noted the majority of children with mental retardation (not caused by Down syndrome) with iris speckling had Brushfield spots (Figure 6.3) (see also Pueschel, chap. 1, this volume).

Although the etiology of Brushfield spots remains unknown, numerous histopathologic reports have noted that they are condensations of collagenous tissue in the anterior iris stroma (Donaldson, 1961; Jaeger, 1980; Menkes, 1980; Purtcher, 1958). Areas between the spots appear to have less than the normal amount of stromal fibers.

Lowe (1949) believed that iris hypoplasia was a more prominent feature of Down syndrome than iris spots, occurring up to 95% of the time and at an early age. Skeller and Öster (1951), however, found only 42% of their patients to have iris hypoplasia.

CATARACTS

More than 80 years ago, Pearce, Rankine, and Ormond (1910) noted flake-like, "coronary-cerulean" lens opacities (Figure 6.4) in individuals with Down syndrome. Numerous subsequent investigators have also noted cataracts in 25%–85% of adults with Down syndrome (Apple, 1974; Ormond, 1912; van der Scheer, 1919; von Tobel, 1933). Ingersheim (1951), in a study of 125 persons, found minute, gray, flake or punctate opacities to be the most common form of cataract in persons with Down syndrome. He believed these opacities began to appear between 6–10 years of age and were almost universally present after 16 years. Jaeger (1980) also found an increased prevalence of flake opacities with a predilection for the peripheral cortex and the anterior and posterior polar areas. Likewise, he found that senile cataracts occur at a younger age and believed that this may be a manifestation of early aging in Down syndrome.

Cogan and Kuwabara (1962) proposed that the characteristic flake opacity was due to the proliferation of wart-like excrescences of the lens capsule that eventually dropped off into the cortex of the lens. In a pathologic study of the lenses of 21 persons with Down syndrome, however, Robb and Marchevsky (1978) were unable to demonstrate this. Homogeneous, slightly granular, periodic acid-Schiff (PAS) staining focal lesions appeared without obvious relation to the lens capsule. On the basis of their findings, Robb

Table 6.2.   Brushfield spots versus Wolfflin nodules

Characteristic	Brushfield spots	Wolfflin nodules
Prevalence	85%–90% in persons with Down syndrome	10%–24% in typical individuals
Size and shape	0.1 to 1.0 mm Variable shape May coalesce	0.1 to 0.2 mm Uniform shape Regular formation
Position in iris	Middle and outer thirds of iris	Outer four fifths of iris
Iris hypoplasia	80%–95% in persons with Down syndrome	0%–9% in typical individuals

Adapted from Williams, R.D.B. (1981). Brushfield spots and Wolfflin nodules in the iris: An appraisal in handicapped children. *Developmental Medicine and Child Neurology, 23,* 647; reprinted with permission.

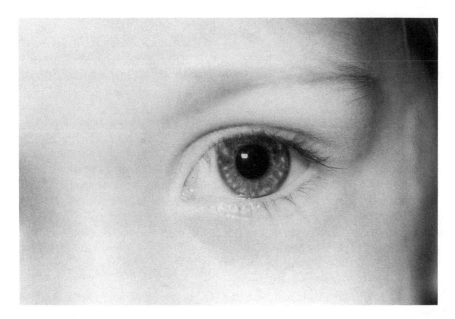

Figure 6.3.   Brushfield spots in a child with Down syndrome.

and Marchevsky also concluded there was no pathologic evidence that the flake opacities were progressive or precursors of more generalized cortical cataracts. The pathogenesis of flake opacities, which are not unique to Down syndrome (Ginsberg et al., 1980; Lowe, 1949), remains unknown.

Although considered rare, congenital cata-racts also occur at a higher rate in persons with Down syndrome than in the general population. In a survey of 386 infants with cataracts, Merin and Crawford (1971) found 4% to have Down syndrome. Howard, Boue, Deluchat, Albert, and Lahav (1974) observed all of the lenses of 4 embryos with trisomy G to have changes compatible with cataract formation, and microscopic

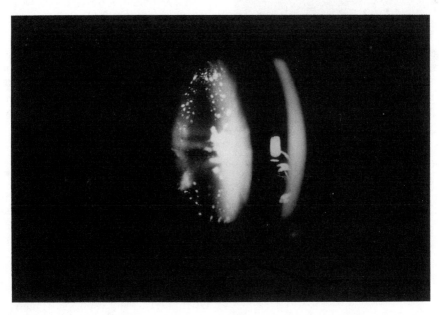

Figure 6.4.   Flake-like lens opacities ("coronary-cerulean cataracts") in a child with Down syndrome.

capsular and subcapsular changes have been noted in a 5th embryo (Ginsberg et al., 1977). Lowe (1949) found a 6% prevalence of congenital cataracts.

RETINAL ANOMALIES

E.J. Williams, McCormick, and Tischler (1973) observed that persons with Down syndrome had an increased number of retinal vessels crossing the disc margin. These were often arranged in a spoke-like distribution (Figure 6.5). Studying photographs of 50 eyes, they found an average of 17.7 vessels crossing the disc margin and extending for at least one disc diameter, as compared with an average of 13.4 vessels in the control population. Jaeger (1980) corroborated these findings in 55 additional individuals and found no correlation between IQ and number of disc vessels.

Ahmad and Pruett (1976) noted myopic fundus changes, including temporal crescents along

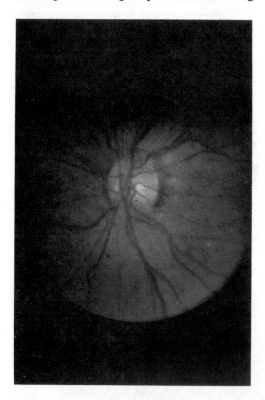

Figure 6.5. Increased number of vessels crossing the disc margin, arranged in a spoke-like pattern, in a child with Down syndrome.

the disc margin, choroidal thinning, and a blond appearance of the fundus in all eyes of individuals with Down syndrome, regardless of the refractive error or degree of iris or skin pigmentation.

Retinoblastoma has been documented in 7 children with Down syndrome (Bentley, 1975; Day, Wright, Koons, & Quigley, 1963; Keith, 1978; Taktikos, 1964). The karyotypes were examined in 2 of these children and both were found to have a double aneuploidy, 48,XXX + 21. Individuals with retinal folds (Day et al., 1963) and retinal dysplasia (Ginsberg et al., 1977) have also been reported.

OPTIC NERVE ANOMALIES

The increased number of retinal vessels crossing the disc margin can give the disc a more hyperemic than normal appearance (Ahmad & Pruett, 1976; E.J. Williams et al., 1973). Optic nerve hypoplasia has been reported in only 3 persons with Down syndrome (Awan, 1977; Catalano, 1990; Ginsberg et al., 1980), and an optic nerve glioma in only 1 (Jonakin & Hensley, 1983).

Five infants with Down syndrome and idiopathic optic nerve head elevation (Figure 6.6) also have been reported (Catalano & Simon, 1990). No child was observed to have retinal vessel dilation, splinter hemorrhages, optic nerve drusen, subsequent optic atrophy, or apparent visual loss. No central nervous system abnormalities were found on enhanced computer tomography, and partial, complete or intermittent resolution occurred in 3 of the 5 children (Catalano & Simon, 1990). The reason for this occurrence remains undetermined.

STRABISMUS

Various investigators have reported a prevalence of strabismus in persons with Down syndrome of between 23%–44% (Cullen & Butler, 1963; Eissler & Longenecker, 1962; Falls, 1970; Gaynon & Schimeck, 1977; Hiles, Hoyme, & McFarlane, 1974; Jaeger, 1980; Lowe, 1949; Ormond, 1912; Shapiro & France, 1985; Skeller & Öster, 1951). Only esotropia (Figure 6.7) had been associated until 1949 when Engler reported

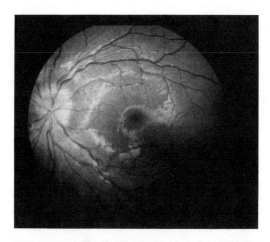

Figure 6.6. Idiopathic optic nerve head elevation in an infant with Down syndrome. (From Catalano, R.A., & Simon, J.W. [1990]. Optic disk elevation in Down syndrome. *American Journal of Ophthalmology, 110,* 29; published with permission from *The American Journal of Ophthalmology;* copyright by The Ophthalmic Publishing Company.)

2 individuals with Down syndrome who had exotropia. The greatest prevalence of exotropia was reported by Hiles et al. (1974), who found 8 of their 123 patients (6%) to have exodeviations. Two of their patients with exotropia had third cranial nerve palsies, 2 had meningomyeloceles, and 1 had dense amblyopia. Most of their patients with exotropia also had hyperdeviations. Accommodative esotropia accounted for most of their esodeviations. Jaeger (1980), however, did not find an association of esotropia and hyperopia, noting that high myopia (− 6.00 diopters [D]) occurred as frequently as high hyperopia in persons with esotropia. Jaeger believed that esotropia in persons with Down syndrome may be due to decreased fusional or visual resolution ca-

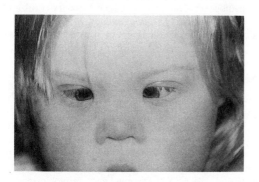

Figure 6.7. Esotropia (inward deviation of the eyes) in an individual with Down syndrome.

pacity, or a failure to develop an adequate accommodative convergence mechanism.

AMBLYOPIA

Although strabismus is very common in children with Down syndrome, amblyopia (unilateral decreased visual acuity) is reported to be uncommon. Hiles et al. (1974) reported that less than 10% of their strabismic patients with Down syndrome had amblyopia and Jaeger (1980) found amblyopia in only 12.5% of his patients with ocular misalignment. Despite these findings, children with Down syndrome who have identified amblyopia should receive occlusive therapy.

NYSTAGMUS

Nystagmus (ocular ataxia) has been reported in 5%–30% of individuals with Down syndrome (Cullen & Butler, 1963; Eissler & Longenecker, 1962; Hiles et al., 1974; Lowe, 1949; Shapiro & France, 1985; Skeller & Öster, 1951; Wagner, Caputo, & Reynolds, 1988). Typically, no ocular pathology contributing to poor retinal image formation is present. Nystagmus is especially prevalent in persons with strabismus, occurring in 33%–73% of persons with Down syndrome who have esotropia (Hiles et al., 1974; Wagner et al., 1988). The nystagmus is typically horizontal (Shapiro & France, 1985; Wagner et al., 1988), although rotatory nystagmus has also been described (Hiles et al., 1974). In over half of such individuals, the nystagmus is fine, rapid, and pendular. Wagner et al. (1988) noted that it is dissociative in 25% of affected individuals.

REFRACTIVE ERRORS

Excessive deviation from emmetropia has been well documented in persons with Down syndrome (Brousseau, 1928; Cullen & Butler, 1963; Gardiner, 1967; Jaeger, 1980; Lowe, 1949; Shapiro & France, 1985; Skeller & Öster, 1951). The prevalence of differing levels of ametropia is difficult to estimate because investigators often report refractive errors differently. It is clear, however, that a substantial number of persons with Down syndrome have high myopia

(>8.00 diopters). Two large studies reported a prevalence of high myopia of between 35%–40% (Jaeger, 1980; Lowe, 1949). Astigmatism of greater than 2.50–3.00 diopters has been reported in 18%–25% of individuals with Down syndrome (Jaeger, 1980; Shapiro & France, 1985). Jaeger (1980) also found a fivefold greater prevalence of lower levels of ametropia ($\geq$ + 4.00 diopter sphere; −2.50 diopter cylinder) as compared to a control group of office patients. At higher levels of ametropia, myopia is predominant, whereas at lower levels a more even distribution of refractive errors occurs.

The etiology of high myopia in individuals with Down syndrome remains unknown. Gardiner (1967) noted that school-age children with cyanotic congenital heart defects had an increased prevalence of myopia. He speculated that the myopia in individuals with Down syndrome may be similarly related, but provided no evidence to support this hypothesis. Ginsberg and associates (1980) noted an increased corneal curvature of the eyes in 1 infant with Down syndrome and suggested that this could be the basis for the high myopia. Shapiro and France (1985) speculated that the high astigmatism may be due to rubbing or to structural abnormalities of the cornea, which are also believed to cause keratoconus.

CONCLUSION

Ocular features are very important in the clinical diagnosis of Down syndrome. They also remain a prominent disability for individuals with Down syndrome. Cataracts and acute keratoconus continue to be the principal causes of visual loss. Strabismus, blepharitis, and high refractive errors, however, are more common and may be functionally debilitating. Fortunately, treatment for all of these conditions exists, and such treatment can significantly affect the quality of life of individuals with Down syndrome.

REFERENCES

Ahmad, A., & Pruett, R.C. (1976). The fundus in mongolism. *Archives of Ophthalmology, 94,* 772–776.

Apple, J. (1974). Chromosome-induced ocular disease. In M.F. Goldberg (Ed.), *Genetic and metabolic eye diseases* (pp. 540–544). Boston: Little, Brown.

Applemans, M., Micheiels, J., Nelis, J., & Massa, J.M. (1961). Keratocone aigu chex la mongoloide [Keratoconus in a mongoloid child]. *Bulletin of the Society of Belgian Ophthalmology, 128,* 249–259.

Awan, K.J. (1977). Uncommon ocular changes in Down's syndrome (mongolism). *Journal of Pediatric Ophthalmology, 14,* 215–216.

Bardelli, A.M., Hadjistilianou, T., & Frezzotti, R. (1985). Etiology of congenital glaucoma. Genetic and extragenetic factors. *Ophthalmic Paediatric Genetics, 6,* 265–270.

Beach, F. (1878). On the diagnosis and treatment of idiocy, with remarks on prognosis. *Lancet, ii,* 764–766.

Bentley, D. (1975). A case of Down's syndrome complicated by retinoblastoma and celiac disease. *Pediatrics, 56,* 131–133.

Bleeker-Wagemakers, E.M., Delleman, J.W., & Van Walbeek, K. (1976). Congenital eversion of the eyelids in a case of Down's syndrome. *Ophthalmologica, 173,* 250–256.

Brousseau, K. (1928). *Mongolism.* Baltimore: Williams & Wilkins.

Brushfield, T. (1924). Mongolism. *British Journal of Children's Diseases, 21,* 241–258.

Catalano, R.A. (1990). Down syndrome. *Survey of Ophthalmology, 34,* 385–398.

Catalano, R.A., & Simon, J.W. (1990). Optic disk elevation in Down syndrome. *American Journal of Ophthalmology, 100,* 28-32.

Cogan, D.G., & Kuwabara, T. (1962). Pathology of cataracts in mongoloid idiocy: A new concept of the pathogenesis of cataracts of the coronary-cerulean type. *Doctrine of Ophthalmology, 16,* 73–80.

Cullen, J.F. (1963). Blindness in mongolism (Down's syndrome). *British Journal of Ophthalmology, 47,* 331–333.

Cullen, J.F., & Butler, H.G. (1963). Mongolism (Down's syndrome) and keratoconus. *British Journal of Ophthalmology, 47,* 321–330.

Dark, A.J., & Kirkham, T.H. (1968). Congenital corneal opacities in a patient with Reiger's anomaly and Down's syndrome. *British Journal of Ophthalmology, 52,* 631–635.

Day, R.W., Wright, S.W., Koons, A., & Quigley, M. (1963). 48XXX21-trisomy and retinoblastoma. *Lancet, ii,* 154–155.

Donaldson, D.D. (1961). The significance of spotting of the iris in mongoloids: Brushfield spots. *Ar-

chives of Ophthalmology, 65, 26–31.

Eissler, R., & Longenecker, J.P. (1962). The common eye findings in mongolism. *American Journal of Ophthalmology, 54*, 398–406.

Erb, A. (1909). Ein fall von doppelseitigem congenitalen ectropion des oberlids [A case of bilateral ectropion of the eyelids]. *Correspondenz Schweizer Aerzte, 39*, 733.

Falls, H.F. (1970). Ocular changes in mongolism. *Annals of the New York Academy of Science, 171*, 627–636.

Francois, J., Berser, R., & Saraux, U. (1975). *Chromosomal aberrations in ophthalmology.* Amsterdam: Van Gorcum.

Gardiner, P.A. (1967). Visual defects in cases of Down's syndrome and in other mentally handicapped children. *British Journal of Ophthalmology, 51*, 469–474.

Gaynon, M.W., & Schimeck, R.A. (1977). Down's syndrome. A ten-year group study. *Annals of Ophthalmology, 9*, 1493–1497.

Gilbert, H.D., Smith, R.E., Barlow, M.H., & Mohr, D. (1973). Congenital upper eyelid eversion and Down's syndrome. *American Journal of Ophthalmology, 75*, 469–472.

Ginsberg, J., Ballard, E.T., Buchind, J.J., & Kinkler, A.K. (1980). Further observations of ocular pathology in Down's syndrome. *Journal of Pediatric Ophthalmology, 17*, 166–171.

Ginsberg, J., Bofinger, M.K., & Roush, J.R. (1977). Pathologic features of the eye in Down's syndrome with relationship to other chromosomal anomalies. *American Journal of Ophthalmology, 83*, 874–880.

Heinmuller, G. (1959). Akuter keratokonus [Acute keratoconus]. *Klinisches Monatsblatt der Augenheilkunde, 134*, 410–413.

Hiles, D.A., Hoyme, S.H., & McFarlane, F. (1974). Down's syndrome and strabismus. *American Orthoptics Journal, 24*, 63–68.

Hofmann, H. (1956). Akuter keratokonus bei mongoloider idiotie [Acute keratoconus of the mongoloid idiot]. *Klinisches Monatsblatt der Augenheilkunde, 129*, 756–762.

Howard, R.O., Boue, J., Deluchat, C., Albert, D.M., & Lahav, M. (1974). The eyes of embryos with chromosome abnormalities. *American Journal of Ophthalmology, 78*, 167–168.

Ingersheim, J. (1951). The relationship of lenticular changes in mongolism. *Transactions of the American Ophthalmologic Society, 49*, 595–624.

Jaeger, E.A. (1980). Ocular findings in Down's syndrome. *Transactions of the American Ophthalmologic Society, 158*, 808–845.

Johnson, C.C., & McGowan, B.L. (1969). Persistent congenital ectropion of all four eyelids with megaloblepharon. *American Journal of Ophthalmology, 67*, 252–256.

Jonakin, W.L., & Hensley, M.F. (1983). Optic glioma and Down's syndrome. *Journal of the American Osteopathic Association, 82*, 806.

Keith, C.G. (1978). *Genetics and ophthalmology.* New York: Churchill Livingston.

Kenyon, K.R., & Kidwell, E.J. (1976). Corneal hydrops and keratoconus associated with mongolism. *Archives of Ophthalmology, 94*, 494–495.

Kerwood, L.A., Lang-Brown, J., & Penrose, L.S. (1954). The interpupillary distance in mentally defective patients. *Human Biology, 26*, 313–323.

Krachmer, J.H., Feder, R.S., & Berlin, M.W. (1984). Keratoconus and related noninflammatory corneal thinning disorders. *Survey of Ophthalmology, 28*, 293–322.

Leffertstra, L.J. (1959). Acute keratoconus in the presence of mongoloid idiocy. *Ophthalmologica, 137*, 432.

Lowe, R. (1949). The eyes in mongolism. *British Journal of Ophthalmology, 33*, 131–154.

Mazhar, M. (1955). Congenital eversion of upper eyelids. *British Journal of Ophthalmology, 39*, 702.

Menkes, J.H. (1980). Chromosomal anomalies. In J.H. Menkes (Ed.), *Textbook of child neurology* (2nd ed., pp. 151–152). Philadelphia: Lea & Febiger.

Merin, S., & Crawford, J.S. (1971). The etiology of congenital cataracts: A survey of 386 cases. *Canadian Journal of Ophthalmology, 6*, 178–182.

Missiroli, A., & Vanni, V. (1970). Sui segni oculari della sindrome di Down [About the ocular signs of Down syndrome]. *Bolletin Oculi, 49*, 123–139.

Ormond, A.W. (1912). Notes on the ophthalmic condition of 43 mongolian imbeciles. *Transactions of the Ophthalmologic Society of the United Kingdom, 32*, 69–76.

Ostriker, P.J., & Lasky, M.A. (1954). Congenital eversion of the upper eyelids. *American Journal of Ophthalmology, 37*, 779–781.

Pearce, F.H., Rankine, R., & Ormond, A.W. (1910). Notes on twenty-eight cases of mongolian imbeciles: With special reference to their ocular condition. *British Medical Journal, 2*, 186–190.

Pierse, D., & Eustace, P. (1971). Acute keratoconus in mongols. *British Journal of Ophthalmology, 55*, 50–54.

Pouliquen, Y. (1987). Keratoconus. *Eye, 1*, 1–14.

Purtcher, E. (1958). Knotenförmige verdichtungen im irisstroma bei mongolismus [Moth-like densities in the iris stroma in mongoloidism]. *Archiv für Ophthalmologie, 160*, 200–215.

Rados, A. (1948). Conical cornea and mongolism. *Archives of Ophthalmology, 40*, 454–478.

Robb, R.M., & Marchevsky, A. (1978). Pathology of the lens in Down's syndrome. *Archives of Ophthalmology, 96*, 1039–1042.

Rogers, G.L., & Poloiteno, R.C. (1964). Autosomal dominant inheritance of megalocornea associated with Down's syndrome. *American Journal of Ophthalmology, 78*, 526–529.

Schirb, M. (1968). Corneal opacities in Down's syndrome with thyrotoxicosis. *Archives of Ophthalmology, 80*, 618–621.

Shapiro, M.B., & France, T.D. (1985). The ocular features of Down's syndrome. *American Journal of Ophthalmology, 99,* 659–663.

Skeller, E., & Öster, J. (1951). Eye symptoms in mongolism. *Acta Ophthalmologica, 29,* 149–161.

Slusher, M.M., Laibson, P.R., & Mulberger, R.D. (1968). Acute keratoconus in Down's syndrome. *American Journal of Ophthalmology, 66,* 1137–1143.

Solomons, G., Zellweger, H., Jahnke, P.G., & Opitz, E. (1965). Four common eye signs in mongolism. *American Journal of Diseases of Children, 110,* 46–50.

Smith, F.G., & Berg, J.M. (1976). *Down's anomaly.* Edinburgh: Churchill Livingston.

Stern, E., Campbell, C.H., & Faulkner, H.W. (1973). Conservative management of congenital eversion of the eyelids. *American Journal of Ophthalmology, 75,* 319–320.

Stillerman, M.L., Emanuel, B., & Padoor, M.P. (1966). Eversion of the eyelids in newborns without an apparent cause. *Journal of Pediatrics, 69,* 656–658.

Sutterle, H., & Gottesleben, H.U. (1967). Konatales ektropium der oberlider und mongolismus [Congenital ectropion of the eyelid and mongoloidism]. *Klinisches Monatsblatt der Augenheilkunde, 150,* 552–556.

Taktikos, A. (1964). Association of retinoblastoma with mental defect and other pathologic manifestations. *British Journal of Ophthalmology, 48,* 495–498.

Traboulsi, E.I., Levine, E., Mets, M.B., Parelhoff, E.S., O'Neill, J.F., & Gaasterland, D.E. (1988). Infantile glaucoma in Down's syndrome (trisomy 21). *American Journal of Ophthalmology, 105,* 389–394.

van der Scheer, W.M. (1919). Cataractis lentis bei mongoloider idiotie [Cataracts of the lens in the mongoloid idiot]. *Klinisches Monatsblatt der Augenheilkunde, 62,* 155–170.

von Tobel, W. (1933). Über linsen und hornhautuntersuchungen an mongoloiden idioten [About the combination of the lens and cornea of the mongoloid idiot]. *Archiv für Ophthalmologie, 130,* 325–338.

Wagner, R.S., Caputo, A.R., & Reynolds, R.D. (1988). The incidence and classification of nystagmus in Down's syndrome [abstract of presentation]. *Ophthalmology, 95* (Suppl. 149).

Wallis, R.E. (1951). The significance of Brushfield's spots in the diagnosis of mongolism in infancy. *Archives of Diseases of Children, 26,* 495–500.

Walsh, S.Z. (1981). Keratoconus and blindness in 469 institutionalized subjects with Down's syndrome and other causes of mental retardation. *Journal of Mental Deficiency Research, 25,* 243–251.

Williams, E.J., McCormick, A.Q., & Tischler, B. (1973). Retinal vessels in Down's syndrome. *Archives of Ophthalmology, 89,* 269–271.

Williams, R.D.B. (1981). Brushfield spots and Wolfflin nodules in the iris: An appraisal in handicapped children. *Developmental Medicine and Child Neurology, 23,* 646–650.

Woillez, M., & Dansaut, C. (1960). Les manifestations oculaires dans le mongolisme [The ocular manifestations of mongolism]. *Archives of Ophthalmology, 20,* 810–828.

Wolfflin, E. (1902). Ein klinischer beitrag zur kenntniss der structur der iris [A clinical contribution to the knowledge of the structure of the iris]. *Archiv der Augenheilkunde, 45,* 1–4.

Young, R.J. (1954). Congenital ectropion of the upper lids. *Archives of Diseases of Children, 29,* 97–100.

CHAPTER
7

Audiologic and Otolaryngologic Concerns

Arthur J. Dahle and Robert L. Baldwin

Individuals with Down syndrome are at increased risk for a number of otolaryngologic and audiologic disorders. These include congenital malformations; increased prevalence of diseases of nose, sinuses, oral cavity, nasopharynx, larynx, and ears; and loss of hearing sensitivity. Children and adults with Down syndrome should be carefully examined for the presence of otolaryngologic problems and hearing disorders and followed on a routine basis. Since they are at increased risk for so many different anomalies, a team of health professionals including the audiologist, speech-language pathologist, dentist, pediatrician, family physician, and otolaryngologist should work together in providing diagnostic and intervention services. Such teamwork has vastly improved the quality of life, as well as the life expectancy, of individuals with Down syndrome.

COMMON VARIANTS IN ANATOMIC AND PHYSIOLOGIC FEATURES

Numerous common physical features are associated with Down syndrome. Some of these occur with a high frequency and are considered typical to the syndrome; others vary in their prevalence. Additionally, some features are noted at birth and in childhood, whereas others present later in life. Many of the anatomic and physiologic variants in Down syndrome are not directly associated with any particular disability or disease process (e.g., the appearance of the nose and the

external ear). Other abnormalities require medical attention and continuous follow-up. (See also Pueschel, chap. 1, this volume.)

Children with Down syndrome are born with a skull smaller than average; the anterior-posterior dimension of the skull is short. Rett (1977) found that brachycephaly was present in approximately 80% of these individuals. However, their heads rarely fall in the microcephalic range, but the circumference is markedly below average (Cronk, 1983). Their typical midfacial features result from hypoplasia of the midfacial bones. There may be mandibular and maxillary underdevelopment, with the mandible set at an obtuse angle (Gerald & Silverman, 1965). Additionally, there may be structural variations in the sella turcica, cribriform plate, and sphenoid bone (Benda, 1969). Hypotelorism (abnormal closeness of the eyes) is associated with the midface hypoplasia due to a decreased distance between the inner canthi.

The child with Down syndrome has a somewhat characteristic nose, being small with a depressed bridge. At birth, the nasal bone may not be ossified and is underdeveloped. The flat facial profile, caused by the depressed nasal bridge, is one of the more frequently observed characteristics in persons with Down syndrome. Pueschel (1984) observed a hypoplastic nose in 83% of newborns with Down syndrome. Other investigators (e.g., Lee & Jackson, 1972) also described the characteristic underdeveloped structure of the nose, with reported occurrence rates

The authors wish to acknowledge the contributions made by Jannis Reeves, Anita Ingram, and Sharon Graham in preparing this manuscript.

between 57%–86%. Deviations of the nasal septum are also common and the paranasal sinuses may be underdeveloped (Benda, 1969).

The oral cavity in individuals with Down syndrome is smaller than average. Although the tongue and lips may be of normal size at birth, progressive enlargement occurs in some individuals. The enlarged tongue may be a true macroglossia or only relatively large in comparison to the small oral cavity. Protrusion of the tongue, fissuring, and hypertrophied papillae also occur in many individuals. The palate is typically narrow and may be high and/or short. The relatively large tongue contributes to mouth breathing and tongue protrusion in some individuals with Down syndrome. Ardron, Harker, and Kemp (1972) assessed the size of the tongue radiographically. They found it to be no larger than average, and tongue protrusion was found to be related to the small oral cavity and underdeveloped maxilla. Tongue fissuring is often observed in youngsters with Down syndrome. Papillary hypertrophy and tongue fissures may be due to excessive sucking and chewing. Eruption of both deciduous and permanent teeth is delayed and some teeth may be missing or smaller than average size (see Vigild, chap. 8, this volume).

There also may be anatomic variants in the nasopharynx and larynx. The nasopharynx may be small due to deviations from normal in the anterior-posterior dimension of the skull and increased vertical growth in the parietal region. Strome (1981) reported the nasopharynx was distinctly abnormal in individuals with Down syndrome. The Eustachian tube tori were found to be cylindrical and firmer than normal, and their position in the nasopharynx was more posterior-superior with a more acute angle of entry. The posterior choanae were reported to be slit like and smaller in overall dimension. Shibahara and Sando (1989) published a histopathologic case report of a congenital Eustachian tube anomaly in a fetus with Down syndrome. They believed that this type of abnormality could be a causative factor in postnatal Eustachian tube dysfunction. In addition to the small oral cavity, many individuals show a lateral compression or narrowing of the pharynx at the faucial pillars.

This results in tonsils positioned at a relatively superior point in a narrow area, which may contribute to a tendency for tongue protrusion.

There are extensive anomalies of the ears associated with Down syndrome, including variants found in the external, middle, and inner ear. One of the most common findings at birth is small pinnae, which may be set somewhat lower and more obliquely than normal. Aase, Wilson, and Smith (1973), Pueschel (1984), and Thelander and Pryor (1966) reported that this finding occurred in 16%–28% of children with Down syndrome. Another typical finding is an overlapping helix, which has been reported to occur at a frequency of 25%–75% (Wahrman & Fried, 1970). Other external ear abnormalities may include a prominent antihelix, projecting pinnae, absent or malformed earlobes, and narrowed or stenotic ear canals (Schmid, 1976).

The middle ear also may be a site of congenital anomalies in individuals with Down syndrome. Balkany, Mischke, Downs, and Jafek (1979) and Igarashi, Takahashi, Alford, and Johnson (1977) reported the occurrence of malformed stapes, typically with distorted crura, and poor development of the mastoid air cells. Balkany, Mischke, et al. also found a high incidence of dehiscent facial nerves. In addition to middle ear dysfunction, Igarashi et al. reported congenital abnormalities of the inner ear, including a shortened cochlea, absence of the utriculo-endolymphatic valve, hypogenesis of the posterior semicircular canal, and an enlarged bony posterior canal ampulla.

CLINICAL OTOLARYNGOLOGIC FINDINGS

There is an increased incidence of infections in individuals with Down syndrome. Levin et al. (1979) reported that respiratory tract infection was 100 times more frequent in individuals with Down syndrome than in age-matched controls. Both respiratory illnesses and ear, nose, and throat infections occur extremely frequently in children with Down syndrome. The susceptibility to infections may be due to a variety of factors. Evidence suggests that individuals with Down syndrome may have a depressed immune function. Studies have shown that these individuals have low T-cell counts, which may be reduced as much as 40% from normal levels and the T cells that are present may not function normally (Levin et al., 1979). Benda and Strassman (1965) reported that individuals with Down syndrome have small and abnormal thymuses. Additionally, these studies indicate that immune functioning may deteriorate with increasing age. The immune system also may be significantly influenced by other sequelae associated with Down syndrome. These include heart disease, pulmonary hypertension, and nutritional problems, which may predispose these individuals to infection. Exposure to infectious organisms in day care centers may be another factor that contributes to the number of infections. The frequency of upper respiratory infection in individuals with Down syndrome is much higher than normal and does decrease with age, as often occurs in the general pediatric population. Persistent rhinorrhea, often purulent, is one of the most persistent, troublesome otolaryngologic problems observed in some persons with Down syndrome.

Nasal obstruction is also common due to factors other than frequent upper respiratory infections. For example, individuals with Down syndrome typically have a small nasopharynx and dysfunctional Eustachian tubes, which can cause significant problems; however, with growth of these structures, function is somewhat improved. Nasopharyngeal obstruction also results from adenoid and tonsil hypertrophy. In some individuals, the adenoids and tonsils may not be significantly hypertrophied but are large in relation to the small size of the nasopharynx. Any increase in the size of the tonsils and adenoids creates an obstruction.

Laryngeal function may be affected by subglottic stenosis (narrowing of the airway below the vocal folds). Miller, Gray, Cotton, Myer, and Netterville (1990) indicated that subglottic stenosis may be more common in persons with Down syndrome. This may be due, in part, to the high rate of surgery for correcting cardiac malformations and gastrointestinal abnormalities (see Marino, chap. 9, and Levy, chap. 11, this volume). With so many significant physical anomalies, children with Down syndrome frequently undergo one or multiple major surgeries during childhood. Endotracheal tubes may aggravate a pre-existing condition of mild to moderate subglottic narrowing. Miller et al. suggested that elective endoscopy be considered in all individuals with a history of stridor (high-pitched, noisy breathing, indicating respiratory obstruction) prior to endotracheal intubation. They also recommended that when intubation is performed, tubes selected should be at least 0.5 mm smaller in diameter than is predicted by the child's age. Miller et al.'s findings indicate that subglottic stenosis is more difficult to repair in persons with Down syndrome and is associated with lower success rates of decannulation.

In the oral cavity, periodontal disease is common. Eruption of both deciduous and permanent teeth is delayed and many teeth may show anomalies. As stated earlier, mouth breathing is common due to enlargement of the tongue in a small oral cavity. Occasionally, a bifid uvula or cleft palate may be present.

Disorders affecting the ears are extremely common in persons with Down syndrome. The external ear, in addition to showing abnormalities of the pinnae, may have a small or stenotic ear canal, which can lead to accumulation and impaction of cerumen (earwax). Schwartz and Schwartz (1978) and Strome (1981) reported that stenotic ear canals are also associated with an increased prevalence of middle ear effusion. The incidence of tympanic membrane retraction, obviously related to Eustachian tube dysfunction, is greatly increased.

Children and adults with Down syndrome have an extremely high prevalence of middle ear effusion. Balkany, Downs, Jafek, and Kraticek (1979) found 64% of 107 individuals with Down syndrome had a significant hearing loss. Of the 64% with loss, 60% showed evidence of middle ear effusion. Balkany, Mischke, Downs, and Jafek (1979) and Igarashi et al. (1977) also identified the presence of congenital stapedial abnormalities with the stapes crura being commonly affected. The malleus and incus may also be abnormal because of congenital anomalies and ossicular erosion as a result of chronic inflammation from middle ear effusion. Similar to the general population, the incidence of cholesteatoma (tumor-like mass in the middle ear) is increased in those individuals with chronic ear disease. Thus, individuals with Down syndrome are at great risk of having some degree of conductive hearing loss due to outer and middle ear disorders.

There is also increased incidence of sensorineural hearing loss in both children and adults with Down syndrome. Whereas the prevalence of sensorineural loss may range from 4% to 10% in children with Down syndrome (Dahle & McCollister, 1986; Davis, 1988), the prevalence is much greater in older individuals. The occurrence of sensorineural hearing loss may be, in part, related to chronic middle ear disease, in which transudate may pass through the round window, allowing pathogens to affect neural structures and function. Additionally, sensorineural loss is undoubtedly associated with the advanced aging seen in individuals with Down syndrome.

CLINICAL AUDIOLOGIC FINDINGS

Considering the numerous outer, middle, and inner ear structural abnormalities just discussed, it is not surprising that there is a high prevalence of hearing impairment in individuals with Down syndrome. Lloyd and Reid (1967) reviewed prevalence studies conducted up to 1965 that reported prevalence of hearing loss among individuals with Down syndrome ranging from 6.8% to 56.7%. The wide discrepancy in findings was attributed to differences in criteria for defining hearing impairment and in the procedures used to assess hearing. In a widely quoted study, Glovsky (1966) reported a high prevalence of perceptive (sensorineural) hearing loss in a sample of 38 individuals with Down syndrome who attended the Vineland Training School. However, as noted by Fulton and Lloyd (1968), Glovsky's conclusions were confounded by the fact that sensorineural hearing impairment was defined by the configuration of the pure tone air conduction audiogram, rather than on the basis of bone conduction results. When Fulton and Lloyd used both air and bone conduction tests to assess children and young adults at the Parsons State Hospital, they found a much lower prev-

alence of hearing loss, and the majority of persons with hearing loss had conductive impairments.

The advent of the use of acoustic impedance audiometry helped clarify the nature of the hearing and otologic problems in persons with Down syndrome. Brooks, Wooley, and Kanjilal (1972) conducted one of the first large-scale studies to include acoustic impedance measures in assessing hearing and middle ear function in persons with Down syndrome. They evaluated 100 institutionalized patients with Down syndrome and an equal number of control subjects consisting of patients with mental retardation due to other etiologies. Of the 78 subjects with Down syndrome who were testable, 77% were found to have some degree of hearing impairment, with 60% exhibiting conductive pathology. The prevalence of hearing loss in the control group was dramatically less (25%), and there was a more even proportion of conductive and sensorineural impairments. Dahle and McCollister (1986) assessed auditory and middle ear function in children with Down syndrome and a group of matched control subjects. They found a significantly lower occurrence of hearing loss and middle ear problems among the control subjects, even though subjects in both groups had similar degrees of mental retardation.

Dahle and McCollister (1986) studied children living with their parents, whereas Brooks et al. (1972) studied an institutionalized population. Thus, it appears that individuals with Down syndrome are much more likely to develop hearing and otologic disorders than individuals with other forms of mental retardation, regardless of whether they reside in an institution or at home with their parents. Other investigations have also demonstrated that both children and adults with Down syndrome are prone to have conductive hearing loss related to middle ear dysfunction (Balkany, Downs, et al., 1979; Davis, 1988; Keiser, Montague, Wold, Manue, & Pattison, 1981).

In relation to language development, it is significant that the majority of individuals were found to have impairments in both ears, with losses occurring frequently in the mild to moderate range of severity. Also of interest is the finding that abnormal middle ear function has been found to correlate with lower cognitive function in children and adolescents with Down syndrome (Libb, Dahle, Smith, McCollister, & McLain, 1985). Several investigators have also reported a decline in measured intelligence with increasing age among children with Down syndrome. Saxon and Witriol (1976) suggested that hearing problems may be a contributing factor to the apparent reduction in cognitive functioning.

Studies that have investigated both the prevalence and type of hearing disorders in persons with Down syndrome are summarized in Table 7.1. With the exception of Fulton and Lloyd (1968), all of the investigators reported that over 50% of the subjects had decreased hearing, and conductive impairments were found to be the most frequent type of loss. In the majority of individuals, hearing impairment was attributed to middle ear effusion.

Although middle ear problems appear to be the major cause of conductive hearing impairment in individuals with Down syndrome, the accumulation of impacted cerumen in the outer ear canal is also a frequent problem (Brooks et al., 1972; Dahle & McCollister, 1986). If left untreated, impacted earwax can cause a significant reduction in hearing sensitivity, as illustrated in Figure 7.1. In this case, hardened earwax resulted in a mild decrease in hearing sensitivity similar to the pattern of attenuation provided by protective ear plugs. After the earwax was softened with mineral oil, removal of the cerumen provided an immediate improvement in hearing across all frequencies. If both ears were to remain impacted over an extended period of time, this degree of loss could cause difficulties in listening and could impede the acquisition of language and cognitive development. As indicated previously, the narrowed or stenotic ear canals found in very young children with Down syndrome likely contribute to the accumulation and impaction of cerumen.

Although prevalence studies list conductive pathology as the most frequent cause of hearing impairment in persons with Down syndrome, a significant percentage of both children and adults have sensorineural impairments and many have mixed losses. As indicated in Table 7.1, the prevalence of sensorineural hearing losses range

from a low of 4% to a high of 29%. If mixed losses are added, the prevalence rate for sensorineural impairments reaches 34%. In many individuals, the sensorineural component is limited to the higher frequencies, similar to the pattern of loss displayed in Figure 7.2. The reasons for a higher than normal prevalence of sensorineural impairments are unclear; however, inner ear structural abnormalities could be a factor. Additionally, premature aging has been documented to occur in adults with Down syndrome (Blackwood, St. Clair, Muir, Oliver, & Dickens, 1988; Brown, 1985), which could lead to presbycusic high-frequency sensorineural impairment. Buchanan (1990) analyzed audiologic data collected on 255 persons with Down syndrome and found that they had an earlier onset of presbycusis than both "normal" individuals and persons with mental retardation due to other etiologies. In many of the individuals, the onset of presbycusis was evident by the 2nd decade of life.

CONSIDERATIONS IN PERFORMING AUDIOLOGIC ASSESSMENTS

The possibility of collapsing ear canals should always be considered when hearing is assessed using standard earphone cushions. This is particularly true when testing individuals with Down syndrome, who are known to have small auditory canals and malformed pinnae. Figure 7.2 illustrates the spurious decrease in hearing that can result from collapsed ear canals when pure tone audiometry is performed using standard audiometric earphones. Audiometric evaluations conducted at several different facilities consistently indicated that this 20-year-old male with Down syndrome had a mild to moderate bilateral conductive hearing impairment along with a high-frequency sensorineural loss (only test results for the left ear are illustrated in Figure 7.2). However, test results were of questionable validity, since tympanograms indicated normal middle ear function, and otologic examinations failed to reveal any active pathology. His hearing for pure tones and speech was subsequently tested in sound field through loudspeakers and was found to be within normal

Table 7.1. Summary of studies of prevalence of hearing loss in individuals with Down syndrome

Study	Sample age range	N	Failure criterion	Percentage[a] of hearing loss		
				Conductive	Sensori-neural	Mixed
Fulton & Lloyd (1968)	7–27 yrs	79	>25 dB	22	9	9
Brooks, Wooley, & Kanjilal (1972)	1–59 yrs	78	>25 dB	41	17	19
Balkany, Downs, Jafek, & Kraticek (1979)	2 mos–60 yrs	107	>15 dB	54	10	—
Keiser, Montague, Wold, Manue, & Pattison (1981)	15–52 yrs	48	>15 dB	21	29	15
Dahle & McCollister (1986)	5–14 yrs	60	>15 dB	31[b]	10[b]	15[b]
Davis (1988)	8 mos–22 yrs	100	>25 dB	58[c]	4	—

[a]Results based on percentage of testable subjects except as noted.
[b]Percentages based upon number of ears tested (9% had undetermined loss).
[c]Included mixed impairments.

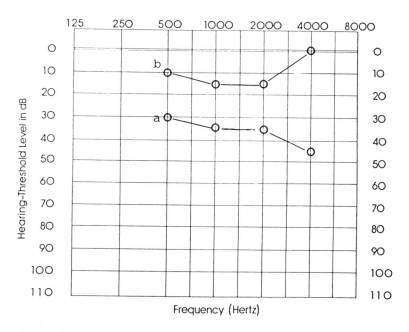

Figure 7.1. Effect of impacted cerumen in a 9-year-old boy with Down syndrome: a) right ear prior to removal of impacted cerumen; b) right ear following removal of impacted cerumen.

limits for the frequencies 250 Hz–4000 Hz. Retesting with insert earphones, which prevent the ear canal from collapsing, indicated near normal hearing except at 6000 Hz and 8000 Hz. Although collapsed ear canals tend to decrease hearing by only 10 dB–25 dB, the misleading results cause unnecessary concern and may lead to inappropriate treatment. As a precaution, it is advisable to use insert earphones routinely when testing both children and adults with Down syndrome.

The high prevalence of hypoplastic and sclerotic mastoid bones in persons with Down syndrome (Glass, Yousefzadeh, & Roizen, 1989) can also influence pure tone bone conduction test results. A poorly developed mastoid process makes it difficult to maintain proper tension on the bone vibrator and increased mastoid density may alter threshold levels. For these reasons, a forehead bone vibrator placement may be advantageous in situations where the mastoid bone appears to be underdeveloped or when test results appear unreliable using a mastoid placement.

Due to their delayed cognitive development, individuals with Down syndrome should have their hearing evaluated by audiologists who are experienced in assessing children and adults

with developmental delays. It is also helpful if they are aware of some of the special problems that may be encountered in assessing individuals with Down syndrome. For example, although visual reinforcement audiometry can be used successfully with "normal" children as young as 6 months of age (Dahle & McCollister, 1983), children with Down syndrome may need to be several months older before they can be conditioned to respond consistently to this procedure. Greenberg, Wilson, Moore, and Thompson (1978) reported that only 1 of 6 infants with Down syndrome under 13 months chronological age were able to complete a threshold task using visual reinforcement audiometric procedures. When the results were based upon developmental age, they found that children with Down syndrome could not be conditioned to respond consistently to the procedure until they had attained a mental age of at least 10–12 months.

The difficulties encountered in utilizing visual reinforcement audiometric procedures with young children with Down syndrome could be due to both the nature of the task (i.e., conditioning children to localize to sound while their attention is diverted by the examiner) and the reported lag in the development of their ability

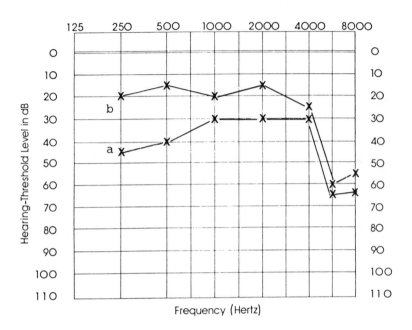

Figure 7.2.   Effect of collapsing left ear canal in a 20-year-old man with Down syndrome: a) standard cushion earphone; b) insert earphone.

to shift attention from a person to an object or event. This process is known as "joint attention" and it has been found to be delayed in infants with Down syndrome (Landry & Chapieski, 1990). These authors defined joint attention as the process of learning to coordinate visual attention with another person in relation to objects in the environment. The ability to shift attention between two or more activities requires complex attentional skills, which are important for the development of cognitive and communication skills.

If a child fails to respond consistently to behavioral audiometry, more objective electrophysiologic procedures may need to be utilized to assess hearing sensitivity accurately. Auditory brainstem response audiometry has proven to be a valuable clinical procedure for objectively evaluating hearing in "normal" infants, and it has also been found to be useful for assessing hearing sensitivity in infants and children with Down syndrome (Folsom, Widen, & Wilson, 1983; Jiang, Wu, & Liu, 1990; Kaga & Marsh, 1986; Maurizi, Ottaviani, Paludetti, & Lungarotti, 1985). Because of the likelihood of conductive impairments, auditory brainstem as-

sessment should include obtaining bone conduction thresholds.

When feasible, middle ear function should be assessed using acoustic impedance or immittance audiometry. However, the presence of small ear canals and impacted earwax may make it difficult to obtain valid tympanograms. Similarly, acoustic reflexes are frequently absent in children with Down syndrome, even when middle ear function is normal. Schwartz and Schwartz (1978) speculated that the absence of acoustic reflexes in the otherwise normal ears of children with Down syndrome could be due to muscular hypotonia, which may reduce tension in the stapedius muscle. They also suggested that there may be subtle differences in the neuronal organization of the reflex arc in children with Down syndrome. Regardless of the reasons, failure to elicit acoustic reflexes in individuals with Down syndrome should be interpreted cautiously.

AUDITORY PROCESSING ABNORMALITIES

As indicated previously, auditory brainstem response audiometry has been found to be useful in assessing hearing sensitivity in infants and young children with Down syndrome. However, investigators (e.g., Folsom et al., 1983; Jiang et al., 1990; Kaga & Marsh, 1986) also reported that, in comparison to "normal" children, children with Down syndrome frequently exhibited waveform abnormalities such as reduced response amplitude, shorter wave V latencies, shorter I-V peak intervals, and steeper latency-intensity functions. Many of these same abnormal findings have also been reported to occur in older individuals with Down syndrome (Squires, Aine, Buckwaid, Norman, & Galbraith, 1980; Squires, Ollo, & Jordon, 1986; Widen, Folsom, Thompson, & Wilson, 1987). Although some of these abnormalities could have been caused by conductive pathology or the presence of high-frequency hearing impairment (Widen et al., 1987), the consistency of these findings raises a question of whether the development and functioning of the auditory brainstem pathways may be abnormal in persons with Down syndrome.

Abnormal findings have also been reported for some higher level central auditory processing functions. For example, Schafer and Peeke (1982) examined cortical evoked potentials in response to repetitive auditory stimuli and found that individuals who were not mentally retarded experienced rapid habituation of their cortical potentials, whereas individuals with Down syndrome failed to show habituation. Differences have also been found for the amplitude of certain components of cortical auditory potentials and for auditory processing time (Lincoln, Courchesne, Kilman, & Galambos, 1985). Differences also have been reported in relation to the performance of infants with Down syndrome in processing the temporal aspects of speech discrimination (Eilers, Moroff, & Turner, 1985). Additionally, dichotic listening studies have suggested that individuals with Down syndrome may have reversed (right) hemispheric dominance for processing speech (Hartley, 1981; Pipe, 1983). The presence of central processing abnormalities may also explain why some researchers have reported that the language skills of children with Down syndrome are delayed beyond what would be expected on the basis of mental age, and the belief that these deficiencies may be unique to this population (Stoel-Gammon, 1990).

MEDICAL, SURGICAL, AND AUDIOLOGIC MANAGEMENT CONSIDERATIONS

Due to the prevalence of otolaryngologic and audiologic disorders, individuals with Down syndrome should be screened routinely and treated aggressively. Although nasal obstruction is generally somewhat relieved due to expansion of the skull as the child grows, some obstruction may be present throughout life. Often in the presence of chronic rhinorrhea, nasal cultures do not reveal a prevalent organism and biopsy of nasal turbinates is often negative. Some children with Down syndrome benefit from being maintained on low-dose antibiotics throughout the winter months until the rhinorrhea disappears. Immunity may improve somewhat with age into adolescence, but may decrease again as they become older.

The surgical decision to perform an adenoidectomy and tonsillectomy should be based on factors particular to the population with Down syndrome. The 1981 study by Strome involving individuals with Down syndrome showed that adenoidectomy had little clinical effect on the course of otologic pathology, including middle ear effusion, mouth breathing, or rhinorrhea. This is quite different from the effects in the general population. Additionally, consideration should be given to determining if the adenoids and tonsils are actually hypertrophied or only appear large in relation to a very small nasopharynx. Removing the tonsils and adenoids will reduce tongue protrusion only when true tonsillar hypertrophy is the contributing problem.

Surgical management, including the postoperative period, may be more difficult than is typical of the general population. Postoperative hydration is not easily assured due to problems in swallowing, and hospitalization may be longer than average. Structural differences, including a high-arched short hard palate and a short soft palate, put this population at significant risk for velopharyngeal incompetence following adenotonsillectomy. The adenoid pad may be important to the normal nasopharyngeal and speech physiologic functions. Following adenotonsillectomy, speech may be hypernasal. This risk should be considered and evaluated prior to surgery. Another surgical consideration involves anesthetic risks. Individuals with Down syndrome also should be carefully examined for the presence of atlantoaxial instability; stress on the neck during intubation could cause permanent damage to the cervical spine.

Disorders of the ear require frequent examinations and often long-term treatment. For individuals with stenotic ear canals, frequent cleaning may be necessary to prevent cerumen impaction, which can cause misleading audiometric results. Cerumen accumulation compounds any hearing loss that may be already present due to either middle ear disorders or sensorineural impairment. Any treatable condition associated with hearing loss requires immediate attention, since the presence of long-term hearing loss may significantly impede the development of language and cognitive skills. Children with obviously stenotic canals also seem to be at greater risk for middle ear effusion and chronic upper respiratory infections and should be monitored accordingly.

Ventilation tubes should be used when middle ear effusion is not responsive to antibiotic medication; however, surgical placement may be difficult in a stenotic canal. For a child with a history of chronic middle ear effusion, the ventilation tubes should be the type designed for long-term placement. Due to the increased risk for chronic infections, myringotomies (incision of tympanic membrane) with ventilation tubes should be performed aggressively to prevent ossicular erosion and other middle and inner ear sequelae.

Surgery for correcting ossicular chain interruption or fixation in individuals with Down syndrome is often not as successful as it is in the general population (Balkany, Mischke, et al., 1979). The stapes may be found to be congenitally anomalous; malleus and incus abnormalities may be due either to congenital anomalies or

to erosion from long-term disease. If tympanoplasty is to be successful, the ear must be dry with some evidence of basic Eustachian tube function. Balkany, Mischke, et al. also pointed out an additional risk associated with middle ear surgery in persons with Down syndrome. They found a significantly increased incidence of facial nerve dehiscence in individuals with Down syndrome undergoing middle ear surgery. Thus, the risk for facial nerve injury must be considered in making surgical decisions.

In view of the risks involved, some individuals with Down syndrome may not be considered good candidates for middle ear surgery. Consequently, they may need to be fitted with a hearing aid. Individuals with sensorineural hearing loss should also be seen by an audiologist for a hearing aid evaluation. Since individuals with Down syndrome have delayed cognitive function, it is critically important that amplification be provided for situations in which the hearing loss does not respond to medical treatment or where surgery is contraindicated. Considering the pervasive nature of their hearing and otologic disorders, it is highly advisable to provide continuous audiologic and otolaryngologic monitoring of all individuals with Down syndrome.

CONCLUSION

The chronic nature of the otolaryngologic problems experienced by individuals with Down syndrome necessitates that parents and health care professionals remain alert for the signs and symptoms of hearing impairment; respiratory illnesses; and ear, nose, and throat infections. Ideally, services should be provided by a team of health care professionals who work together to provide the most appropriate intervention. In particular, it is critical that middle ear functioning and hearing sensitivity be routinely monitored. If hearing has not been screened in the hospital nursery, infants with Down syndrome should receive an audiologic evaluation within the first few months of life, preferably using auditory brainstem evoked potential audiometry. Even if the initial test results are normal, children with Down syndrome should have their hearing checked every 6–12 months. If a conductive hearing loss is detected, the child's hearing and middle ear function should be monitored in accordance with the needs dictated by the treatment regimen. It is important that otologic problems be treated aggressively and hearing aid amplification should be considered whenever a hearing impairment cannot be corrected through medical treatment or surgery. When required, amplification should be provided as soon as the type, degree, and configuration of the loss can be determined. For very young children, auditory brainstem response assessment using toneburst stimuli may be required in order to determine the appropriate type of hearing aid. The goal in treating hearing and otolaryngologic problems should be to maximize the person's ability to hear so as to enhance his or her potential to achieve.

REFERENCES

Aase, J.M., Wilson, A.C., & Smith, D.W. (1973). Small ears in Down syndrome: A helpful diagnostic aid. *Journal of Pediatrics, 82,* 845.

Ardron, G.M., Harker, P., & Kemp, F.H. (1972). Tongue size in Down syndrome. *Journal of Mental Deficiency, 16,* 160–166.

Balkany, T.J., Downs, M.P., Jafek, B.W., & Kraticek, M.J. (1979). Hearing loss in Down's syndrome. *Clinical Pediatrics, 18,* 116–118.

Balkany, T.J., Mischke, R.E., Downs, M.P., & Jafek, B.W. (1979). Ossicular abnormalities in Down's syndrome. *Otolaryngology Head Neck Surgery, 87,* 372–384.

Benda, C.E. (1969). *Down syndrome: Mongolism and its management.* New York: Grune & Stratton.

Benda, C.E., & Strassman, G.S. (1965). The thymus in mongolism. *Journal of Mental Deficiency Research, 9,* 109.

Blackwood, D.H., St. Clair, D.M., Muir, W.J., Oliver, C.J., & Dickens, P. (1988). The development of Alzheimer's disease in Down's syndrome assessed by auditory event-related potentials. *Journal of Mental Deficiency Research, 32,* 439–453.

Brooks, D.M., Wooley, H., & Kanjilal, G.C. (1972). Hearing loss and middle ear disorders in patients with Down's syndrome (mongolism). *Journal of Mental Deficiency Research, 16,* 21–29.

Brown, W.T. (1985). Genetics of aging. In M.P. Janicki & H.M. Wisniewski (Eds.), *Aging and developmental disabilities* (pp. 185–194). Baltimore: Paul H. Brookes Publishing Co.

Buchanan, L.H. (1990). Early onset of presbycusis in Down syndrome. *Scandinavian Audiology, 19,* 103–110.

Cronk, C.E. (1983). Anthropometric studies. In S.M. Pueschel (Ed.), *A study of the young child with Down syndrome* (pp. 22–23). New York: Human Science Press.

Dahle, A.J., & McCollister, F.P. (1983). Considerations and implications for assessing hearing in multiply handicapped children. In G. Mencher & S. Gerber (Eds.), *The multiply handicapped hearing impaired child* (pp. 171–205). New York: Grune & Stratton.

Dahle, A.J., & McCollister, F.P. (1986). Hearing and otologic disorders in children with Down syndrome. *American Journal of Mental Deficiency, 90,* 636–642.

Davis, B. (1988). Auditory disorders in Down's syndrome. *Scandinavian Audiology, 30,* 65–68.

Eilers, R.E., Moroff, D.A., & Turner, R.H. (1985). Discrimination of formant transitions by Down syndrome and normally developing infants. *Human Communication Canada, 9,* 99–103.

Folsom, R.C., Widen, J.E., & Wilson, W.R. (1983). Auditory brain-stem responses in infants with Down's syndrome. *Archives of Otolaryngology, 109,* 607–610.

Fulton, R.T., & Lloyd, L.L. (1968). Hearing impairment in a population of children with Down's syndrome. *American Journal of Mental Deficiency, 73,* 298–302.

Gerald, B.E., & Silverman, F.C. (1965). Normal and abnormal interorbital distances with special reference to mongolism. *American Journal of Roentgenology, 95,* 154–161.

Glass, R.B., Yousefzadeh, D.K., & Roizen, N.J. (1989). Mastoid abnormalities in Down syndrome. *Pediatric Radiology, 19,* 311–312.

Glovsky, L. (1966). Audiological assessment of a mongoloid population. *Training School Bulletin, 83,* 27–36.

Greenberg, D.B., Wilson, W.R., Moore, J.M., & Thompson, G. (1978). Visual reinforcement audiometry (VRA) with young Down's syndrome children. *Journal of Speech & Hearing Disorders, 43,* 446–458.

Hartley, X.Y. (1981). Lateralisation of speech stimuli in young Down's syndrome children. *Cortex, 17,* 241–248.

Igarashi, M., Takahashi, M., Alford, B.R., & Johnson, P.E. (1977). Inner ear morphology in Down's syndrome. *Acta Otolaryngologica, 83,* 175–181.

Jiang, Z.D., Wu, Y.Y., & Liu, X.Y. (1990). Early development of brainstem auditory evoked potentials in Down's syndrome. *Early Human Development, 23,* 41–51.

Kaga, K., & Marsh, R.R. (1986). Auditory brainstem responses in young children with Down's syndrome. *International Journal of Pediatric Otorhinolaryngology, 11,* 29–38.

Keiser, H., Montague, J., Wold, D., Manue, S., & Pattison, D. (1981). Hearing loss of Down syndrome adults. *American Journal of Mental Deficiency, 85,* 467–472.

Landry, S.H., & Chapieski, M.L. (1990). Joint attention of six-month old Down syndrome and preterm infants: Attention to toys and mother. *American Journal on Mental Retardation, 94,* 488–497.

Lee, L., & Jackson, J. (1972). Diagnosis of Down's syndrome: Clinical vs laboratory. *Clinical Pediatrics, 11,* 353–356.

Levin, S., Schlesinger, M., Handzel, A., Hand, T., Altman, Y., Czernobilsky, B., & Boss, J. (1979). Thymic deficiency in Down's syndrome. *Pediatrics, 63,* 80–86.

Libb, J.W., Dahle, A.J., Smith, K., McCollister, F.P., & McLain, C. (1985). Hearing disorder and cognitive function of individuals with Down syndrome. *American Journal of Mental Deficiency, 90,* 353–356.

Lincoln, A.J., Courchesne, E., Kilman, B.A., & Galambos, R. (1985). Neuropsychological correlates of information-processing by children with Down syndrome. *American Journal of Mental Deficiency, 89,* 403–414.

Lloyd, L.L., & Reid, M.J. (1967). The incidence of hearing impairment in an institutional mentally retarded population. *American Journal of Mental Deficiency, 71,* 746–763.

Maurizi, M., Ottaviani, F., Paludetti, G., & Lungarotti, S. (1985). Audiological findings in Down's children. *International Journal of Pediatric Otorhinolaryngology, 9,* 227–232.

Miller, R., Gray, S.D., Cotton, R.T., Myer, C.M., & Netterville, J. (1990). Subglottic stenosis and Down syndrome. *American Journal of Otolaryngology, 11,* 274–277.

Pipe, M.E. (1983). Dichotic-listening performance following auditory discrimination training in Down's syndrome and developmentally retarded children. *Cortex, 19,* 481–491.

Pueschel, S.M. (1984). *The young child with Down syndrome.* New York: Human Science Press.

Rett, A. (1977). *Mongolismus* [Mongolism]. Bern: Huber.

Saxon, S.A., & Witriol, E. (1976). Down's syndrome and intellectual development. *Journal of Pediatric Psychology, 1,* 45–57.

Schafer, E.W., & Peeke, H.V. (1982). Down syndrome individuals fail to habituate cortical evoked potentials. *American Journal of Mental Deficiency, 87,* 332–337.

Schmid, F. (1976). *Das mongolismus syndrome* [The mongolism syndrome]. Muensterdorf: Hansen and Hansen.

Schwartz, D.M., & Schwartz, R.H. (1978). Acoustic impedance and otoscopic findings in young children with Down's syndrome. *Archives of Otolaryngology, 104,* 652–656.

Shibahara, Y., & Sando, I. (1989). Congenital anomalies of the Eustachian tube in Down syndrome. *Annals of Otology, Rhinology, & Laryngology, 98,* 543–547.

Squires, N., Aine, C., Buchwaid, J., Norman, R., & Galbraith, G. (1980). Auditory brain stem response abnormalities in severely and profoundly retarded adults. *Electroencephalography Clinical Neurophysiology, 50,* 172–185.

Squires, N., Ollo, C., & Jordan, R. (1986). Auditory brainstem responses in the mentally retarded: Audiometric correlates. *Ear & Hearing, 7,* 83–92.

Stoel-Gammon, G.S. (1990). Down syndrome. Effects on language development. *Asha, 32,* 42–44.

Strome, M. (1981). Down's syndrome: A modern otorhinolaryngologic perspective. *Laryngoscope, 91,* 1581–1594.

Thelander, H.E., & Pryor, H.B. (1966). Abnormal patterns of growth and development in mongolism: An anthropometric study. *Clinical Pediatrics, 5,* 493–498.

Wahrman, J., & Fried, L.T. (1970). The Jerusalem Prospective Newborn Survey of Mongols. *Annals of the New York Academy of Science, 171,* 341–360.

Widen, J.E., Folsom, R.C., Thompson, G., & Wilson, W.R. (1987). Auditory brainstem responses in young adults with Down syndrome. *American Journal of Mental Deficiency, 91,* 472–479.

CHAPTER
8

Oral Health Conditions

Merete Vigild

Individuals with Down syndrome exhibit a variety of characteristic anomalies in the cranial morphology and in the oral cavity (Gorlin, Cohen, & Levin, 1990). The oral anomalies are related to both bony and soft structures such as the tongue, oral mucosa, lips, salivary glands, soft palate, and dentition; and, in particular, to the occurrence of malocclusions, periodontal disease, and dental caries.

Most studies of persons with Down syndrome have been carried out within younger age groups, simply because of the previous high mortality rate that has made it difficult to select representative groups of older individuals with Down syndrome (Dupont, Vaeth, & Videbech, 1986; Thase, 1982). However, as the number of older persons with Down syndrome is increasing, it would be relevant and desirable to describe their special oral health problems. Although the present chapter deals mainly with a review of the orofacial characteristics and problems of children and younger adults with Down syndrome, most of these problems are also relevant to older persons with Down syndrome. The last section of the chapter is devoted to recommendations for oral health care for persons with Down syndrome.

CRANIAL MORPHOLOGY

The maxilla and the mandible are considerably smaller in persons with Down syndrome than in the general population (Cohen & Winer, 1965; Frostad, Cleall, & Melosky, 1971; Kisling, 1966), and the width, length, and height of the palate are also less. This is in part caused by a general growth deficiency related to Down syndrome (see Cronk & Anneren, chap. 3, this volume). Some authors have reported that all the craniofacial dimensions in individuals with Down syndrome are small (Jensen, Cleall, & Yip, 1973; Kisling, 1966); others have indicated that the height of the palate is not different from normal, but that it is shorter and narrower (B.L. Shapiro, Gorlin, Redman, & Bruhl, 1967).

The differences in the dimensions and shape of the cranial base and in the relations between the various regions of the cranium account for the phenotypic characteristics in persons with Down syndrome (Frostad et al., 1971; Kisling, 1966; see also Pueschel, chap. 1, this volume). Furthermore, the mandible often protrudes markedly in relation to the cranial base and to the maxilla, and the freeway space (the difference between the face height at rest and the face height during occlusion) is about three times greater than the normal value of 2 mm–3 mm (Frostad et al., 1971; Kisling, 1966). The size of the upper jaw in adults with Down syndrome is considerably less than the lower jaw, and this is suggested to be one of the reasons for the malocclusions often found in these individuals (Kisling, 1966).

ORAL CAVITY

The soft structures that surround the oral cavity include the tongue, the oral mucosa, the lips, the salivary glands, and the soft palate. As a consequence of the small oral cavity, the tongue appears to be larger than normal in individuals with Down syndrome. True macroglossia exists, however, only in a small percentage of these persons (Ardran, Harker, & Kemp, 1972; Cohen & Cohen, 1971); although frequencies as high as 60% have been reported (Gullikson, 1973), these reports do not distinguish between true and relative macroglossia. The tongue enhances oral dysfunctions because the individual presses the tongue against the lower front teeth. The relatively large tongue makes cleaning of the teeth difficult. Previously, almost all persons with Down syndrome presented with a protruded tongue and open mouth. Today, many children are taught early in life to keep the tongue inside the mouth. The tongue position is probably the main cause of the enlarged freeway space in persons with Down syndrome, but other important factors such as specific malocclusions, the skeletal development, malfunction of the masticatory apparatus, and the shape of the lower face also may be explanatory factors for the enlargement of the freeway space (Kisling, 1966).

Many individuals with Down syndrome exhibit a furrowing of the tongue, but the criteria for this phenomenon vary considerably, which accounts for the variation in its reported prevalence (Cohen & Cohen, 1971; Cohen & Winer, 1965). In most individuals with Down syndrome, however, it is necessary to brush the tongue during the daily oral hygiene procedure in order to remove food remnants and bacteria.

Most persons with Down syndrome breathe through the mouth, which causes dryness of the oral mucosa and the lips. The lips are often fissured, and cheilitis angularis (split, inflamed corners of the lips) is quite common (Butterworth, 1960). Some reports suggest that mouth dryness is also caused by a reduced parotid salivary flow in persons with Down syndrome (Cutress, 1972). The protruded mandible, the protruded and relatively large tongue, and the dry mouth are all complicating factors for the preparation and wearing of full dentures for adults with Down syndrome.

Finally, it has been reported that the prevalence of bifid uvula and cleft palate is increased in persons with Down syndrome. The prevalence of soft cleft palate has been found to be 0.7%, compared to 0.04% among the general population (Schendel & Gorlin, 1974; B.L. Shapiro et al., 1967).

MALOCCLUSIONS

One of the characteristics of persons with Down syndrome is the high prevalence of malocclusions. Almost 100% have one or more occlusal anomalies (Cohen, Arvystos, & Baum, 1970; Gullikson, 1973; Kisling, 1966, Vigild, 1985b). Several reports have dealt with the prevalence of various types of malocclusions in persons with Down syndrome (Cohen & Winer, 1965; Gullikson, 1973; Jensen et al., 1973; Kisling, 1966; Swallow, 1964). All have agreed that mandibular overjet, mesial molar occlusion, and crossbite occur far more frequently in persons with Down syndrome than among persons with mental retardation of other etiologies and "normal" individuals. The reported prevalence varies considerably because different scoring criteria are used and because of differences in the age of the study groups. A study of 6- to 19-year-olds with Down syndrome showed that 41% had mandibular overjet, 54% had mesial molar occlusion, 38% had frontal open bite, and 65% had a crossbite (Vigild, 1985b). Kisling (1966) reported even higher frequencies among 19- to 25-year-old males with Down syndrome. However, because of the longer growth period of the mandible compared to other facial bone structures, the prevalence of mandibular overjet can be expected to increase with age. It can be concluded that individuals with Down syndrome, children as well as adults, have frequencies of mandibular overjet, frontal inversion, frontal open bite, and crossbite that are significantly higher than observed in the general population. A Swedish study found that children with Down syndrome who had severe mental retardation had the highest prevalence of, and often the most severe, malocclusions (Oreland, Heijbel, & Jagell, 1987).

The high frequency of occlusal anomalies in the front region may be explained by the cranial morphology, but functional anomalies of the tongue and the perioral muscles probably also play a role. Some individuals with Down syndrome have great difficulty chewing their food; the occlusal conditions are often so poor that only a few teeth occlude during the chewing process.

In children and young adults with Down syndrome, there are no biologic factors that contraindicate orthodontic treatment per se. But lack of cooperation from the child or from the parents may make this treatment difficult or impossible, just as it may with "normal" children. The increased risk and early onset of periodontal disease should also be taken into consideration. Finally, one must recall that dysfunctions such as the pressing of the tongue against the front teeth and other oral habits can be complicating factors.

DENTITION

Individuals with Down syndrome have numerous anomalies in the shedding and eruption of the teeth. In the majority of children with Down syndrome, the deciduous and permanent teeth erupt 1–2 years later than in "normal" children (Barkla, 1966; Cutress; 1971a; Le Clerch, Journel, Roussey, & Marec, 1986; Orner, 1973; Orner, 1975b; Roche & Barkla, 1964, 1967), and

the sequence of the erupting teeth is often different from normal (Barkla, 1966; Cutress, 1971a; Jensen et al., 1973; Roche & Barkla, 1964; Swallow, 1964). Due to the late eruption of the permanent teeth, the shedding of the primary teeth is delayed. The permanent teeth may sometimes erupt anteriorly or posteriorly to the primary teeth as in "normal" children.

Many studies of persons with Down syndrome have revealed an extremely high prevalence of congenitally missing teeth (Cohen, Blitzer, Arvystos, & Bonneau, 1970; Jensen et al., 1973; Kisling, 1966; Orner, 1971; Roche & Barkla, 1967). Orner (1971) reported, for example, that 53% of a group of children with Down syndrome had congenitally missing teeth (excluding the third molars). The tooth that is most frequently missing is the lateral upper incisor followed by the mandibular second bicuspid, the maxillary second bicuspid, and the lateral and central mandibular incisors (Orner, 1971) (see Figure 1). There is also a high prevalence of peg-shaped incisors and slender-pointed canines, and the permanent teeth sometimes display microdontia (Cohen, Blitzer, et al., 1970; Jensen et al., 1973; Kisling, 1966; Prahl-Andersen & Oerlemans, 1976).

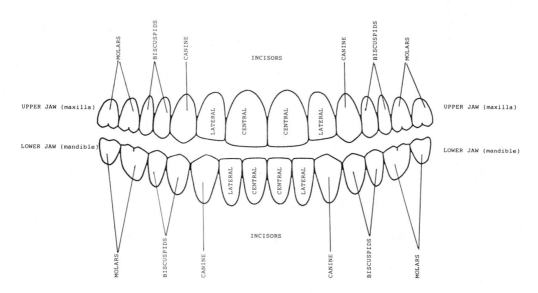

Figure 8.1.   Anatomical drawing of typical adult teeth.

PERIODONTAL CONDITIONS

Periodontal disease is defined as gingivitis with loss of attachment and loss of alveolar bone. This condition appears in practically all persons with Down syndrome, depending mainly on the age of the individuals and the level of their oral hygiene. Several reports have dealt with the periodontal conditions in persons with Down syndrome, and although the studies were carried out within different age groups and employed different oral health scoring criteria, it has generally been agreed that persons with Down syndrome are characterized by a marked, rapid, and early onset of severe periodontal disease (Cohen, Winer, Schwartz, & Shklar, 1961; Modéer, Barr, & Dahllöf, 1990; Orner, 1976; Reuland-Bosma & Van Dijk, 1986; Ulseth, Hestnes, Stovner, & Storhaug, 1991). The prevalence of periodontal disease is highest in the older age groups, but the incidence is highest among the younger (Brown, 1978; Miller & Ship, 1977). The most frequently affected teeth are the mandibular incisors and the maxillary molars (Kisling & Krebs, 1963; Modéer et al., 1990; Reuland-Bosma & Van Dijk, 1986; Saxèn & Aula, 1982).

Some studies have suggested that institutionalized children with Down syndrome suffer more from severe periodontal disease than those who live at home (Cutress, 1971b; Johnson & Young, 1963; Swallow, 1964). According to these studies, the reason is that the institutionalized individuals have more deposits, probably due to environmental differences in diet or in oral hygiene. However, if oral hygiene is assessed by measuring the amount of soft deposit (plaque), there arises a methodologic problem with regard to the validity of the clinical scoring. If the institutional staff and/or the parents know the time of the dental examination, it is almost inevitable that they clean the children's teeth prior to the examination; therefore, the scoring of the soft deposits on the teeth becomes misleading. However, there are other factors that could explain the difference between the two groups of children. The altered immune response combined with larger amounts of calculus may explain the difference in the severity

of periodontal disease between the institutionalized children and the children living at home (Reuland-Bosma & Van Dijk, 1986). It should be noted here that, to date, research focusing on persons with Down syndrome living in the community has been rather scarce. However, as more and more children with Down syndrome are now living in the community, future research may therefore focus on their oral health to a greater extent than was done previously.

Recent studies of children with mental retardation have shown that children with Down syndrome have less plaque and calculus than individuals with mental retardation of other etiologies (Reuland-Bosma & Van Dijk, 1986; M.J. Shaw, Shaw, & Foster, 1990; Vigild, 1985a). It seems surprising that children with Down syndrome have better oral hygiene than other mentally retarded children. The explanation could well be that parents are informed about the high susceptibility to periodontal disease related to Down syndrome and therefore are particularly careful with daily oral hygiene for their children. In spite of this, children with Down syndrome often have more gingivitis than other children. In one study, 91% of the children with Down syndrome between 6–19 years had gingival bleeding. Twenty-two percent had pocket formation, compared to a prevalence of only 0.1% among "normal" individuals (Vigild, 1985a).

A number of reports exist on the occurrence of acute necrotizing ulcerative gingivitis in children with Down syndrome (Brown, 1973; Reuland-Bosma & Van Dijk, 1986). Today, this type of gingivitis is rare in the Western world and is almost never seen prior to puberty. However, among persons with Down syndrome, necrotizing gingivitis has been reported to occur quite frequently, with a prevalence up to 84% (Brown, 1978; Reuland-Bosma & Van Dijk, 1986). Some studies even found the highest prevalence among 15- to 19-year-olds. More recent studies, however, have failed to demonstrate necrotizing ulcerative gingivitis among persons with Down syndrome (Barnett, Press, Friedman, & Sonnenberg, 1986; Vigild, 1985a). This apparent discrepancy is probably due to generally improved oral hygiene among persons with Down syndrome.

It has been suggested that local factors such as

true or false macroglossia, tooth morphology, habits such as bruxism and tongue thrusting, lack of lip seal, and lack of masticatory functions are etiologic factors for the onset of periodontal disease among persons with Down syndrome (Cutress, 1971b; Reuland-Bosma & Van Dijk, 1986; Shaw & Saxby, 1986). These factors are important because they may affect oral hygiene, but the effect on the periodontal tissues is indirect (Reuland-Bosma & Van Dijk, 1986). Studies on oral bacteria in persons with Down syndrome are scarce and generally there is no difference in the plaque flora between persons with Down syndrome and "normal" individuals within the same environments. There is a tendency for institutionalized individuals with Down syndrome to have higher levels of aerobic bacteria and streptococci (cf. review by Reuland-Bosma & Van Dijk, 1986).

There have been several attempts to identify systemic etiologic factors and pathogenetic mechanisms that may explain the high susceptibility toward periodontal disease among persons with Down syndrome. The factors suggested include: poor blood circulation and differences in connective tissue (Reuland-Bosma & Van Dijk, 1986); elevated blood levels of citric acid (S. Shapiro, Gedalia, Hofman, & Miller, 1969); metabolic blocks in the collagen maturation (Claycomb, Summers, Hall, & Hart, 1970); vitamin A malabsorption or malnutrition (Cutress, 1976); and a three times higher concentration of cyclic amino-monophosphate, which has been demonstrated in inflamed gingival tissue from persons with Down syndrome (Schaeffer, 1977). However, in recent years, there seems to be agreement that the main reason for the high prevalence and the severity of periodontal disease in persons with Down syndrome is a general low resistance caused by immunodeficiency (Barkin, Weston, Humbert, & Marie, 1980; Barkin, Weston, Humbert, & Sunada, 1980; Reuland-Bosma & Van Dijk, 1986; L. Shaw & Saxby, 1986; Ugazio et al., 1978).

The number of fibroblasts, macrophages, plasma cells, and mast cells in persons with Down syndrome are in the same range as in "normal" controls (Reuland-Bosma, Liem, Jansen, Van Dijk, & Wiele, 1988). The main immunologic defect occurs in the thymus-dependent system, which may result in a reduced number of mature T cells and a relatively large proportion of immature cells. According to Whittingham, Pitt, Sharma, and MacKay (1977), the immune system is under stress. The antigenic stimulus is so heavy that the system becomes overloaded. Together with the larger amount of calculus and of soft deposits and bacteria in the plaque among institutionalized individuals, this may explain some of the previously reported differences in the severity of periodontitis between persons living in institutions and those living in the community (Reuland-Bosma & Van Dijk, 1986).

It can be concluded that persons with Down syndrome constitute a special risk group with respect to periodontal disease. Meticulous oral hygiene is one of the most important methods of minimizing the prevalence and severity of periodontal disease. Unfortunately, good oral hygiene is not enough to stop the onset and progression of periodontal disease completely. Further research within this field is still badly needed.

DENTAL CARIES

Most studies of children with Down syndrome show that the prevalence of dental caries is lower than in children with mental retardation of other etiologies and in "normal" children (Barnett et al., 1986; Creighton & Wells, 1966; Gullikson, 1973; Johnson, Young, & Gallios, 1960; Orner, 1975a; Steinberg & Zimmerman, 1978), and for many years it has been widely believed that individuals with Down syndrome are inherently resistant toward caries. However, a number of studies have failed to demonstrate any difference in caries prevalence between persons with Down syndrome and others (Cutress 1971a; Kroll, Budnick, & Kobren, 1970; Shaw et al., 1990; Ulseth et al., 1991).

Many factors must be taken into consideration when the results from different studies are compared. First of all, the living conditions are important. It has been shown that children with Down syndrome residing in institutions have very little dental caries, but this is probably because they have a lower consumption of sweets and more regular meals than children living at home. Second, the number of teeth is important, and also the time these teeth have been erupted and thus exposed to decay. Third, it is important to take into account whether the decay is scored as the number of decayed, missing, and filled teeth or as the number of decayed, missing, and filled tooth surfaces. Both these indices express the caries experience, which is the sum of untreated and treated decay. When the tooth is used as the unit of measurement, a tooth is scored as decayed or filled regardless of the number of surfaces involved, whereas when the surface is used as the scoring unit, all of the numerous affected surfaces are identified. In other words, when the number of surfaces is used, the seriousness of the decay is taken into account—in particular, whether or not the approximal surfaces are involved. The problem was illustrated in a study by Steinberg and Zimmerman (1978). They found no difference in the number of decayed, missing, and filled teeth between children with Down syndrome and "normal" children, whereas the number of decayed, missing, and filled tooth surfaces was significantly lower in the children with Down syndrome.

Some authors have considered the late eruption of the permanent teeth (Barkla, 1966; Cutress, 1971a; Swallow, 1964), while other studies focused on the higher frequency of missing teeth in children with Down syndrome (Creighton & Wells, 1966; Cutress, 1971a; Orner, 1975a; Vigild, 1986). Only Cutress (1971a) and Vigild (1986) took into consideration the living conditions (at home or in institution), the number of erupted teeth and tooth surfaces, and the time these teeth (surfaces) have been erupted. The studies by Cutress (1971a) and Vigild (1986) both show that youngsters with Down syndrome residing in institutions have a significantly lower caries prevalence than those living at home. Among the 6- to 12-year-olds with Down syndrome, however, there was no significant difference between institutionalized children and non-institutionalized children either with respect to the number of caries-free individuals or to the distribution of caries. This was probably due to

the overall low caries prevalence in both groups of youngsters (Vigild, 1986). However, in 13- to 19-year-olds with Down syndrome, 71% of the institutionalized Danish individuals were caries free compared to only 22% of those who were not institutionalized. This illustrates that the caries experience among children and young adults with Down syndrome is affected by environmental factors just as it is in other individuals.

When the children and young adults with Down syndrome were compared to persons with mental retardation of other etiologies from the same environments, the individuals with Down syndrome had less caries than the others, but they also had fewer erupted teeth. In order to correct for the differences in the number of teeth and the period of time during which the teeth had been exposed to caries, the persons with Down syndrome were compared to persons with mental retardation of other etiologies who were 1 year younger. After this correction, the difference in the caries experience between the persons with Down syndrome and persons with mental retardation of other etiologies was still significant in the older age group. When the analysis was based on the number of teeth instead of the number of tooth surfaces no differences were found in any of the age groups, even without the 1-year age correction. This observation is in agreement with the findings of Steinberg and Zimmerman (1978) and Swallow (1964), and indicates that subjects with Down syndrome have less caries on the approximal surfaces than persons with mental retardation of other etiologies (Barnett et al., 1986; Vigild, 1986).

This can be explained by the increased interdental spacing in persons with Down syndrome due to hypodontia. Even though some persons with Down syndrome present crowding of the permanent dentition just as do "normal" individuals, it has been demonstrated that interdental spacing in persons with Down syndrome increases with age, even when there is no hypodontia. Contrary to this, there is an overall decrease of the interdental space with age in "normal" controls (Jensen et al., 1973). The morphologic deviations in the dentition in persons with Down syndrome (e.g., the peg-shaped front teeth) may also play a role when their caries pattern is compared to that of others.

It has been suggested that the high concentration of cyclic adenosine monophosphate in the saliva of persons with Down syndrome (Schaeffer, 1977) and the increased pH and sodium level in the saliva (Cutress, 1972; Winer & Feller, 1972) may be of importance for the susceptibility to dental caries. It has also been noted that the decreased flow from the parotid gland (Cutress, 1972) and the habit of mouth breathing causes mouth dryness, which normally results in more decay due to the low level of natural self-rinsing.

It can be concluded that individuals with Down syndrome are not resistant to dental caries, although they have a low frequency of approximal caries. Therefore, caries-preventive measures should not be neglected. This is particularly important for individuals living in the community.

CONCLUSION AND RECOMMENDATIONS FOR ORAL HEALTH CARE

The oral health problems specific to persons with Down syndrome are caused by the congenital anomalies in the cranial morphology, particularly the jaws and the dentition. Prosthodontic or orthodontic measures toward these problems are sometimes difficult, and the dentist must always be absolutely certain that the patient will benefit from a denture or an orthodontic appliance before such treatment is instituted.

With respect to dental caries and periodontal disease, it is important to bear in mind that because of the mental retardation and the difficulties in controlling the tongue, traditional dental treatment is often more difficult and time consuming than in "normal" patients. General anesthesia is, however, seldom necessary.

The following guidelines for dental care for patients with Down syndrome are recommended:

1. Dental visits with emphasis on preventive activities should be scheduled three to four times per year, starting when the child is 18 to 24 months old.
2. The aim of the preventive measures should be to prevent the onset of dental caries, especially on the occlusal surfaces, and to minimize the progression of periodontal disease. The desired level of oral hygiene can rarely be obtained by means of traditional mechanical plaque control. It is therefore recommended that the mechanical methods be supplemented by chemical plaque control (e.g., chlorhexidine).
3. Parents and teachers must be informed and sufficiently trained in daily oral hygiene procedures. The proper oral health care can only be implemented if a confident relationship and an adequate coordination are established between the dentist, the teachers, and the parents. Even though more children with Down syndrome are now living in the community, some persons with Down syndrome, especially adults, are still living in institutions. The staff should therefore also be informed and trained.
4. In some countries, the dentist must obtain informed consent from the legal guardian of the individual with Down syndrome before any treatment is instituted.

REFERENCES

Ardran, G.M., Harker, P., & Kemp, F.H. (1972). Tongue size in Down's syndrome. *Journal of Mental Deficiency Research, 16,* 160–166.

Barkin, R.M., Weston, W.L., Humbert, J.R., & Marie, F. (1980). Phagocytic function in Down syndrome: I. Chemotaxis. *Journal of Mental Deficiency Research, 24,* 243–250.

Barkin, R.M., Weston, W.L., Humbert, J.R., & Sunada, K. (1980). Phagocytic function in Down syndrome: II. Bactericidal activity and phagocytosis. *Journal of Mental Deficiency Research, 24,* 251–256.

Barkla, D.H. (1966). Ages of eruption of permanent teeth in mongols. *Journal of Mental Deficiency Research, 10,* 190–197.

Barnett, M.L., Press, K.P., Friedman, D., & Sonnenberg, S.M. (1986). The prevalence of periodontitis and dental caries in a Down's syndrome population. *Journal of Periodontology, 57,* 288–293.

Brown, R.H. (1973). Necrotizing ulcerative gingivitis

in mongoloid and non-mongoloid retarded individuals. *Journal of Periodontology, 8,* 290–295.

Brown, R.H. (1978). A longitudinal study of periodontal disease in Down's syndrome. *New Zealand Dental Journal, 74,* 137–144.

Butterworth, T. (1960). Cheilitis of mongolism. *Journal of Investigative Dermatology, 35,* 347–351.

Claycomb, C.K., Summers, G.W., Hall, W.B., & Hart, R.W. (1970). Gingival collagen biosynthesis in mongolism. *Journal of Periodontal Research, 5,* 30–35.

Cohen, M.M., Arvystos, M.G., & Baum, B.J. (1970). Occlusal disharmonies in trisomy G (Down's syndrome, mongolism). *American Journal of Orthodontics, 58,* 367–372.

Cohen, M.M., Blitzer, F.J., Arvystos, M.G., & Bonneau, R.H. (1970). Abnormalities of the permanent dentition in trisomy G. *Journal of Dental Research, 49* (Suppl. 6), 1386–1396.

Cohen, M.M., Sr., & Cohen, M.M., Jr. (1971). The oral manifestations of trisomy G (Down syndrome). *Birth Defects, 7,* 241–251.

Cohen, M.M., & Winer, R.A. (1965). Dental and facial characteristics in Down's syndrome (mongolism). *Journal of Dental Research, 44,* 197–208.

Cohen, M.M., Winer, R.A., Schwartz, S., & Shklar, G. (1961). Oral aspects of mongolism: Part I. Periodontal diseases in mongolism. *Oral Surgeon, 14,* 92–107.

Creighton, W.E., & Wells, H.B. (1966). Dental caries experience in institutionalized mongoloid and non-mongoloid children in North Carolina and Oregon. *Journal of Dental Research, 45,* 66–75.

Cutress, T.W. (1971a). Dental caries in trisomy 21. *Archives of Oral Biology, 16,* 1329–1344.

Cutress, T.W. (1971b). Periodontal disease and oral hygiene in trisomy 21. *Archives of Oral Biology, 16,* 1345–1355.

Cutress, T.W. (1972). Composition, flow rate and pH of mixed and parotid saliva from trisomic and other mentally retarded subjects. *Archives of Oral Biology, 17,* 1081–1094.

Cutress, T.W. (1976). Vitamin A absorption and periodontal disease in trisomy G. *Journal of Mental Deficiency Research, 20,* 17–23.

Dupont, A., Vaeth, M., & Videbech, P. (1986). Mortality and life expectancy of Down's syndrome in Denmark. *Journal of Mental Deficiency Research, 30,* 111–120.

Frostad, W.A., Cleall, J.F., & Melosky, L.C. (1971). Craniofacial complex in the trisomy 21 syndrome (Down's syndrome). *Archives of Oral Biology, 16,* 707–722.

Gorlin, R.J., Cohen, M.M., Jr., & Levin, L.S. (1990). *Syndromes of the head and neck.* New York: Oxford University Press.

Gullikson, J.S. (1973). Oral findings in children with Down syndrome. *Journal of Dentistry for Children, 41,* 293–297.

Jensen, G.M., Cleall, J.F., & Yip, A.S.G. (1973). Dentoalveolar morphology and developmental changes in Down's syndrome (trisomy 21). *American Journal of Orthodontics, 64,* 607–618.

Johnson, N.P., & Young, M.A. (1963). Periodontal disease in mongols. *Journal of Periodontology, 34,* 41–47.

Johnson, N.P., Young, M.A., & Gallios, J.A. (1960). Dental caries experience of mongoloid children. *Journal of Dentistry for Children, 27,* 292–294.

Kisling, E. (1966). *Cranial morphology in Down's syndrome. A comparative roentgencepholometric study in adult males.* Copenhagen: Munksgaard.

Kisling, E., & Krebs, G. (1963). Periodontal conditions in adult patients with mongolism. *Acta Odontologica Scandinavica, 21,* 391–405.

Kroll, R.G., Budnick, J., & Kobren, A. (1970). Incidence of dental caries and periodontal disease in Down's syndrome. *New York Dental Journal, 36,* 151–156.

Le Clerch, G., Journel, H., Roussey, M., & Marec, B.L. (1986). La première dentition du trisomique 21 [Primary dentition in Down syndrome]. *Annales de Pédiatrie, 33,* 795–798.

Miller, M.F., & Ship, I.I. (1977). Periodontal disease in the institutionalized mongoloid. *Journal of Oral Medicine, 32,* 9–13.

Modéer, T., Barr, M., & Dahllöf, G. (1990). Periodontal disease in children with Down's syndrome. *Scandinavian Journal of Dental Research, 98,* 228–234.

Oreland, A., Heijbel, J., & Jagell, S. (1987). Malocclusions in physically and/or mentally handicapped children. *Swedish Dental Journal, 11,* 103–119.

Orner, G. (1971). Congenitally absent permanent teeth among mongols and their sibs. *Journal of Mental Deficiency Research, 15,* 292–302.

Orner, G. (1973). Eruption of permanent teeth in mongoloid children and their sibs. *Journal of Dental Research, 52,* 1202–1208.

Orner, G. (1975a). Dental caries experience among children with Down's syndrome and their sibs. *Archives of Oral Biology, 20,* 627–634.

Orner, G. (1975b). Posteruptive tooth age in children with Down's syndrome and their sibs. *Journal of Dental Research, 54,* 581–587.

Orner, G. (1976). Periodontal disease among children with Down's syndrome and their siblings. *Journal of Dental Research, 55,* 778–782.

Prahl-Andersen, B., & Oerlemans, J. (1976). Characteristics of permanent teeth in persons with trisomy G. *Journal of Dental Research, 55,* 633–638.

Reuland-Bosma, W., & Van Dijk, L.J. (1986). Periodontal disease in Down's syndrome: A review. *Journal of Clinical Periodontology, 13,* 64–73.

Reuland-Bosma, W., Liem, R.S.B., Jansen, H.W.B., Van Dijk, L.J., & Wiele, L. (1988). Cellular aspects of effects on the gingiva in children with Down's syndrome during experimental gingivitis. *Journal of Clinical Periodontology, 15,* 303–311.

Roche, A.F., & Barkla, D.H. (1964). The eruption of deciduous teeth in mongols. *Journal of Mental Deficiency Research, 8,* 54–64.

Roche, A.F., & Barkla, D.H. (1967). The development of the dentition in mongols. *Australian Dental Journal, 12,* 12–16.

Saxèn, L., & Aula, S. (1982). Periodontal bone loss in patients with Down's syndrome: A follow-up study. *Journal of Periodontology, 53,* 158–162.

Schaeffer, L.A. (1977). Cyclic AMP in saliva, salivary glands and gingival tissue. *Advanced Cyclic Nucleotide Research, 3,* 283–293.

Schendel, S.A., & Gorlin, R.J. (1974). Frequency of cleft uvula and submucous cleft palate in patients with Down's syndrome. *Journal of Dental Research, 53,* 840–843.

Shapiro, B.L., Gorlin, R.J., Redman, R.S., & Bruhl, H.H. (1967). The palate and Down's syndrome. *New England Journal of Medicine, 276,* 1460–1463.

Shapiro, S., Gedalia, I., Hofman, A., & Miller, M. (1969). Periodontal disease and blood citrate levels in patients with trisomy 21. *Journal of Dental Research, 48,* 1231–1233.

Shaw, L., & Saxby, M.S. (1986). Periodontal destruction in Down's syndrome and in juvenile periodontitis. How close a similarity? *Journal of Periodontology, 57,* 709–715.

Shaw, M.J., Shaw, L., & Foster, T.D. (1990). The oral health in different groups of adults with mental handicaps attending Birmingham (UK) adult training centres. *Community Dental Health, 7,* 135–141.

Steinberg, A.D., & Zimmerman, S. (1978). The Lincoln dental caries study: A three-year evaluation of dental caries in persons with various mental disorders. *Journal of American Dental Association, 97,* 981–984.

Swallow, J.N. (1964). Dental disease in children with Down's syndrome. *Journal of Mental Deficiency Research, 8,* 102–118.

Thase, M.E. (1982). Longevity and mortality in Down's syndrome. *Journal of Mental Deficiency Research, 26,* 177–192.

Ugazio, A.G., Anzavecchia, A.L., Jayakar, S., Plebani, A., Duse, M., & Burgio, G.R. (1978). Immunodeficiency in Down syndrome. *Acta Paediatric Scandinavica, 67,* 705–708.

Ulseth, J.O., Hestnes, A., Stovner, J.L., & Storhaug, K. (1991). Dental caries and periodontitis in persons with Down syndrome. *Special Care in Dentistry, 11,* 71–73.

Vigild, M. (1985a). Periodontal conditions in mentally retarded children. *Community Dentistry and Oral Epidemiology, 13,* 180–182.

Vigild, M. (1985b). Prevalence of malocclusion in mentally retarded young adults. *Community Dentistry and Oral Epidemiology, 13,* 183–184.

Vigild, M. (1986). Dental caries experience among children with Down's syndrome. *Journal of Mental Deficiency Research, 30,* 271–276.

Winer, R.A., & Feller, R.P. (1972). Composition of parotid and submandibular saliva and serum in Down's syndrome. *Journal of Dental Research, 51,* 449–455.

Whittingham, S., Pitt, D.B., Sharma, D.L.B., & MacKay, I.R. (1977). Stress deficiency of the T-C lymphocyte system exemplified by Down syndrome. *Lancet, i,* 163–166.

CHAPTER
9

Cardiac Aspects

Bruno Marino

Congenital heart malformations in persons with Down syndrome were first described by Garrod (1894). The frequency of congenital heart diseases in persons with Down syndrome is very high: About 50% of children with trisomy 21 have congenital heart malformations (Martin, Rosenbaum, & Sardegna, 1989), compared to 0.3% of children with normal chromosomes (Ferencz et al., 1985). It has recently been reported that the prevalence of these defects is higher in females than in males with Down syndrome (Pinto, Nunes, Ferraz, & Sampayo, 1990). Furthermore, cardiac anomalies are the main cause of death in children with Down syndrome (30%–35%) (Thase, 1982), especially in the first 2 years of life. In a study carried out by Fabia and Drolette in 1970, only 40%–60% of children with Down syndrome and congenital heart disease survived after 10 years of age. Due to recent developments in pediatric cardiology and cardiac surgery, and the more appropriate medical care provided to persons with Down syndrome in general, the life expectancy has markedly improved (Bell, Pearn, & Firman, 1989). In spite of these positive changes, cardiologic concerns are still a central problem for the survival and the quality of life of persons with Down syndrome.

TYPES OF CONGENITAL CARDIAC DEFECTS

Many studies have addressed the analysis of the types of congenital heart disease in persons with Down syndrome (Berg, Crome, & France, 1960; Cullum & Liebman, 1969; Ferencz et al., 1989; Greenwood & Nadas, 1976; Laursen, 1976; Liu

& Corlett, 1959; Park et al., 1977; Rainsford Evans, 1950; Rowe, 1962; Rowe & Uchida, 1961; Sharer, Farina, Porter, & Bishop, 1972; Tandon & Edwards, 1973; Warkany, Passarge, & Smith, 1966). There is no doubt that children with trisomy 21 display certain congenital heart defects and seem to be "protected" from others.

The great majority of congenital cardiac defects affect the region of the membranous septum, the valves, and the atrioventricular junction. Atrioventricular canal (atrioventricular septal defects or endocardial cushion) defects represent the "classic" congenital heart anomaly in children with Down syndrome, accounting for about 60% of all cardiac malformations (Ferencz et al., 1989). The complete form of atrioventricular canal is frequently observed (Park et al., 1977). It has been suggested that the high prevalence of this cardiac defect is due to the increased adhesiveness of trisomy 21 cells, causing the failure of endocardial cushion-to-septum fusion, hence resulting in the persistence of the atrioventricular canal (Kurnit, Aldridge, Matsuoka, & Matthysse, 1985). There are also other types of cardiac defects that may result in increased pulmonary blood flow, such as atrial septal defect, ventricular septal defect, and patent ductus arteriosus, which together represent about 30% of all congenital heart defects (Ferencz et al., 1989; Park et al., 1977).

The only cono-truncal malformation with reduced pulmonary blood flow is tetralogy of Fallot (Ferencz et al., 1989; Park et al., 1977; Rowe & Uchida, 1961; Tandon & Edwards, 1973), which is observed in almost 7% of persons with Down syndrome. The pathogenesis of tetralogy

The author is grateful to Miss Orietta Castellacci for the editing of the manuscript.

of Fallot is different from that of atrioventricular canal and may be related to maldevelopment of neural crest cells, similar to that observed in persons with DiGeorge anomaly (Van Mierop & Kutsche, 1986). Furthermore, it is of interest that some congenital heart malformations in persons with Down syndrome are extremely rare, and even virtually absent. Such cardiac defects include anomalies of viscero-atrial situs and pulmonary venous connections, atrioventricular valve atresia, ventricular inversions (L-ventricular loop), transposition of great arteries, and truncus arteriosus (Cullum & Liebman, 1969; Ferencz et al., 1989; Greenwood & Nadas, 1976; Laursen, 1976; Liu & Corlett, 1959; Park et al., 1977; Rainsford Evans, 1950; Rowe, 1962; Rowe & Uchida, 1961; Sharer et al., 1972; Tandon & Edwards, 1973; Warkany et al., 1966). Also, coarctation (constriction) of the aorta and the muscular-type ventricular septal defect are less often seen in children with Down syndrome than in persons with normal chromosomes (De Biase et al., 1986; Marino, 1989; Marino, Corno, Guccione, & Marcelletti, 1991). The reasons for the rare occurrence of these congenital cardiac anomalies in persons with Down syndrome are unknown. It has been suggested that the complete absence of inversion at visceral, ventricular, and arterial levels in persons with trisomy 21 could be the consequence of an overexpression of specific genes on chromosome 21 (Van Praagh et al., 1989).

Moreover, recent reports have indicated that even among the more frequent anomalies observed in children with trisomy 21 (atrioventricular canal, ventricular septal defect, tetralogy of Fallot), there are certain anatomic subgroups and associated malformations different from those found in children with normal chromosomes. For example, in children with Down syndrome who have atrioventricular canal (De Biase et al., 1986; Marino, 1989; Marino, Vairo, et al., 1990) it is rare to find left-side obstructions, whereas this defect is often associated with tetralogy of Fallot (Table 9.1). In persons with ventricular septal defect (Marino, 1989; Marino, Papa, et al., 1990), the muscular and restrictive defects are rare, whereas the perimembranous posterior defect with cleft of the mitral valve is quite prevalent (Tables 9.2., 9.3). Thus, a specific pattern of congenital heart diseases is observed in persons with Down syndrome. Usu-

Table 9.1. Types of atrioventricular canal and associated cardiac anomalies in 220 persons with and without Down syndrome

Associated cardiac anomaly	Partial	Complete	DS	Non DS	Total
Left superior vena cava	7	8	7	8	15
Double outlet atrium	3	0	0	3	3
Double mitral orifice	4	0	0	4	4
"Parachute" mitral valve	8	2	2	8	10
Additional ventricular septal defects	2	7	1	8	9
Hypoplastic ventricle: left	8	10	5	13[a]	18
right	0	1	1	0	1
Subaortic stenosis	6	7	4	9	13
Aortic coarctation	12	13	5	20[a]	25
Patent ductus arteriosus	5	7	6	6	12
Peripheral pulmonary stenosis	0	1	0	1[b]	1
Tetralogy of Fallot	0	19[c]	14[d]	5	19
Double outlet right ventricle	0	3	2	1	3
Congenitally corrected transposition of great arteries	0	1	0	1	1

From Marino, B., Vairo, U., Corno, A., Nava, S., Guccione, P., Calabró, R., & Marcelletti, C. (1990). Atrioventricular canal in Down syndrome. Prevalence of associated cardiac malformations compared with patients without Down syndrome. *American Journal of Diseases of Children, 144*, 1121. Copyright 1990, American Medical Association. Reprinted with permission.

DS = Down syndrome.
[a]$p < 0.01$.
[b]Person had DiGeorge syndrome.
[c]$p < 0.000$.
[d]$p < 0.05$.

Table 9.2.   Types of ventricular septal defect in 376 patients

Type of defect	Down syndrome (Group I)	Non-Down syndrome (Group II)
Perimembranous subaortic	49 (67%)	233 (76%)
Perimembranous inlet	21 (28%)	7 (2%)[a]
Trabecular muscular	0	31 (10%)[b]
Subarterial	0	7 (2%)
Multiple	3 (4%)	25 (8%)

From Marino, B., Papa, M., Guccione, P., Corno, A., Marasini, M., & Calabró, R. (1990). Ventricular septal defect in Down syndrome. Anatomic types and associated malformations. *American Journal of Diseases of Children, 144,* 545. Copyright 1990, American Medical Association. Reprinted with permission.

[a]$p < 0.001$.

[b]$p < 0.05$.

ally the anatomic defects are simple and the associated cardiac malformations are rare and predictable.

Interesting data are derived from cardiac assessments of persons with mosaic Down syndrome (De Zorzi et al., 1991). This subgroup of children seems to have a lower prevalence and less severe types of congenital heart defects compared with those observed in trisomy 21. In particular, the complete form of atrioventricular canal, frequently seen in trisomy 21, is rare in mosaic Down syndrome (De Zorzi et al., 1991). Thus, we can postulate that phenotypic expression at the cardiac level is attenuated in these individuals.

PULMONARY IMPLICATIONS

Pulmonary artery hypertension and pulmonary vascular obstructive disease, in association with congestive heart failure, are the major complica-

tions of cardiac defects in children with Down syndrome (Chi & Krovetz, 1975; Clapp et al., 1990; R.W. Clark, Schmidt, & Schuller, 1980; Cooney & Thurlbeck, 1982; Frescura, Thiene, Franceschini, Talenti, & Mazzucco, 1987; Haworth, 1986; Loughlin, Wynne, & Victorica, 1981; Rowland, Nordstrom, Bean, & Burkhardt, 1981; Soudon, Stijns, Tremouroux-Wattiez, & Vliers, 1975; S.K. Wilson, Hutchins, & Neill, 1979; Yamaki, Horiuschi, & Sekino, 1983). The increased pulmonary blood flow, caused by the septal defects, leads to early irreversible damage to the pulmonary vascular bed (Chi & Krovetz, 1975; Soudon et al., 1975; S.K. Wilson et al., 1979). Persons with Down syndrome who have a complete atrioventricular canal frequently have a significant degree of pulmonary vascular resistance starting in the 1st year and sometimes even in the first 6 months of life (Clapp et al., 1990; Frescura et al., 1987; Haworth, 1986; S.K. Wilson et al., 1979; Yamaki et al., 1983) (see

Table 9.3.   Associated cardiac malformations in 376 patients with ventricular septal defect

Cardiac malformation	Down syndrome (Group I)	Non-Down syndrome (Group II)
Patent ductus arteriosus	15 (20%)	33 (11%)
Atrial septal defect	4 (5%)	21 (7%)
Left ventricular outflow tract obstruction	0	53 (17%)[a]
Right ventricular outflow tract obstruction	1 (1%)	9 (3%)
Cleft of the mitral valve	15 (20%)	2 (0.7%)[a]
Straddling tricuspid valve	0	6 (2%)
Mitral stenosis	0	18 (6%)

From Marino, B., Papa, M., Guccione, P., Corno, A., Marasini, M., & Calabró, R. (1990). Ventricular septal defect in Down syndrome. Anatomic types and associated malformations. *American Journal of Diseases of Children, 144,* 545. Copyright 1990, American Medical Association. Reprinted with permission.

[a]$p < 0.001$.

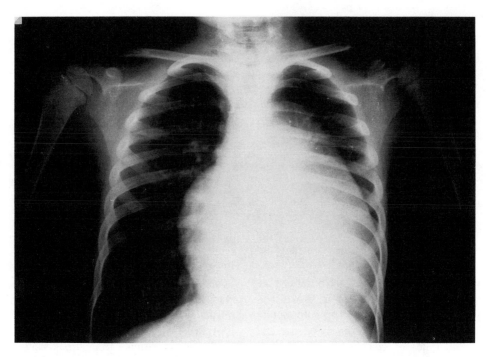

Figure 9.1.   Chest X ray of a 9-year-old child with Down syndrome, complete atrioventricular canal, and pulmonary hypertension. Note the cardiomegaly—in particular, the enlargement of the pulmonary artery and reduction of the pulmonary flow due to the vascular obstructive disease.

Figure 9.1). This progression to irreversible pulmonary vascular obstructive disease in children with Down syndrome is more rapid than in children with the same heart defects and normal chromosomes (Clapp et al., 1990; Frescura et al., 1987; Haworth, 1986) (see Figures 9.2 and 9.3).

The reason for this early complication is unclear. It may be related to associated upper airway obstruction with subsequent chronic hypercarbia (R.W. Clark et al., 1980; Loughlin et al., 1981; Rowland et al., 1981) or to intrinsic abnormalities of the vascular bed—that is, pulmonary hypoplasia with a reduced number of alveoli and thus a smaller alveolar surface area (Cooney & Thurlbeck, 1982). To avoid this irreversible complication of pulmonary artery hypertension, early diagnosis of congenital heart disease and surgical treatment of cardiac defects are mandatory and should be accomplished in early life (Frescura et al., 1987). (For further discussion of pulmonary implications, see Howenstine, chap. 10, this volume.)

CLINICAL PRESENTATION AND DIAGNOSIS

The major problem in early recognition of congenital heart defects in infants with Down syndrome is that often a newborn with complete atrioventricular canal or a large ventricular septal defect may have just a soft murmur or no murmur at all. Therefore, it is not rare for a child with Down syndrome to be evaluated for the first time by a pediatric cardiologist after 1 year of age, when the pulmonary complications of the cardiac defect have become irreversible (Sondheimer, Byrum, & Blackman, 1985). Therefore, it seems particularly important for the prognosis that the earliest signs of heart involvement in children with Down syndrome be recognized by parents or pediatricians in the first days, weeks, or months of life (E.B. Clark, 1989; Hallidie-Smith, 1985; Schneider, Kenneth, Clark, & Neill, 1989; Spicer, 1984). Failure to thrive, tachycardia, tachypnea, sweating, and paleness of skin may be important features of congestive heart

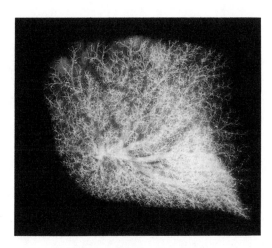

Figure 9.2. Postmortem injection of the pulmonary arterial circulation of a lung in a 9-month-old infant with Down syndrome and complete atrioventricular canal. Note the "winter tree" pattern of the pulmonary vasculature.

failure. In the presence of a large septal defect (atrioventricular canal or ventricular septal defect) and increased pulmonary resistance, the infant may appear intermittently cyanotic because of a bidirectional shunt. Permanent cyanosis may be due to irreversible pulmonary disease (usually after 1 year of age) if the child has an isolated septal defect or if tetralogy of Fallot is present with a right-to-left shunt caused by the pulmonary stenosis.

In children with pulmonary hypertension,

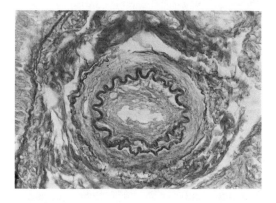

Figure 9.3. Histology of a pulmonary vessel in the same infant as in Figure 9.2. Note the small pulmonary artery with concentric obstructive intimal fibrosis. This picture was kindly provided by Professor Gaetano Thiene, Cardiac Pathology, University of Padua, Italy.

the intensity of the second heart sound may be increased and cardiac enlargement due to the congestive heart failure may produce a typical convex deformity of the anterior chest wall.

Moreover, the clinical examination may be confounded by the presence of tachycardia and tachypnea, which may erroneously be ascribed to primary pulmonary disease; the marked hypotonia often seen in infants with congestive heart failure may be thought of as being part of the delay in motor development. Children with Down syndrome may also present increased mottling of the skin and cyanosis of the extremities. However, these are not related to the cardiac defect, and are probably due to a peripheral vasomotor regulatory effect.

Since the clinical recognition of congenital heart disease may be difficult, each infant with Down syndrome, including those without heart murmurs or other cardiac signs, should be evaluated by a pediatric cardiologist, preferably in the newborn nursery. The cardiologic evaluation should include: 1) an electrocardiogram to look for an abnormal frontal plane loop and axis deviation, which are suggestive of atrioventricular canal (Figures 9.4 and 9.5); 2) a chest X ray to identify cardiomegaly and signs of increased pulmonary blood flow (Figure 9.6); and 3) a two-dimensional echocardiographic examination (Tubman, Shields, Craig, Mulholland, & Nevin, 1991). The latter diagnostic tool has revolutionized the management of infants with congenital heart disease. Utilizing this noninvasive equipment, it is possible to visualize the entire morphology of the heart simply by placing the transducer on the chest wall. The diagnostic accuracy of echocardiography is so high that the current trend is to avoid hospitalization and cardiac catheterization before surgical intervention (Marino, Corno, et al., 1990) (Figures 9.7, 9.8, 9.9). This approach is possible in the majority of children with congenital heart disease and Down syndrome, including those with atrioventricular canal, atrial or ventricular septal defect, and tetralogy of Fallot (Marino, Corno, et al., 1990).

The current outpatient management of these individuals may reduce the risks of respiratory infections so frequent in persons with Down

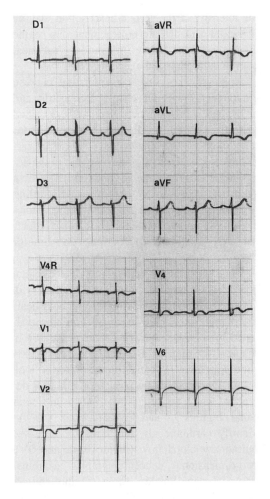

Figure 9.4.   Electrocardiogram of person with Down syndrome and partial atrioventricular canal.

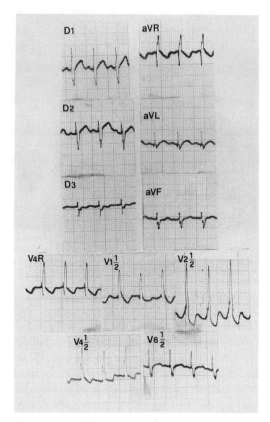

Figure 9.5.   Electrocardiogram of person with Down syndrome and complete atrioventricular canal.

syndrome who have congenital heart disease (McDonald et al., 1982).

Another contribution of echocardiography is in the follow-up of children with Down syndrome who have ventricular septal defect and aneurysm of the membranous septum (Ramaciotti, Keren, & Silverman, 1986). It has been demonstrated that the defect is usually large in persons with Down syndrome and its spontaneous closure or reduction of size is extremely rare (Marino, Corno, et al., 1991; Ramaciotti et al., 1986).

CARDIAC SURGERY

"Children with treatable medical conditions should not be denied routine care because of other handicapping conditions" (Sondheimer et al., 1985, p. 68). Recent experiences have shown that when comparable cardiac care is received (i.e., age at diagnosis and timing of surgery), both children with Down syndrome and "normal" children having similar heart defects have similar surgical outcome (Katlic, Clark, Neill, & Haller, 1977; Schneider et al., 1989; Sondheimer et al., 1985; Vet & Ottenkamp, 1989). The earlier concept that the presence of trisomy 21 increases the mortality of heart surgery (Greenwood & Nadas, 1976; Normand, Sassolas, Bozio, Jocteur-Monrozier, & André, 1981) is not confirmed by reports from the recent literature (Katlic et al., 1977; Schneider et al., 1989; Sondheimer et al., 1985; Vet & Ottenkamp, 1989). Although persons with Down syndrome can present anesthesiologic and immediate postoperative problems due to airway anomalies, increased pulmonary vasoconstric-

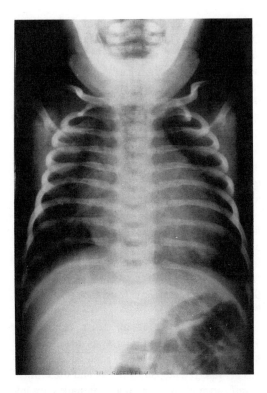

Figure 9.6. Chest X ray in a 4-month-old infant with Down syndrome and complete atrioventricular canal. Note the cardiac enlargement and the pulmonary plethora.

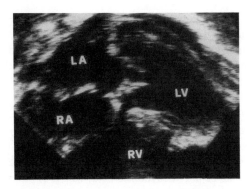

Figure 9.8. Two-dimensional echocardiogram in the subcostal "four chambers" view in a child with Down syndrome and posterior ventricular septal defect.

tion, and an increased susceptibility to infections (Kobel, Creighton, & Steward, 1982; Morray, MacGillivray, & Duker, 1986; Park et al., 1977), this morbidity does not seem to influence the mortality significantly. On the contrary, in particular in persons with complete atrioventricular canal, the surgical outcome of children with

Down syndrome seems better compared to those with normal chromosomes (Giamberti, Marino, Di Donato, Grazioli, & Marcelletti, 1990; Sondheimer et al., 1985; Vet & Ottenkamp, 1989). In addition, the need of reoperation for mitral valve regurgitation is definitively less in persons with trisomy 21 (Marino, 1990; Weintraub, Brawn, Venables, & Mee, 1990). This fact may be due to the associated left-side cardiac malformations observed in persons with atrioventricular canal who do not have Down syndrome (De Biase et al., 1986, Marino, Vairo, et al., 1990; Van Praagh et al., 1989) (see Table 9.1). In spite of this, it has been suggested that because survival at 15 years of age for unoperated children with Down syndrome who have atrioventricular canals seems comparable with that of the operative results, surgical repair may be discouraged (Bull, Rigby, & Shinebourne, 1985). This point

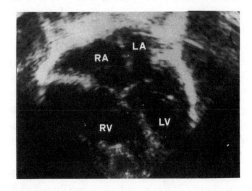

Figure 9.7. Two-dimensional echocardiogram in the apical "four chambers" view in a child with Down syndrome and complete atrioventricular canal.

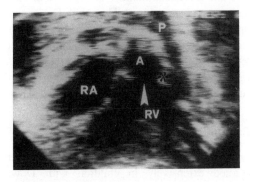

Figure 9.9. Two-dimensional echocardiogram in the right oblique subcostal view in a child with Down syndrome and tetralogy of Fallot. Note the ventricular septal defect (arrow) and the pulmonary stenosis (*).

of view is not shared by the majority of centers dealing with pediatric cardiology and cardiac surgery, since early diagnosis and surgery at an optimal time will result in 80%–90% survival of these children (Kirklin, Blackstone, Bargeron, Pacifico, & Kirklin, 1986; Vet & Ottenkamp, 1989; Weintraub et al., 1990; N.J. Wilson, Gavalaki, & Newman, 1985). It is generally agreed that cardiac surgery for children with atrioventricular canal and Down syndrome should be provided the same way as it is to other children without this chromosome disorder. Similar favorable results have also been obtained in persons with ventricular septal defect, tetralogy of Fallot, and both atrioventricular canal and tetralogy of Fallot (Alonso et al., 1990; Pacifico et al., 1988; Vargas, Otero Coto, Mayer, Jonas, & Castaneda, 1986).

Successful surgery prevents having to care for an infant in cardiac failure, with feeding problems, and with repeated respiratory infections. Obviously, before heart surgery, every infant with Down syndrome requires individual consideration with regard to the existing cardiac defect and other medical and social circumstances.

Postoperative follow-up care has not been thoroughly studied. Information regarding the need for reoperation, cardiac performance, and the quality of life after heart surgery in persons with Down syndrome is needed. A recent paper reported on the increased mortality in the late postoperative period in persons with trisomy 21 (Pozzi, Reming, Fimmers, & Urban, 1991).

Moreover, an increase in cardiac muscle fiber size and a reduced number of myocardial cells have been observed in children with Down syndrome (Recalde, Landing, & Lipsey, 1986). How these cardiac muscular changes influence left ventricular function (Simon-Lamuela et al., 1988) and long-term outcome must be studied further.

CARDIAC ANOMALIES IN ADULTS

Although congenital heart defects have been studied extensively in children with Down syndrome, little attention has been paid to the cardiac structural aspects and their clinical manifestations in adults with trisomy 21. It is note-worthy that the cardiac anatomy of persons with Down syndrome, also in the absence of congenital heart disease, shows some specific manifestation. For example, the membranous ventricular septum is significantly enlarged as compared to that found in the general population (Rosenquist, Sweeney, Amsel, & McAllister, 1974). In addition, the commissure between the anterior and medial leaflets of the tricuspid valve is commonly absent in persons with trisomy 21 (Rosenquist, Sweeney, & McAllister, 1975). Moreover, a recent echocardiographic study in children with Down syndrome who did not have congenital heart disease has shown specific morphologic aberrations of the atrioventricular valves as they insert at the same level in the ventricular septum (Ammirati et al., 1991) (see Figures 9.10 and 9.11), which is different from that observed in "normal" children.

Furthermore, a high incidence of aberrant vertebral and subclavian arteries has been described in this aneuploidy (Rathore & Sreenivasan, 1989). The pathogenesis and the clinical significance of these "minor" anomalies are unknown, but they may represent the internal cardiovascular phenotype of Down syndrome.

Recent studies have revealed a high frequency of aortic regurgitation and mitral valve prolapse among asymptomatic adults with Down syndrome (Goldhaber et al., 1986; Goldhaber, Brown, Robertson, Rubin, & St. John Sutton, 1988; Goldhaber, Brown, & St. John Sutton, 1987). The connective tissue abnormalities occurring in persons with Down syndrome (Pueschel, Scola, Perry, & Pezzullo, 1981) or the congenital or acquired commissural fenestrations of the aortic valve (Sylvester, 1974) may explain these valvular dysfunctions. Abnormalities in collagen formation and deposition may cause a weakness and laxity of connective tissue (Pueschel et al., 1981) affecting the supporting structures of the aortic and mitral valve leaflets (Malcom, 1985) and consequently may be responsible for the increased frequency of mitral valve prolapse and aortic regurgitation.

These unsuspected cardiac anomalies are usually without clinical manifestations (Pueschel & Werner, in press), but if detected in persons with Down syndrome, regular follow-up, the use of

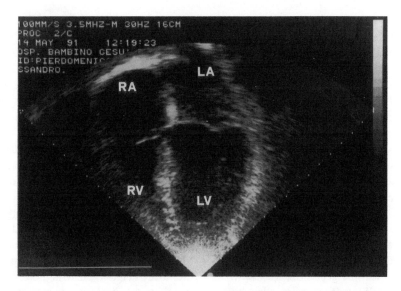

Figure 9.10. Two-dimensional echocardiogram in the apical "four chambers" view in an individual with normal chromosomes.

antibiotic prophylaxis prior to dental or surgical procedures has been recommended (Goldhaber et al., 1986). It is assumed that these associated valvular anomalies have not been previously observed, because, until recently, few persons with Down syndrome survived to adulthood (Bell et al., 1989; Fabia & Drolette, 1970; Thase, 1982). It is not known whether these cardiac abnormalities, including mitral valve prolapse and aortic regurgitation, described in persons without congenital heart disease are also present in persons with Down syndrome and congenital heart defects.

Interestingly, it has been reported that the mean systolic and diastolic blood pressure of persons with Down syndrome are consistently lower than those of controls in all age groups of both sexes (Murdoch, Rodger, Rao, Fletcher, &

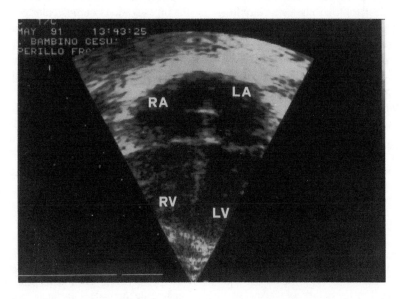

Figure 9.11. Two-dimensional echocardiogram in the apical "four chambers" view in an individual with Down syndrome and without congenital heart disease. Note the tendency of the atrioventricular valves to insertion at the same level.

Dunnigan, 1977; Richards, 1979). In adults with Down syndrome, the rise of blood pressure with age is slight and the reported sex difference noted in the general population has not been observed in persons with this chromosome disorder (Richards, 1979). The cause of these observations is unclear, but it may be related to the absence of atherosclerotic lesions noted during postmortem examination in adults with Down syndrome (Murdoch et al., 1977). Since the gene for cystathionine synthase has been located on chromosome 21 (Skovby, Krassikoff, & Francke, 1984) and since the deficiency of this enzyme results in homocystinuria and precocious atherosclerosis (Mudd & Levy, 1983), it has been suggested that the excess of cystathionine synthase due to a triple gene dose may protect persons with Down syndrome from atherosclerotic lesions (Brattstrom, England, & Brun, 1987; Murdoch et al., 1977). If these findings should be confirmed by further studies, adults with Down syndrome may be considered a population at low cardiovascular risk in terms of hypertension, myocardial infarction, and cerebrovascular strokes.

Pueschel, Craig, and Haddow (in press) observed in their patients with Down syndrome low levels of high-density lipoprotein cholesterol, low apo AI levels, and a decreased high-density lipoprotein cholesterol:total cholesterol ratio—all of which are associated with an increased risk for coronary artery disease. They concluded that any decreased prevalence of coronary artery disease in individuals with Down syndrome cannot be explained by the lipid and lipoprotein levels observed in their study population.

CONCLUSION

Both life expectancy and quality of life for persons with Down syndrome have improved

dramatically since the early 1970s. Many more individuals with Down syndrome with or without congenital heart defects are surviving to adulthood.

It is now well known that cardiac problems are common in children with Down syndrome and this is important for the overall management of these children. The patterns of cardiac defects in this aneuploidy have been well studied. Today we have improved noninvasive diagnostic techniques that allow outpatient management of children with Down syndrome. Preoperative hospitalization and invasive diagnostic procedures can be avoided in the majority of children. Optimal cardiac surgery is now available, and the results of cardiac surgery for persons with Down syndrome are comparable with those for the general population. In addition, postoperative follow-up care will enhance their quality of life.

Early diagnosis and treatment, appropriate interdisciplinary service provision, and a positive approach toward overall care, including cardiac care, will favorably influence the long-term prognosis of children with Down syndrome. Moreover, further studies on the extracellular matrix of the heart and its role in the morphogenesis of endocardial cushions, the analysis of cardiovascular malformations of mouse trisomy 16 (an animal model for human trisomy 21), and the investigations in molecular genetics will improve our understanding of the causes and processes of cardiac defects in persons with Down syndrome. Studies of adolescents and adults with Down syndrome will provide us with increased knowledge of their specific cardiac problems during this time period in life.

Finally, more information is needed regarding the cardiac anatomy and function in persons with Down syndrome without congenital heart defect. Confirmation of the associated low risk of atherosclerosis is also needed.

REFERENCES

Alonso, J., Nunez, P., Perez de Leon, J., Sanchez, P.A., Villagra, F., Gomez, R., Lopez Checa, S., Vellibre, D., & Brito, J.M. (1990). Complete atrioventricular canal and tetralogy of Fallot: Surgical management. *European Journal of Cardiothoracic Surgery, 4,* 297–299.

Ammirati, A., Marino, B., Annicchiarico, M., Ferrazza, A., Affinito, V., & Ragonese, P. (1991). Sindrome di Down senza cardiopatia congenita: E' realmente normale l'anatomia ecocardiografica? *Giornale Italiano di Cardiologia, 21,* 55.

Bell, J.A., Pearn, J.H., & Firman, D. (1989). Childhood deaths in Down's syndrome. Survival curves and causes of death from a total population study in Queensland, Australia, 1976 to 1985. *Journal of Medical Genetics, 26,* 764–768.

Berg, J.M., Crome, L., & France, N.E. (1960). Congenital cardiac malformations in mongolism. *British Heart Journal, 22,* 331–346.

Brattstrom, L., England, E., & Brun, A. (1987). Does Down syndrome support homocysteine theory of arteriosclerosis? *Lancet, i,* 391–392.

Bull, C., Rigby, M.L., & Shinebourne, E.A. (1985). Should management of complete atrioventricular canal defect be influenced by coexistent Down syndrome? *Lancet, i,* 1147–1149.

Chi, T.P.L., & Krovetz, J. (1975). The pulmonary vascular bed in children with Down syndrome. *Journal of Pediatrics, 86,* 533–538.

Clapp, S., Perry, B.L., Farooki, Z.Q., Jackson, W.L., Karpawich, P.P., Hakimi, M., Arciniegas, E., Green, E.W., & Pinsky, W.W. (1990). Down's syndrome, complete atrioventricular canal, and pulmonary vascular obstructive disease. *Journal of Thoracic and Cardiovascular Surgery, 100,* 115–121.

Clark, E.B. (1989). Congenital cardiovascular defects in infants with Down syndrome. *Pediatrics in Review, 11,* 99–100.

Clark, R.W., Schmidt, H.S., & Schuller, D.E. (1980). Sleep-induced ventilatory dysfunction in Down's syndrome. *Archives of Internal Medicine, 140,* 45–50.

Cooney, T.P., & Thurlbeck, W.M. (1982). Pulmonary hypoplasia in Down's syndrome. *New England Journal of Medicine, 307,* 1170–1173.

Cullum, L., & Liebman, J. (1969). The association of congenital heart disease with Down's syndrome (mongolism). *American Journal of Cardiology, 24,* 354–357.

De Biase, L., Di Ciommo, V., Ballerini, L., Bevilacqua, M., Marcelletti, C., & Marino, B. (1986). Prevalence of left-sided obstructive lesions in patients with atrioventricular canal without Down's syndrome. *Journal of Thoracic and Cardiovascular Surgery, 91,* 467–469.

De Zorzi, A., Marino, B., Calabró, R., Milanesi, O., Grazioli, S., & De Simone, G. (1991). Cardiopatie congenite nella sindrome di Down con mosaicismo. *Giornale Italiano di Cardiologia, 21,* 31.

Fabia, J., & Drolette, M. (1970). Life tables up to age 10 for mongols with and without congenital heart defect. *Journal of Mental Deficiency Research, 14,* 235–242.

Ferencz, C., Neill, C.A., Boughman, J.A., Rubin, J.D., Brenner, J.I., & Perry, L.W. (1989). Congenital cardiovascular malformations associated with chromosome abnormalities: An epidemiologic study. *Journal of Pediatrics, 114,* 79–86.

Ferencz, C., Rubin, J.D., McCarter, R.J., Brenner, J.I., Neill, C.A., Perry, L.W., Hepner, S.I., &

Downing, J.W. (1985). Congenital heart disease: Prevalence at live birth: The Baltimore–Washington infant study. *American Journal of Epidemiology, 121,* 31–36.

Frescura, C., Thiene, G., Franceschini, E., Talenti, E., & Mazzucco, A. (1987). Pulmonary vascular disease in infants with complete atrioventricular septal defect. *International Journal of Cardiology, 15,* 91–100.

Garrod, A.E. (1894). On the association of cardiac malformations with other congenital defects. *St. Bartholomew's Hospital Report, 39,* 53.

Giamberti, A., Marino, B., Di Donato, R., Grazioli, S., & Marcelletti, C. (1990). Canale atrioventricolare parziale: Fattori di deterioramento clinico e risultati chirurgici nel primo anno di vita. *Giornale Italiano di Cardiologia, 20,* 19.

Goldhaber, S.Z., Brown, W.D., Robertson, N., Rubin, I.L., & St. John Sutton, M.G. (1988). Aortic regurgitation and mitral valve prolapse with Down's syndrome: A case-control study. *Journal of Mental Deficiency Research, 32,* 333–336.

Goldhaber, S.Z., Brown, W.D., & St. John Sutton, M.G. (1987). High frequency of mitral valve prolapse and aortic regurgitation among asymptomatic adults with Down's syndrome. *Journal of the American Medical Association, 258,* 1793–1795.

Goldhaber, S.Z., Rubin, I.L., Brown, W., Robertson, N., Stubblefield, F., & Sloss, L.J. (1986). Valvular heart disease (aortic regurgitation and mitral valve prolapse) among institutionalized adults with Down syndrome. *American Journal of Cardiology, 57,* 278–281.

Greenwood, R.D., & Nadas, A.S. (1976). The clinical course of cardiac disease in Down's syndrome. *Pediatrics, 58,* 893–897.

Hallidie-Smith, K.A. (1985). Current approaches to Down syndrome. In D. Lane & B. Stratford (Eds.), *The heart* (pp. 52–70). New York: Holt, Rinehart & Winston.

Haworth, S.G. (1986). Pulmonary vascular bed in children with complete atrioventricular septal defect: Relation between structural and hemodynamic abnormalities. *American Journal of Cardiology, 57,* 833–839.

Katlic, M.R., Clark, E.B., Neill, C., & Haller, A., Jr. (1977). Surgical management of congenital heart disease in Down's syndrome. *Journal of Thoracic and Cardiovascular Surgery, 74,* 204–209.

Kirklin, J.W., Blackstone, E.H., Bargeron, L.M., Jr., Pacifico, A.D., & Kirklin, J.K. (1986). The repair of atrioventricular septal defects in infancy. *International Journal of Cardiology, 13,* 333–351.

Kobel, M., Creighton, R.E., & Steward, D.J. (1982). Anaesthetic considerations in Down's syndrome: Experience with 100 patients and a review of the literature. *Canadian Anaesthetists' Society Journal, 29,* 593–599.

Kurnit, D.M., Aldridge, J.F., Matsuoka, R., &

Matthysse, S. (1985). Increased adhesiveness of trisomy 21 cells and atrioventricular canal malformations in Down syndrome: A stochastic model. *American Journal of Medical Genetics, 20,* 385–399.

Laursen, H.B. (1976). Congenital heart disease in Down's syndrome. *British Heart Journal, 38,* 32–38.

Liu, M.C., & Corlett, K. (1959). A study of congenital heart defect in mongolism. *Archives of Disease in Childhood, 12,* 410–419.

Loughlin, G.M., Wynne, J.W., & Victorica, B.E. (1981). Sleep apnea as a possible cause of pulmonary hypertension in Down syndrome. *Journal of Pediatrics, 98,* 435–437.

Malcom, A.D. (1985). Mitral valve prolapse associated with other disorders: Casual coincidence, common link, or fundamental genetic disturbance? *British Heart Journal, 53,* 353–362.

Marino, B. (1989). Left-sided cardiac obstruction in patients with Down syndrome. *Journal of Pediatrics, 115,* 834–835.

Marino, B. (1990). Valve insufficiency after atrioventricular septal defect repair: Differences between patients with and without Down's syndrome. *Annals of Thoracic Surgery, 50,* 854–860.

Marino, B., Corno, A., Carotti, A., Pasquini, L., Giannico, S., Bevilacqua, M., De Simone, G., & Marcelletti, C. (1990). Pediatric cardiac surgery guided by echocardiography. Established indications and new trends. *Scandinavian Journal of Thoracic and Cardiovascular Surgery, 24,* 197–201.

Marino, B., Corno, A., Guccione, P., & Marcelletti, C. (1991). Ventricular septal defect and Down's syndrome. *Lancet, 337,* 245–246.

Marino, B., Papa, M., Guccione, P., Corno, A., Marasini, M., & Calabró, R. (1990). Ventricular septal defect in Down syndrome. Anatomic types and associated malformations. *American Journal of Diseases of Children, 144,* 544–545.

Marino, B., Vairo, U., Corno, A., Nava, S., Guccione, P., Calabró, R., & Marcelletti, C. (1990). Atrioventricular canal in Down syndrome. Prevalence of associated cardiac malformations compared with patients without Down syndrome. *American Journal of Diseases of Children, 144,* 1120–1121.

Martin, G.R., Rosenbaum, K.N., & Sardegna, K.M. (1989). Prevalence of heart disease in trisomy 21: An unbiased population [Abstract]. *Pediatric Research, 25,* 225.

McDonald, N.E., Breese Hall, C., Suffin, S.C., Alexon, C., Harris, P.J., & Manning, J.A. (1982). Respiratory syncytial viral infection in infants with congenital heart disease. *New England Journal of Medicine, 307,* 397–400.

Morray, J.P., MacGillivray, R., & Duker, G. (1986). Increased perioperative risk following repair of congenital heart disease in Down's syndrome. *Anesthesiology, 65,* 221–224.

Mudd, S.H., & Levy, H.L. (1983). Disorders of transsulfuration. In J.B. Stanbury, J.B. Wyngaarden, D.S. Frederickson, J.L. Goldstein, & M.S. Brown (Eds.), *The metabolic basis of inherited disease* (pp. 522–529). New York: McGraw-Hill.

Murdoch, J.C., Rodger, J.C., Rao, S.S., Fletcher, C.D., & Dunnigan, M.G. (1977). Down's syndrome: An atheroma-free model? *British Medical Journal, 2,* 226–228.

Normand, J., Sassolas, F., Bozio, A., Jocteur-Monrozier, D., & André, M. (1981) [Congenital heart disease and Trisomy 21]. *Archive des Maladies du Coeur, 12,* 1427–1436.

Pacifico, A.D., Ricchi, A., Bargeron, L.M., Jr., Colvin, E.C., Kirklin, J.W., & Kirklin, J.K. (1988). Corrective repair of complete atrioventricular canal defects and major associated cardiac anomalies. *Annals of Thoracic Surgery, 46,* 645–651.

Park, S.C., Mathews, R.A., Zuberbuhler, J.R., Rowe, R.D., Neches, W.H., & Lenox, C.C. (1977). Down syndrome with congenital heart malformation. *American Journal of Diseases of Children, 131,* 29–33.

Pinto, F.F., Nunes, L., Ferraz, F., & Sampayo, F. (1990). Down's syndrome: Different distribution of congenital heart diseases between the sexes. *International Journal of Cardiology, 27,* 175–178.

Pozzi, M., Reming, J., Fimmers, R., & Urban, A.E. (1991). Atrioventricular septal defects. Analysis of short- and medium-term results. *Journal of Thoracic and Cardiovascular Surgery, 101,* 138–142.

Pueschel, S.M., Craig, W.Y., & Haddow, J.E. (in press). Lipids and lipoproteins in persons with Down syndrome. *Journal of Mental Deficiency Research.*

Pueschel, S.M., Scola, F.H., Perry, C.D., & Pezzullo, J.C. (1981). Atlanto-axial instability in children with Down syndrome. *Pediatric Radiology, 10,* 129–132.

Pueschel, S.M., & Werner, J.C. (in press). Mitral valve prolapse in persons with Down syndrome. *Journal of Mental Deficiency Research.*

Rainsford Evans, P. (1950). Cardiac anomalies in mongolism. *British Heart Journal, 12,* 258–262.

Ramaciotti, C., Keren, A., & Silverman, N.H. (1986). Importance of (perimembranous) ventricular septal aneurysm in the natural history of isolated perimembranous ventricular septal defect. *American Journal of Cardiology, 57,* 268–272.

Rathore, M.H., & Sreenivasan, V.V. (1989). Vertebral and right subclavian artery abnormalities in Down syndrome. *American Journal of Cardiology, 63,* 1528–1529.

Recalde, A.I., Landing, B.H., & Lipsey, A.I. (1986). Increased cardiac muscle fiber size and reduced cell number in Down syndrome. Heart muscle cell number in Down syndrome. *Pediatric Pathology, 6,* 47–53.

Richards, B.W. (1979). Blood pressure in Down's syndrome. *Journal of Mental Deficiency Research, 23,* 123–135.

Rosenquist, G.C., Sweeney, L.J., Amsel, J., & McAllister, H.A. (1974). Enlargement of the membranous ventricular septum: An internal stigma of Down's syndrome. *Journal of Pediatrics, 85,* 490–493.

Rosenquist, G.C., Sweeney, L.J., & McAllister, H.A. (1975). Relationships of the tricuspid valve to the membranous ventricular septum in Down's syndrome without endocardial cushion defect: Study of 28 specimens, 14 with a ventricular septal defect. *American Heart Journal, 90,* 458–462.

Rowe, R. (1962). Cardiac malformation in mongolism. *American Heart Journal, 64,* 567–569.

Rowe, R.D., & Uchida, I.A. (1961). Cardiac malformation in mongolism. A prospective study of 184 mongoloid children. *American Journal of Medicine, 31,* 726–735.

Rowland, T.W., Nordstrom, L.G., Bean, M.S., & Burkhardt, H. (1981). Chronic upper airway obstruction and pulmonary hypertension in Down's syndrome. *American Journal of Diseases of Children, 135,* 1050–1052.

Schneider, D.S., Kenneth, G.Z., Clark, E.B., & Neill, C.A. (1989). Patterns of cardiac care in infants with Down syndrome. *American Journal of Diseases of Children, 143,* 363–365.

Sharer, R.M., Farina, M.A., Porter, J.H., & Bishop, M. (1972). Clinical aspects of congenital heart disease in mongolism. *American Journal of Cardiology, 29,* 497–503.

Simon-Lamuela, J., Roca, J., Lozano Sainz, C., Sanmartí, J., Girona, J.M., & Casaldaliga, J. (1988). Pediatric cardiology. Atrioventricular septal defects. In M.Q. Jimenez & M.A. Martinez (Eds.), *Ventricular function in atrioventricular septal defects with Down's syndrome* (pp. 232–238). Madrid: Ediciones Norma.

Skovby, F., Krassikoff, N., & Francke, U. (1984). Assignment of the gene for cystathionine beta-synthase to human chromosome 21 in somatic cell hybrids. *Human Genetics, 65,* 291–294.

Sondheimer, H.M., Byrum, C.J., & Blackman, M.S. (1985). Unequal cardiac care for children with Down's syndrome. *American Journal of Diseases of Children, 139,* 68–70.

Soudon, P., Stijns, M., Tremouroux-Wattiez, M., & Vliers, A. (1975). Precocity of pulmonary vascular obstruction in Down's syndrome. *European Journal of Cardiology, 2,* 473–476.

Spicer, R.L. (1984). Cardiovascular disease in Down syndrome. *Pediatric Clinics of North America, 31,* 1331–1343.

Sylvester, P.E. (1974). Aortic and pulmonary valve fenestrations as aging indices in Down syndrome. *Journal of Mental Deficiency Research, 18,* 367–378.

Tandon, R., & Edwards, J.E. (1973). Cardiac malformations associated with Down's syndrome. *Circulation, 47,* 1349–1355.

Thase, M.E. (1982). Longevity and mortality in Down's syndrome. *Journal of Mental Deficiency Research, 26,* 177–192.

Tubman, T.R.J., Shields, M.D., Craig, B.G., Mulholland, H.C., & Nevin, N.C. (1991). Congenital heart disease in Down's syndrome: Two year prospective early screening study. *British Medical Journal, 302,* 1425–1427.

Van Mierop, L.H.S., & Kutsche, L.M. (1986). Cardiovascular anomalies in DiGeorge syndrome and importance of neural crest as a possible pathogenetic factor. *American Journal of Cardiology, 58,* 133–137.

Van Praagh, S., Truman, T., Firpo, A., Bano-Rodrigo, A., Fried, R., McManus, B., Engle, M.A., & Van Praagh, R. (1989). Cardiac malformations in trisomy 18: A study of 21 postmortem cases. *Journal of the American College of Cardiology, 13,* 1586–1597.

Vargas, F.J., Otero Coto, E., Mayer, J.E., Jonas, R.A., & Castaneda, A.R. (1986). Complete atrioventricular canal and tetralogy of Fallot: Surgical considerations. *Annals of Thoracic Surgery, 42,* 258–263.

Vet, T.W., & Ottenkamp, J. (1989). Correction of atrioventricular septal defect. Results influenced by Down syndrome? *American Journal of Diseases of Children, 143,* 1361–1365.

Warkany, J., Passarge, E., & Smith, L.B. (1966). Congenital malformations in autosomal trisomy syndromes. *American Journal of Diseases of Children, 112,* 502–517.

Weintraub, R.G., Brawn, W.J., Venables, A.W., & Mee, R.B.B. (1990). Two-patch repair of complete atrioventricular septal defect in the first year of life. *Journal of Thoracic and Cardiovascular Surgery, 99,* 320–326.

Wilson, N.J., Gavalaki, E., & Newman, C.G.H. (1985). Complete atrioventricular canal defect in presence of Down syndrome. *Lancet, ii,* 834–835.

Wilson, S.K., Hutchins, G.M., & Neill, C.A. (1979). Hypertensive pulmonary vascular disease in Down syndrome. *Journal of Pediatrics, 95,* 722–726.

Yamaki, S., Horiuschi, T., & Sekino, Y. (1983). Quantitative analysis of pulmonary vascular disease in simple cardiac anomalies with Down syndrome. *American Journal of Cardiology, 51,* 1502–1506.

CHAPTER 10

Pulmonary Concerns

Michelle S. Howenstine

Respiratory problems in persons with Down syndrome have been recognized more frequently in recent years. This increased awareness of pulmonary complications has occurred concurrently with the discovery of phenotypic respiratory structural abnormalities and functional difficulties. Many of the pulmonary problems in Down syndrome are closely intertwined with the well-recognized cardiac, immunologic, and neurologic complications and are often secondary to more than one dysfunctional system. This chapter attempts to define anatomic basic abnormalities and to explore the major pulmonary complications.

STRUCTURAL ABNORMALITIES

Structural abnormalities of the respiratory tract are often observed in persons with Down syndrome. The well-recognized features of Down syndrome have a major impact on the respiratory system. The midfacial region is noted to be small with short nasal passages, a narrowed hypopharynx, a small oral cavity, and mandibular, as well as maxillary, hypoplasia. Relative macroglossia is noted in most individuals. The tongue extends backward with further compromise of the small oropharynx. Several airway abnormalities have been reported in persons with Down syndrome with varying frequencies. Graham, Wertelecki, O'Connor, and Cohen (1981) reported 4 patients with Down syndrome and choanal stenosis (narrowing of the nasal passages) and hypothesized that the frequency of this obstruction was significantly greater than in the general population. Subglottic stenosis or narrowing of the cricoid area, tracheal narrowing, and/or vas-

cular rings have been reported to occur with varying frequency (Strome, 1981). Although laryngomalacia (presence of soft laryngeal cartilage) has not been reported to occur at an increased frequency, Aggarwal, Rastogi, and Singhi (1981) reported 1 infant with Down syndrome with laryngomalacia to have a significant airway obstruction and resultant cor pulmonale (hypertrophy of right ventricle).

In persons with Down syndrome, the thoracic cage is usually normally shaped. There is an increased frequency of 12th rib abnormalities with either complete absence or a rudimentary 12th rib noted. Pueschel (1983) reported an 18% prevalence of pectus excavatum and an 11% prevalence of pectus carinatum. Other studies have shown varying percentages of these chest wall abnormalities; however, there is no evidence of any cardiopulmonary dysfunction.

The lung is abnormal both in gross appearance and on histologic evaluation. Cooney and Thurlbeck (1982) evaluated 7 persons with Down syndrome, some of whom had congenital heart disease. Although the population size in this study was limited, a striking similarity in the pathology of the lungs was noted. Alveolar maturation was observed to be well advanced; however, the alveolar number was reduced to approximately 36% of the predicted value. The radial alveolar count, a measure of alveolar complexity, was found to be reduced. This diminished alveolarization of the terminal lung unit was seen in all age groups (from 4 months to 63 years of age) and was approximately 72% of the predicted value. The defect was felt to be secondary to deficient alveolar multiplication or acinar hypoplasia. This abnormal radial count was observed in persons with Down syndrome irrespective of whether or not they had congenital heart disease. The alveoli were noted to be well formed, but larger. By comparison, persons with congenital heart disease who did not have Down syndrome had a similar, but not as significant, reduction in lung volume without evidence of acinar hypoplasia or reduced radial counts.

Prenatal microscopic examination of lung tissue of persons with Down syndrome has shown normal or accelerated radial counts in late gestation, suggesting this abnormality was acquired during the postnatal period (Cooney & Thurlbeck, 1982). The radial counts were noted to fall below normal in the immediate postnatal period. They persisted without change throughout childhood and adulthood, with no further change in alveolar number or reduction in internal surface area noted. These abnormalities were felt to be secondary to a lack of development rather than atrophy because of lack of progression with age.

The characteristic gross appearance of the lungs as described by Cooney, Wentworth, and Thurlbeck (1988) was observed postnatally and was not seen at 34 weeks gestation. As seen in Figure 10.1, the lung had a diffuse and uniform porous appearance secondary to enlargement of the alveoli and alveolar ducts as well as the related diminished acinar complexity. These distended alveolar ducts and alveoli were beginning to be apparent in 1 infant evaluated at the gestational age of 37 weeks.

These observations led Cooney's group to believe that lung growth may be normal in fetuses with Down syndrome and is altered following birth. Cooney et al. (1988) hypothesized that intrauterine growth and postnatal development may be governed by a different genetic control with the latter being abnormal in their study group. An alternative mechanism would place intrauterine lung growth under the influence of maternal placental control and perhaps as independent of altered fetal genetics. Neither mech-

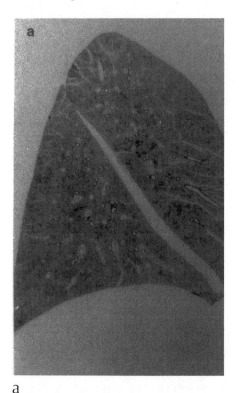 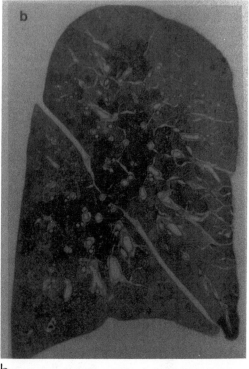

a   b

Figure 10.1.   Gross appearance of the lung: (a) velvety appearance of a normal lung, (b) uniform porous pattern of a lung of a person with Down syndrome. (From Cooney, T.P., Wentworth, P.J., & Thurlbeck, W.M. [1988]. Diminished radial count is found only postnatally in Down's syndrome. *Pediatric Pulmonology, 5,* 206. Copyright 1988: Alan R. Liss, Inc. Reprinted by permission of Wiley-Liss, a division of John Wiley & Sons, Inc.)

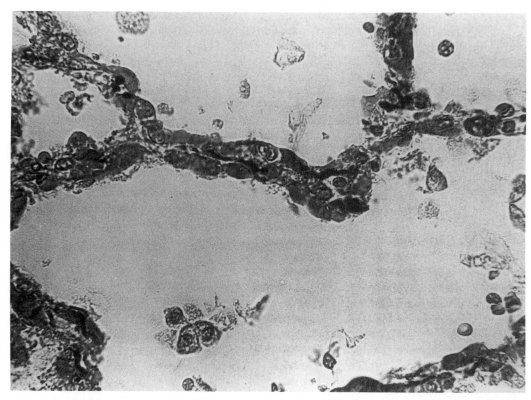

Figure 10.2. The persistent alveolar double capillary network in Down syndrome with alveolar walls containing a central strand of elastic and parallel adjoining capillaries. Humberstone elastic stain (X400). (From Cooney, T.P., Wentworth, P.J., & Thurlbeck, W.M. [1988]. Diminished radial count is found only postnatally in Down's syndrome. *Pediatric Pulmonology, 5*, 207. Copyright 1988: Alan R. Liss, Inc. Reprinted by permission of Wiley-Liss, a division of John Wiley & Sons, Inc.)

anism has been fully elucidated. If, however, lung growth is found to be abnormal during the intrauterine period, further investigation of altered or abnormal fetal respiration may be necessary, since the two accepted causes of pulmonary hypoplasia, oligohydramnios and chest wall abnormalities, are not recognized as typical complications of Down syndrome. It is of note that Cooney et al.'s (1988) 1 patient with Down syndrome with normal morphology and morphometry was born following a pregnancy complicated by polyhydramnios (excessive amniotic fluid).

A persistent alveolar double capillary network was observed in 20 out of 23 (86%) patients with Down syndrome evaluated in this same study (Cooney et al., 1988). As seen in Figure 10.2, the abnormality consisted of an alveolar wall, a central area of fibrous tissue, and parallel adjoining capillaries. This abnormality was felt to be similar to the normal intrauterine pattern of development that usually disappears during the

first 18 months of life. The double capillary network was not related to areas of parenchymal abnormalities or to the degree of acinar hypoplasia. It was visible regardless of the presence of congenital heart disease. Cooney et al. felt the defect could be attributed to an abnormality in the proteolytic system responsible for the remodeling of the vasculature and could be representative of a separately determined genetic defect that caused failure of fusion in the two layers. The possible role of the double capillary network and the precocious pulmonary artery hypertension seen in persons with Down syndrome is discussed later in this chapter.

An increased frequency of postoperative respiratory complications has been observed in children with Down syndrome. Yamaki, Horiuchi, and Takahashi (1985) evaluated 28 children with Down syndrome, ages 3 months to 10 years, with open-lung biopsy in an effort to determine the etiology of the increased postoperative difficulties. The findings were compared with children with congenital heart disease. The authors noted substantial changes after surgery with significant interstitial emphysema, overdistention of peripheral air sacs, and alveolar hypoplasia that were not evident in the control group. Alveolar septitis or thickened alveolar septa infiltrated with lymphoid cells were seen equally in both groups. The changes of interstitial emphysema and overdistention of peripheral air sacs were seen only after surgery. In 2 patients who were biopsied before and after surgery, only alveolar hypoplasia was present before the procedure. This abnormality was also the only significant alteration seen in 2 patients undergoing lung biopsy alone and in 2 patients undergoing postmortem evaluation without surgery. It was noted that the severity of the lesions worsened proportional to the duration of the artificial respiratory support, suggesting that the interstitial emphysema and overdistention of the air sacs were secondary to the surgery and artificial positive pressure ventilation. As stated earlier, the alveolar hypoplasia is probably intrinsic to persons with Down syndrome.

Yamaki et al. (1985) also suggested that the varying degrees of congenital alveolar hypoplasia in children with Down syndrome are characterized by a deficiency of elastic fibers in the entrance rings of the alveoli. These fibers would be responsible for maintaining normal alveolar structure in the lung. The potentially increased airway pressure utilized in surgery could overdistend alveolar ducts and sacs, causing either rupture of the poorly reinforced air sacs or, ultimately, interstitial emphysema.

Less frequently described disorders in persons with Down syndrome include congenital pleural effusions (Foote & Vickers, 1986) and chylothorax (Yoss & Lipsitz, 1977). Joshi, Kasznica, Ali Khan, Amato, and Levine (1986) reported cystic lung disease in 2 children with Down syndrome who had atrioventricular canal. Progressive symptoms and X-ray changes were seen during the first 2 years of life in these children. The peripheral location of these cystic lesions was also reported by Stocker, McGill, and Orsini (1985) in a patient with Down syndrome. Suggested etiologies for these cystic peripheral changes included persistence of a bronchopulmonary artery system, thromboembolism or occlusion of the pulmonary artery, and compensatory dilation of the alveoli.

LOWER RESPIRATORY TRACT INFECTIONS

Infections continue to cause significant morbidity and mortality in persons with Down syndrome despite the use of antibiotics. Pneumonia remains one of the major causes of death throughout the various age groups. The predisposition to infectious diseases in the lower respiratory tract is related to both structural and functional disorders associated with Down syndrome. As is well known, many children with Down syndrome have significant difficulty with chronic rhinitis and problems with nasal and oral secretion control. Sinus infections are common and may be the antecedent infection to a lower respiratory illness (see Dahle & Baldwin, chap. 7, this volume). Many children with Down syndrome appear to have a poor cough, which may compromise the ability to clear secretions. An airway obstructive lesion such as subglottic stenosis or vascular rings can also reduce mucociliary clearance. Similar findings have been observed in children with congenital heart disease and left atrial hypertrophy: The enlarged heart chamber causes compression of the left mainstem bronchus and results in impairment of clearance. These structural and functional abnormalities, when added to the strong likelihood of either cellular and/or humoral immunologic defects, contribute to a greater risk for frequent and perhaps more serious lower respiratory illnesses.

Signs and symptoms of lower respiratory infection in persons with Down syndrome parallel those of the general population. Bacterial pneumonia usually is more acute in its presentation and is associated with fevers and often leukocytosis. Viral infections, however, especially in infants, may also present with acute respiratory distress and be associated with significant morbidity, especially in children with Down syndrome who have congenital heart disease. The evaluation of an individual with respiratory distress should include a detailed history of complicating past medical problems, course of the current illness, and any previous respiratory illness. A chest X ray is valuable and should be compared to all previous radiographs, especially in persons with preexisting pulmonary or cardiac disease. Evaluation of white-cell counts as well as investigations of immune function should be done on an individual basis. The individual's oxygenation status should be evaluated on presentation. If the person is in significant distress, an arterial blood gas may be necessary to evaluate fully the status of the patient's ventilation.

The treatment of lower respiratory tract infection in persons with Down syndrome again parallels that of the general population. There is, however, a need to be quite attentive to certain viral infections such as respiratory syncytial virus, parainfluenza, adeno and influenza virus, especially in young infants with congenital heart disease. Individuals with heart defects such as ventriculoseptal defect, atrioventricular canal, patent ductus arteriosus, or any defect with a large left-to-right shunt are especially at risk for severe respiratory complications with bronchiolitis. This increased work of breathing is secondary to the added inflammation and edema of the airways superimposed to a chronic state of increased interstitial fluid.

The treatment of respiratory infections in children and adults with Down syndrome includes the following:

1. Supportive care
   a. Adequate fluids
   b. Monitoring
   c. Oximetry
2. Oxygen
3. Antiviral agents (e.g., ribavirin)
4. Antibiotics
5. Chest physiotherapy
6. Diuretics
7. Bronchodilators
8. Mechanical ventilation

Monitoring is especially important in the very small infant during a respiratory syncytial virus infection because of the increased risk for apnea. Oxygen is an extremely important drug for children and adults in respiratory distress.

Broad-spectrum antibiotics should be used to cover appropriate organisms in the patient's age group if bacterial pneumonia is suspected. Careful pulmonary toilet is essential for all infections and should include nasal evacuation when necessary. Hall, McBride, Gala, Hildreth, and Schnabel (1985) utilized ribavirin for treatment of respiratory syncytial virus infection in patients with congenital heart disease and found an improved clinical course and oxygenation status. Ribavirin may also be indicated in sick patients with Down syndrome without congenital heart disease because of the abnormal pulmonary histology. Bronchodilator aerosols with beta-agonists such as albuterol have been assessed in trials with varied results (Wohl, 1985).

In 1987, Cant, Gibson, and West reported on 4 children with Down syndrome and hemophilus influenza bacterial tracheitis. This limited study reported an increased prevalence of tracheitis in persons with Down syndrome, as well as the uniqueness of the hemophilus organism. Typically, *Staphylococcus aureus* is the primary organism in bacterial tracheitis.

Care should be taken to avoid high peak inspiratory pressure as well as significant end expiratory pressure in patients who require mechanical ventilation for respiratory failure. Barotrauma from positive pressure may cause the changes observed in the tissues of postoperative patients.

Evaluation of recurrent or persistent pneumonia in persons with Down syndrome should include a work-up of immune deficiency, cystic fibrosis, or possible foreign body. Sweat osmolality in persons with Down syndrome has been reported to be increased when compared to the general population (Symon, Stewart, & Russell, 1985); therefore, cautious interpretation of test results must be done and correlated with clinical symptoms. There is no definite proof that the incidence of cystic fibrosis in Down syndrome is increased, although such an increased frequency has been reported (Milunsky, 1968). If an individual's history is remarkable for recurrent emesis, coughing or choking, or an uncoordinated swallowing mechanism, then evaluation for recurrent aspiration and/or gastroesophageal reflux may be necessary. Hillemeier, Buchin, and Gryboski (1982) reported an increased incidence of esophageal dysfunction in children with Down syndrome and stressed early intervention prior to stricture formation and chronic respiratory damage. Evaluation for recurrent or persistent sinus disease may also be helpful if the person continues to have lower respiratory problems. Although reactive airway disease or asthma may present as recurrent or persistent pneumonia, the incidence of bronchial asthma in persons with Down syndrome has been reported by Rasore-Quatino, Acutis, and Strigini (1990) to be significantly lower than in age-matched siblings. Chronic congestive heart failure may also masquerade as recurrent pneumonia. Hordof, Mellins, Gersony, and Sterg (1977) reported 10 infants in whom symptoms of airway obstruction and abnormal chest X rays were present and were felt to be related to a ventriculoseptal defect and large left-to-right shunts.

The influenza virus vaccine is indicated for persons with chronic underlying respiratory problems and for those persons maintained on daily cardiopulmonary medications. In infants and small children, avoidance of large day-care centers with exposure to multiple children may also be helpful in decreasing the incidence of recurrent viral respiratory infections.

PULMONARY ARTERY HYPERTENSION

The association of congenital heart disease and Down syndrome has been well recognized for almost a century. Hypertensive pulmonary vascular disease has been a well-recognized complication of structural heart lesions associated with an increased left-to-right shunt. Whether or not persons with Down syndrome are predisposed to the development of precocious and more severe pulmonary artery hypertension despite the absence or presence of congenital heart disease has been the subject of multiple studies.

An accurate diagnosis of pulmonary artery hypertension is an important precursor for determining etiology and initiating treatment. A history suggestive of pulmonary artery hypertension may include the following: episodes of cyanosis or persistent cyanosis, easy fatigability, poor feeding, or subtle signs such as changes in the child's activity. On physical examination, the findings suggestive of increased pulmonary artery pressures would include a right ventricular heave, increased sound of the second heart sound, increased intensity of the pulmonary valve closure, or disappearance of the split second sound. There may be a diminishment of systolic murmurs and the disappearance of a diastolic rumble. Increased pulmonary hypertension decreases pulmonary blood flow and pulmonary interstitial fluid such that signs and symptoms of previous congestive heart failure may improve. Electrocardiographic (EKG) changes would include right ventricular hypertrophy, but this may be difficult to quantitate with the degree of hypertension. Echocardiographic changes may suggest an increased gradient across the pulmonary valve as well as some regurgitation. The chest X ray in persons with early pulmonary hypertension may not show significant changes. In the presence of severe pulmonary hypertension, the X ray may show a dilated main pulmonary artery with very small or pruned peripheral pulmonary arteries. Measurement of pulmonary artery pressures can be accurately assessed by cardiac catheterization. In the presence of pulmonary hypertension, pulmonary artery pressures would exceed the normal values of one-fourth to one-third systemic blood pressure. Lung biopsy specimens may also be evaluated and categorized according to several pulmonary vascular staging systems to quantitate further the degree of pulmonary vascular disease. The development of right-to-left shunting with persistent cyanosis or auscultation of more significant pulmonary regurgitation may signify Eisenmenger phenomenon or evidence of severely compromised pulmonary blood flow. This is a late sign of pulmonary artery disease and is ominous in regard to its reversibility.

Multiple studies have attempted to define the nature of the pulmonary vascular disease in persons with Down syndrome. As early as 1971, Somerville noted that pulmonary artery hypertension was apparently occurring earlier in persons with Down syndrome with atrioventricular canal than in persons with atrioventricular canal who did not have Down syndrome. In 1974, Tandon, Moller, Plett, and Edwards compared the histologic appearance of the pulmonary vasculature in persons with atrioventricular canal both with and without Down syndrome. The pulmonary vessels in this study were classified according to the grade of pulmonary artery small vessel hypertensive changes as designated by Heath and Edwards (1988). This study failed to demonstrate that persons with Down syndrome had an increased incidence of pulmonary artery hypertension. It was felt that the severe pulmonary vascular changes were related to the atrioventricular canal and worsened with increasing age.

Later, in 1975, Chi and Krovetz evaluated 69 children with Down syndrome by cardiac catheterization. These hemodynamic studies of children with Down syndrome with various heart defects were compared with control children with similar cardiac abnormalities. They noted that only 10% of children with Down syndrome had pulmonary artery pressures within the normal range as compared to 76% of the control children with similar cardiac abnormalities. They did not feel that the increased frequency correlated with the severity of the heart defect or the pulmonary blood flow, but rather was secondary to increased pulmonary vascular resistance. They also felt that children with Down syndrome appeared to develop pulmonary artery hypertension at an earlier age than the control group (3.6 years versus 6.2 years). Chi and Krovetz also suggested that the propensity toward pulmonary artery hypertension and the Eisenmenger reaction could be related to the abnormal capillary morphology that had been described in persons with Down syndrome. Soudon, Stijns, Tremouroux-Wattiez, and Vliers (1975) also utilized hemodynamic studies and showed similar significantly increased pulmonary artery pressure in children with Down syndrome when compared to controls.

Wilson, Hutchins, and Neill (1979) studied 82 persons with Down syndrome both with and without heart disease at autopsy. They studied histologic specimens from lungs, utilizing the grading system proposed by Hutchins and Ostrow (1976) for pulmonary vascular disease. They compared these persons first to age- and sex-matched controls without cardiovascular problems and then to persons with the same

heart lesions but without Down syndrome. In general, they did not notice any difference between children with Down syndrome either with or without congenital heart disease and their age- and sex-matched controls. Based on their histologic studies, they concluded that children with Down syndrome were not predisposed to the development of hypertensive pulmonary vascular disease. They felt that the cause of clinically observed pulmonary vascular hypertension in Down syndrome was unknown. The proposal of abnormal pulmonary vascular morphology (Chi & Krovetz, 1975), prolonged retention of fetal pulmonary vascular resistance, and increased prevalence of patient ductus arteriosus with elevated pulmonary blood flow (Noonan & Walters, 1974) could not be substantiated.

In 1983, Yamaki, Horiuchi, and Sekino undertook a complex study utilizing both histologic and hemodynamic investigations. They compared 21 children with Down syndrome who had simple cardiac abnormalities including ventriculoseptal defect, patient ductus arteriosus, and atrioseptal defect, or a combination of these lesions, with control children who had simple congenital heart disease without Down syndrome as well as 17 children with transposition of the great vessels. Yamaki et al. (1983) investigated the mechanism of early development of severe pulmonary vascular disease in complete transposition of the great arteries in a similarly designed study. Yamaki et al.'s (1983) results were three-fold. First, they noted that when the pulmonary artery changes were plotted against age, that intimal changes in the vessels were noted to occur at an earlier age in children with Down syndrome with congenital heart disease than in the control group. Second, they noted that although the changes in the intima were more severe in children with Down syndrome than in those with simple congenital heart disease, they were, in comparison, milder than those seen in transposition of great vessels. Finally, they noted that the children with Down syndrome and simple cardiac abnormalities had thinner media of the small pulmonary arteries than the children without Down syndrome; however, the media were thicker than in transposition of the great arteries. Yamaki et al. (1983)

concluded that there was evidence of intimal and medial changes in the pulmonary arteries of children with Down syndrome that were different from those of children with similar heart lesions without Down syndrome. They also suggested that the delayed development of the medial hypertrophy in response to pulmonary artery hypertension may cause the pulmonary artery to be more susceptible to pressure loads and be responsible for the early development of the severe intimal changes. Yamaki et al. (1983) hypothesized that a congenital underdevelopment of the smooth muscle fibers of the medial layer may be the probable cause of pulmonary hypertension in children with Down syndrome.

Further evaluations of the propensity of children with Down syndrome to develop either precocious or more severe pulmonary artery hypertension are necessary in view of the varied results. Inconsistencies may be due to different grading systems as well as different methods of comparison. It does, however, appear to be the consensus of the majority of investigators and caregivers that persons with Down syndrome should be closely watched for any evidence of pulmonary artery hypertension. Multiple mechanisms may contribute to increased pulmonary artery pressures including an abnormal capillary network as well as pulmonary hypoplasia, which would cause a decreased alveolar surface area. Yamaki et al. (1983) also suggested that the smooth muscle fibers may be underdeveloped and contribute to progression of pulmonary vascular disease. Complicating medical problems causing chronic hypoxia or pulmonary vascular damage could also contribute to pulmonary artery hypertension. These would include either acute or chronic obstructive sleep apnea, gastroesophageal reflux with subsequent aspiration, and chronic infection. The current treatment of pulmonary artery hypertension includes supplemental oxygen and calcium channel blockers such as nifedipine. Hypothetically, the addition of supplemental oxygen may dilate the pulmonary vascular bed and subsequently increase pulmonary blood flow. Whether this may in turn increase pulmonary vascular resistance has not been determined.

Further elucidation of pulmonary vascular disease in persons with Down syndrome will be necessary to determine if early surgical intervention is necessary for repair of cardiac lesions. If there is no evidence of precocious development of pulmonary artery hypertension, then early corrective surgery with its increased risk may not be necessary.

OBSTRUCTIVE SLEEP APNEA

Concerns regarding obstructive sleep apnea in individuals with Down syndrome have been documented since the early 1970s. Obstructive sleep apnea occurs when inspiratory air flow from the upper airways to the lungs is impeded, usually for 10 seconds or greater, resulting in hypoxemia ($Po_2 < 60$ mm Hg) or hypercarbia ($Pco_2 > 45$ mm Hg). During interruption of air flow, respiratory effort continues, differentiating this disorder from central apnea in which respiratory effort and air flow ceases. Obstructive breathing occurs most often in sleep when activation of pharyngeal dilator muscles decreases, causing relaxation of the airway. Airway collapse occurs when the airway is exposed to negative pressure during the inspiratory effort and an anatomical or functional airway exists, impeding air flow.

Similar to persons with other craniofacial abnormalities, persons with Down syndrome are predisposed to obstructive sleep apnea. The pathogenesis is multifactorial, consisting of anatomic, functional, and neurologic difficulties. As noted earlier, the midfacial region in Down syndrome is relatively small, with the tongue contributing to the diminished oropharyngeal area. Even relatively small tonsils may have an increased effect in the small oral cavity. Choanal stenosis and subglottic or tracheal narrowing may also contribute to a compromised airway that is conducive to obstructive breathing. Chronic rhinitis, lymphoid hyperplasia, and obesity are added risk factors. Maintenance of a patent airway is also dependent on the hypopharyngeal muscle tone, which is felt to be diminished in individuals with Down syndrome as a component of the generalized hypotonia. The use of sedative drugs and perhaps antihistamines may also contribute to hypotonia and subsequent airway collapse.

Clark, Schmidt, and Schuller (1980) described 3 individuals with sleep-induced ventilatory dysfunction and hypothesized that occult sleep apnea may contribute to the development of the unexplained pulmonary hypertension in persons with Down syndrome. They also suggested that cardiopulmonary complications of airway obstruction may explain the rapid respiratory deterioration of persons with Down syndrome who have respiratory illnesses as well as the prominent role of pneumonia as a major cause of death.

In 1981, Loughlin, Wynne, and Victorica reported on 5 children with Down syndrome referred for evaluation of right ventricular hypertrophy and pulmonary hypertension. Upper airway obstruction secondary to inspiratory collapse was diagnosed by cinefluoroscopy and several patients had hypoxemia, hypercarbia, and elevated pulmonary arterial pressures documented during sleep. The authors raised concern that sleep-induced upper airway obstruction in this pediatric population could be a significant cause of the accelerated pulmonary hypertension seen in some individuals with Down syndrome. Rowland, Nordstrom, Bean, and Burkhardt (1981) suggested that hypoxia and acidosis from chronic hypoventilation were synergistic in creating the pulmonary artery hypertension and subsequent cor pulmonale in persons with Down syndrome. Levine and Simpser (1982) evaluated 4 infants with Down syndrome who developed cor pulmonale and heart failure in association with a respiratory illness and a past history suggestive of chronic airway obstruction. They emphasized the functional component to these infants' obstruction and documented the frequent failure of tonsillectomy and adenoidectomy when compared to the general population. During their investigation, they also noted a worsening of lethargy and somnolence when supplemental oxygen was added to the therapy prior to relief of the underlying obstruction.

In 1987, Southall et al. investigated 12 children with Down syndrome ages 4 weeks to 6 years with polysomnography in a controlled study. Of the 12 children, 8 had congenital heart disease with over one half having pulmonary hypertension, which was felt to be excessive in relationship to their congenital heart disease. Six of the children evaluated were found to have sleep-related upper airway obstruction. Five of these children were noted to have hypoxemia secondary to obstructed or partially obstructed breathing with elevation of their end tidal carbon dioxide. The majority of the hypoxic episodes occurred with active or discordant sleep. Two thirds of the children were noted to have lower baseline awake saturations when compared to controls. These children were further evaluated by barium swallow, X ray of the airway, and fiberoptic endoscopy. The latter modality was utilized to locate the dynamic source of the obstruction. Eleven children had obstruction at the pharyngeal level, and 1 was diagnosed with bilateral choanal atresia. Southall et al. concluded that obstructive apnea presents as a complication of Down syndrome in all age groups studied and that screening of these patients can be done with overnight recording of oxygen saturations, expiratory CO_2, and respiratory movements.

Marcus, Keens, Bautista, Von Pechmann, and Davidson Ward (1991) recently evaluated 53 persons with Down syndrome between the ages of 2 weeks and 51 years. Nap polysomnograms were abnormal in 77% of the persons, with approximately one half of those studied demonstrating obstructive sleep apnea and two thirds showing hypoventilation. Overnight studies were abnormal in all children evaluated with over one half demonstrating O_2 desaturation. Most children had multiple respiratory abnormalities and hypoventilation was present in 81% of all persons. In this study, the incidence of obstructive sleep apnea was independent of age, obesity, and diagnosis of congenital heart disease. As in Stebbens, Dennis, Croft, and Southall's (1989) study, the history of the individual correlated with obstruction in that all persons with history suggestive of obstructive sleep apnea had abnormal studies. Sixty percent of persons with negative histories also had abnormal polysomnograms (Marcus et al., 1991). In the 8 children who underwent tonsillectomy and adenoidectomy, only 3 had normalization of the polysomnogram in the postoperative period. Further treatment modalities were not extensively investigated.

Children with obstructive sleep apnea have

varying degrees of difficulty breathing at night. The symptoms of obstructive sleep apnea include:

Snoring
Interrupted breathing with sleep
Restless sleep
Difficulty awakening
Chronic nocturnal cough
Daytime somnolence
Mouth breathing
Failure to thrive
Morning headaches
Behavioral changes
School problems
Developmental delay

Snoring is a frequent symptom, although observed periods of interrupted breathing, gasping, respirations, and increased work of breathing are more suggestive of a serious obstruction. Persons with obstructed airways are often restless sleepers, assuming unusual positions that may involve neck extension in an attempt to maintain airway patency. Frequent awakenings are common as are difficulty awakening in the morning and daytime somnolence. Enuresis has been related to a poor sleep pattern and the frequent arousals. During obstruction, intermittent aspiration of pharyngeal secretions may occur, causing a chronic nocturnal cough or aggravation of asthma symptoms. During the day, mouth breathing, morning headaches, frequent rhinorrhea, and a decreased energy level may be observed, often with somnolence or the need for frequent daytime napping. Behavioral changes, decline in school performance, and additional developmental delay are secondary to poor sleep or clinical hypoxia and are frequently described. Poor growth and weight loss may be related to daytime changes or more frequently to difficulty feeding and to breathing with an obstructed airway. Concerns have also been raised regarding alterations in the effectiveness of growth hormone and subsequent delays in growth. Long-standing obstruction affects the cardiopulmonary system causing progressive pulmonary hypertension and cor pulmonale. Symptoms at end stage include progressive shortness of breath and fatigue. Left heart failure as well as cardiopulmonary arrest may also occur.

The diagnosis of obstructive sleep apnea in persons with Down syndrome begins with the recognition of altered nocturnal or daytime behavior. As with all persons with obstructive sleep apnea, symptoms may have been present for some time and therefore have been accepted as a normal pattern or have a slowly progressive course that is unrecognized by caregivers. Often a parent's tape recording of the altered nighttime breathing can help substantiate a suggestive history. Parents may confuse respiratory changes with symptoms of underlying congenital heart disease and dismiss behavioral changes as difficulty related to the effects of trisomy 21.

The initial evaluation should include a complete physical examination. Obstruction of the airway is suspected if a person does not appear to breath comfortably and breathes primarily through the mouth. An evaluation of the airway includes evaluation of bilateral nasal patency and tonsil and adenoid size, as well as size and position of the tongue in relationship to the hypopharynx. Inspiratory stridor and/or expiratory wheezing are auscultated with upper airway obstruction such as subglottic stenosis, tracheal stenosis, or tracheal malacia. A loud second heart sound (S_2) is suggestive of pulmonary hypertension and potential cor pulmonale whereas systolic murmurs and/or gallops are indicative of underlying abnormal cardiac structure and/or function, including congestive heart failure. Hepatomegaly (enlarged liver) is found secondary to the passive congestion of right heart failure. The examination, however, of an individual with significant airway obstruction may be within normal limits especially if completed soon after the condition ensues.

X rays are not always helpful in defining the obstruction, although a lateral neck radiograph may help correlate pharyngeal findings and the amplitude of obstruction. An enlarged heart size on chest X ray is seen with cor pulmonale and often with underlying congenital heart disease. Right ventricular hypertrophy and pulmonary hypertension can be more fully evaluated with an electrocardiogram and echocardiogram. Recurrent aspiration during obstructive events may cause scattered pulmonary infiltrates and/or hyperinflation. Cinefluoroscopy and video nasopharyngoscopy, although technically difficult, can help visualize the area and degree of obstruction. Southall et al. (1987) were able to check the dynamic source of obstruction in infants and children with fiberoptic endoscopy. Home recordings of the obstructive breathing can be obtained with an anesthesia stethoscope and a condenser microphone.

Currently, the most accepted method for evaluating, documenting, and quantitating sleep apnea is the polysomnogram, a study that measures various cardiopulmonary parameters during stages of sleep. This study usually entails a simultaneous multichannel recording of nasal and oral air flow, pulse rate and electrocardiography pattern, thoracic and abdominal impedance, oximetry, and end tidal CO_2. Electronystagmography and electromyography are often utilized as well as electroencephalographic tracings to help define sleep staging. The majority of the studies are done in sleep laboratories and care must be taken to provide surroundings that are conducive to normal sleep staging. Figure 10.3

is an example of a polysomnogram taken in the child with suspected sleep apnea. This example illustrates obstructive apnea as evidenced by the flattening of the nasal oral flow thermistor pattern and increased thoracic and abdominal movement. Desaturation is noted to follow after the obstructed event. More recently, these studies have been carried out in the home, utilizing fewer and less complex monitors with successful documentation of airway obstruction and O_2 desaturation without altering the individual's normal sleep routine (Southall et al., 1987).

Treatment modalities for obstructive sleep apnea include:

1. Management of acute airway obstruction
    a. Oxygen
    b. Pulmonary toilet
    c. Antibiotics
    d. Steroids
    e. Diuretics
2. Surgery
    a. Uvulopalatopharyngoplasty

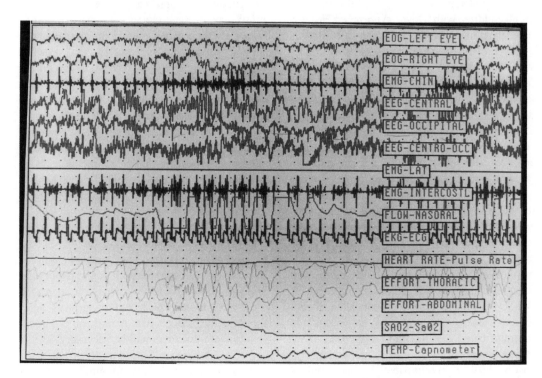

Figure 10.3. Copy of a polysomnogram tracing in a 1-year-old child with Down syndrome. Repeated obstructed episodes occur with cessation of airflow and increased thoracoabdominal breathing. Desaturation ensues within seconds of obstructed events.

b. Tonsillectomy and adenoidectomy
c. Tracheostomy (rare)
3. Continuous   positive   airway   pressure/
    chronic oxygen therapy

Of note, oxygen should be used cautiously if an airway has not been established: Improving the oxygenation without alleviating the obstruction may cause loss of the hypoxic arousal response and subsequent worsening obtundation secondary to hypercarbia. As a rule, children with Down syndrome do not benefit from a tonsillectomy and adenoidectomy as well as do "normal" children, probably related to the complicating airway size and hypotonia. Donaldson and Redmond (1988) reported complete relief of obstruction in 5 out of 6 patients undergoing uvulopalatopharyngoplasty. The remaining patient's course was apparently complicated by central apnea. One half of these patients also underwent tongue reduction surgery with an increase in postoperative morbidity recognized and no definitive role in maintaining airway patency observed. Strome (1981) also suggested using uvulopalatopharyngoplasty and reported 12 successful operations in 14 children with Down syndrome. He also noted the minor role of adenoidal hypertrophy as a source of obstruction. Tracheostomy to alleviate obstruction is rarely used as an initial procedure. When such treatment is necessary, the tracheostomy tube may often remain capped during the day, allowing for normal activities.

The postoperative course is frequently more complicated for children with Down syndrome and adequate airway monitoring in an intensive care unit setting is recommended. Careful attention to secretions and pulmonary toilet is essential because of the risk for frequent infections and poor cough secondary to pain. Often, ventilatory support, and therefore endotracheal intubation, is required. Care should be taken to monitor leak pressures surrounding the airway because of the reported smaller laryngeal size. Whenever possible, duration of intubation should be restricted to a minimum. When surgery is contraindicated or if the acute trigger of airway obstruction is felt to be self-limited, continuous positive airway pressure may be beneficial in maintaining airway patency.

CONCLUSION

The lungs of persons with Down syndrome appear to have a unique microarchitecture, gross anatomic structure, and an abnormal functional response to pulmonary artery hypertension and perhaps infection. Because of structural abnormalities of the upper airway as well as hypotonia, persons with Down syndrome are also susceptible to problems with airway patency and subsequent obstructive sleep apnea. The probable immunologic defects in persons with Down syndrome may contribute to the increased risk of pneumonia and perhaps other infectious complications and may also predispose them to the increased frequency of postoperative complications. Overall, persons with Down syndrome require meticulous attention to pulmonary care, when complications such as atelectasis arise, and careful observation of even subtle changes of the cardiopulmonary system. Cyanosis may signify changes in the pulmonary artery pressures. This in turn may lead to further identification of complicating medical factors such as obstructive sleep apnea and/or gastroesophageal reflux, as well as changes in cardiac status. When children with Down syndrome appear to have regression in their development, or when additional developmental delays are recognized after allowing for effects of trisomy 21, then evaluation of complicating medical factors such as obstructive sleep apnea should be elicited.

For the most part, the diagnosis and treatment of signs and symptoms in children with Down syndrome should be similar to procedures done in "normal" children. One should not assume that a problem exists without a prompt and full diagnostic evaluation, as would be completed in the general population. Reduced airway pressure during and following surgical procedures should be used with all forms of mechanical ventilation in view of the apparent pulmonary hypoplasia and possibly fragile alveoli. With the increased incidence of atelectasis and congestive heart failure in the postoperative period, careful attention to these disorders will be necessary.

Further studies are needed to define better the anatomic, functional, and immunologic abnormalities in persons with Down syndrome. More complete information of such differences will lead to improved treatment for the pulmonary concerns and complications, as well as provide

more insight into the proper timing of surgery for congenital heart disease.

REFERENCES

Aggarwal, K.C., Rastogi, A., & Singhi, S. (1981). Cor pulmonale due to laryngomalacia in Down's syndrome. *Indian Pediatrics, 18,* 914–916.

Cant, A.J., Gibson, P.J., & West, R.J. (1987). Bacterial tracheitis in Down's syndrome. *Archives of Disease in Childhood, 62,* 962–963.

Chi, T.L., & Krovetz, L.J. (1975). The pulmonary vascular bed in children with Down syndrome. *Journal of Pediatrics, 86,* 533–538.

Clark, R.W., Schmidt, H.S., & Schuller, D.E. (1980). Sleep-induced ventilatory dysfunction in Down's syndrome. *Archives of Internal Medicine, 140,* 45–50.

Cooney, T.P., & Thurlbeck, W.M. (1982). Pulmonary hypoplasia in Down's syndrome. *New England Journal of Medicine, 307,* 1170–1173.

Cooney, T.P., Wentworth, P.J., & Thurlbeck, W.M. (1988). Diminished radial count is found only postnatally in Down's syndrome. *Pediatric Pulmonology, 5,* 204–209.

Donaldson, J.D., & Redmond, W.M. (1988). Surgical management of obstructive sleep apnea in children with Down syndrome. *Journal of Otolaryngology, 17* (5), 398–403.

Foote, K.D., & Vickers, D.W. (1986). Congenital pleural effusion in Down's syndrome. *British Journal of Radiology, 59,* 609–610.

Graham, J., Wertelecki, W., O'Connor, J., & Cohen, M. (1981). Choanal atresia with Down syndrome. *Journal of Pediatrics, 98,* 664.

Hall, C.B., McBride, J.T., Gala, C.L., Hildreth, S.W., & Schnabel, K.C. (1985). Ribavarin treatment of respiratory syncytial viral infection in infants with underlying cardiopulmonary disease. *Journal of the American Medical Association, 254,* 3047–3051.

Heath, D.S., & Edwards, J.E. (1988). Pathology of hypertensive pulmonary vascular disease. *Circulation, 18,* 533.

Hillemeier, C., Buchin, P.J., & Gryboski, J. (1982). Esophageal dysfunction in Down's syndrome. *Journal of Pediatric Gastroenterology and Nutrition, 1,* 101–104.

Hordof, A.J., Mellins, R.B., Gersony, W.M., & Sterg, C.N. (1977). Reversibility of chronic obstructive lung disease in infants following repair of ventricular septal defect. *Journal of Pediatrics, 90*(2), 187–191.

Hutchins, G.M., & Ostrow, P.T. (1976). The pathogenesis of the two forms of hypertensive pulmonary vascular disease. *American Heart Journal, 92,* 797.

Joshi, V.V., Kasznica, J., Ali Khan, M.A., Amato, J.J., & Levine, O.R. (1986). Cystic lung disease in Down syndrome. *Pediatric Pathology, 5,* 79–86.

Levine, O.R., & Simpser, M. (1982). Alveolar hypoventilation and cor pulmonale associated with chronic airway obstruction in infants with Down syndrome. *Clinical Pediatrics, 21,* 25–29.

Loughlin, G.M., Wynne, J.W., & Victorica, B.E. (1981). Sleep apnea as a possible cause of pulmonary hypertension in Down syndrome. *Journal of Pediatrics, 98* (3), 435–437.

Marcus, C.L., Keens, T.G., Bautista, D.B., Von Pechmann, W.S., & Davidson Ward, S.L. (1991). Obstructive sleep apnea in children with Down syndrome. *Pediatrics, 88*(1), 132–140.

Milunsky, A. (1968). Cystic fibrosis and Down's syndrome. *Pediatrics, 42,* 501–504.

Noonan, J.A., & Walters, L.R. (1974). Hemodynamic studies in Down's syndrome patients with congenital heart disease. *Pediatric Research, 8,* 353.

Pueschel, S.M. (1984). *A study of the young child with Down syndrome.* New York: Human Science Press.

Rasore-Quatino, A., Acutis, M.S., & Strigini, P. (1990). Incidence of bronchial asthma in Down syndrome. *Journal of Pediatrics, 5,* 487.

Rowland, T.W., Nordstrom, L.G., Bean, M.S., & Burkhardt, H. (1981). Chronic upper airway obstruction and pulmonary hypertension in Down's syndrome. *American Journal of Diseases of Children, 135,* 1050–1052.

Somerville, J. (1971). Atrioventricular defects. *Modern Concepts in Cardiovascular Disease, 40,* 33–38.

Soudon, P., Stijns, M., Tremouroux-Wattiez, M., & Vliers, A. (1975). Precocity of pulmonary vascular obstruction in Down syndrome. *European Journal of Cardiology, 2,* 473.

Southall, D.P., Stebbens, V.A., Mirza, R., Lang, M.H., Croft, C.B., & Shinebourne, E.A. (1987). Upper airway obstruction with hypoxemia and sleep disruption in Down syndrome. *Developmental Medicine and Child Neurology, 29,* 734–742.

Stebbens, V.A., Dennis, J., Croft, C.B., & Southall, D.P. (1989). Incidence of sleep related upper airway obstruction in Down syndrome. *Pediatric Pulmonology, 7,* 281.

Stocker, J.T., McGill, L.C., & Orsini, E.N. (1985). Post-infarction peripheral cysts of the lung in pediatric patients. *Pediatric Pulmonology, 1,* 7–18.

Strome, M. (1981). Down's syndrome: A modern

otorhinolaryngological   perspective.   *Laryngo-scope, 91,* 1581–1594.

Symon, D.N., Stewart, L., & Russell, G. (1985). Abnormally high sweat osmolality in children with Down syndrome. *Journal of Mental Deficiency Research, 29,* 257–261.

Tandon, R., Moller, J.H., Plett, J.A., & Edwards, J.E. (1974). Hypertensive pulmonary vascular disease. *Archives of Pathology, 97,* 187–188.

Wilson, S.K., Hutchins, G.M., & Neill, C.A. (1979). Hypertensive pulmonary vascular disease in Down syndrome. *Journal of Pediatrics, 95*(5), 722–726.

Wohl, M.E. (1985). Bronchiolitis. *Pediatric Annals, 15,* 307–313.

Yamaki, S., Horiuchi, T., & Sekino, Y. (1983). Quantitative analysis of pulmonary vascular disease in simple cardiac anomalies with the Down syndrome. *American Journal of Cardiology, 51,* 1502–1506.

Yamaki, S., Horiuchi, T., & Takahashi, T. (1985). Pulmonary changes in a congenital heart disease with Down's syndrome: Their significance as a cause of post operative respiratory failure. *Thorax, 40,* 380–386.

Yoss, B.S., & Lipsitz, P.J. (1977). Chylothorax in two mongoloid infants. *Clinical Genetics, 12,* 357–360.

CHAPTER
11

Gastrointestinal Concerns

Joseph Levy

Anomalies of the gastrointestinal tract are a common occurrence in persons with Down syndrome. Interestingly, there is no lesion specifically linked to trisomy 21. Effective surgical treatment of the various conditions is available, and results are not too different from those expected in a "normal" child. The associated cardiac defects will often have a more serious impact on the outcome—but even in this respect, cardiovascular surgery has made great strides and the results are very gratifying (see Marino, chap. 9, this volume). Appropriate surgical management of the intestinal lesions in children with Down syndrome greatly improves their quality of life. Recognition of the eventual positive outcome should lead to effective interventions in rehabilitation of gastrointestinal function.

CONGENITAL ANOMALIES

The most common gastrointestinal anomalies are presented in Table 11.1. Esophageal atresia with tracheoesophageal fistula, duodenal atresia or stenosis, and Hirschsprung disease are the most prevalent in reported series. Additional lesions included: annular pancreas, pyloric stenosis, and imperforate anus. The association with cardiac disease—most commonly, endocardial cushion defects—was also high in a retrospective study of children with Down syndrome treated at Babies Hospital, Columbia Presbyterian Medical Center, New York, during the years 1971–1982: More than 70% of infants diagnosed with various gastrointestinal defects had congenital heart disease (Buchin, Levy, & Schullinger, 1986).

ETIOLOGIC CONSIDERATIONS

Interesting insights are emerging in the understanding of the lesions found in the gastrointestinal tract. Embryologic considerations place the defect in a failure to recanalize the lumen of the esophagus or the duodenum during the 4th–6th weeks of gestation. Interference in the normal separation between the trachea and the esophagus is thought to be responsible for the close association of defects, as the respiratory tract develops as an outgrowth of the ventral aspect of the foregut. Normally, a phase of epithelial proliferation causes closure of the lumen. In a process involving recanalization and vacuolar degeneration, a patent lumen is reestablished. Failure to recanalize will result in atresia of the affected structure. This mechanism was postulated by Boyden, Cope, and Bill (1967) after careful reconstruction of duodenal specimens obtained at various stages of development, and it provides an explanation of the preferential location of the stenosis or atresia at the level of the ampulla of Vater. At this level, the complete occlusion takes place and remnants of the epithelium that fail to vacuolate will grow into muscle or connective tissue. An abnormality in cell-to-cell adhesiveness has been found in cultured trisomy 21 fibroblasts (Wright, Orkin, Destrempes, & Kurnit, 1984). This enhanced adhesiveness is not found in skin fibroblasts but is present in lung fibroblasts. The hypothesis that trisomy 21 results in a specific membrane change, which in turn explains the morphogenetic consequences, is indeed very attractive and offers an opportunity to pinpoint a more unique molecular marker of Down syndrome. Furthermore, the associa-

Table 11.1.   Reported gastrointestinal anomalies in persons with Down syndrome

Anomaly	Carter (1958) N = 136	Rowe and Uchida (1961) N = 184	Fabia and Drolette (1970) N = 2,421	Knox and Ten Bensel (1972) N = 110
Tracheoesophageal fistula or esophageal atresia	1	3	7	1
Hiatal hernia	1	1	0	0
Pyloric stenosis	1	0	4	3
Duodenal stenosis or atresia	1	1	63	2
Annular pancreas	0	0	2	1
Hypoplasia of small intestine	0	0	2	1
Meckel's diverticulum	0	0	0	1
Bile duct atresia	0	0	5	0
Imperforate anus	2	4	17	3
Hirschsprung disease	2	0	9	2
Malrotation	0	0	5	0

tion with anorectal malformations has begun to be understood in light of discoveries of the cellular and molecular events determining neural crest development and the ganglion population of the myenteric plexus (Rothman, Tennyson, & Gershon, 1986).

CLINICAL PRESENTATIONS

Esophageal Atresia and Tracheoesophageal Fistula

According to a survey of over 1,000 cases conducted by the surgical section of the American Academy of Pediatrics, certain types of esophageal atresia and tracheoesophageal fistula were identified (see Figure 11.1) (Holder, Cloud, Lewis, & Pilling, 1964, cited in Franken, 1975). As can be gathered from the diagrams in Figure 11.1, many of the clinical features will be determined by the level of obstruction and by the degree of communication between the airway and the stomach. The infant with esophageal atresia might present initially with respiratory distress resulting from accumulated oropharyngeal secretions. Drooling is prominent and feedings will precipitate acute decompensation from respiratory compromise. In such circumstances, the index of suspicion for an underlying esophageal abnormality should be high. Prenatal diagnosis of esophageal atresia is now possible (Barss, Benacerraf, & Frigoletto, 1985). In addition, early intervention will help prevent

more serious respiratory compromise and restore structural continuity without unnecessary delays. Passage of a firm nasogastric tube will encounter resistance and immediate measures should be taken to prevent further respiratory problems. X-ray evaluation will reveal the level of atresia and the most likely location of the fistula, if one is present. A pediatric surgeon should be involved from the early stages of management, as the child will need emergency surgery. A transthoracic or extrapleural approach is the norm and will be determined by the type of fistula and the degree of separation of the blind ends. If the separation between the atretic segments allows it, a primary anastomosis is carried out. In more severe cases, approximation cannot be done without seriously compromising the anastomosis, so a staged operation is planned. Placement of a gastrostomy provides a route of decompression for the air that gets to the stomach from the commonly associated tracheal fistula, and it is also a means for nutritional support. Retrograde (via the gastrostomy) and antegrade dilatations are performed until the two stumps are in sufficient apposition to allow a primary repair.

The most common problems associated with tracheoesophageal fistulas and esophageal atresia are anastomotic leak, chronic lung disease, tracheomalacia (weakness of the tracheal wall), esophageal dysmotility, esophageal stricture, and gastroesophageal reflux. Barky cough and stridor (high-pitched, noisy respiration) are com-

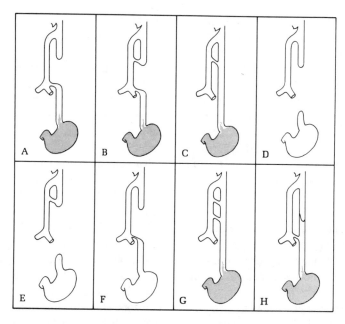

Figure 11.1.   Types of esophageal atresia and tracheoesophageal fistula: a) esophageal atresia with distal tracheoesophageal fistula; b) esophageal atresia with proximal and distal tracheoesophageal fistula; c) tracheoesophageal fistula without esophageal atresia; d) esophageal atresia without tracheoesophageal fistula; e) esophageal atresia with proximal tracheoesophageal fistula; f) esophageal atresia with tiny distal tracheoesophageal fistula; g) multiple tracheoesophageal fistulas without esophageal atresia; h) membranous esophageal atresia with distal tracheoesophageal fistula. (From Holder, T.M., Cloud, D.T., Lewis, J.E., Jr., & Pilling, G.P. [1964]. Esophageal atresia and tracheoesophageal fistula: A survey of its members by the surgical section of the American Academy of Pediatrics. *Pediatrics, 34,* 542–549.)

mon in children, often for years. These symptoms are exacerbated by intercurrent respiratory infections (see Howenstine, chap. 10, this volume), which are more common in children with Down syndrome (Biller, Allen, Schuster, Treves, & Winter, 1987). Tracheomalacia can be demonstrated fluoroscopically. Anastomotic leak is a dreaded complication that can result in significant morbidity and mortality, with mediastinitis, empyema, and chronic drainage. Ischemia from excessive tension and the repair technique contribute to this complication.

Gastroesophageal Reflux

Gastroesophageal reflux frequently accompanies tracheoesophageal fistulas and esophageal atresia (Holder, Ashcraft, Sharp, & Amoury, 1987). Distortion of the lower esophageal sphincter area by tension, laxity of the diaphragmatic crura, loss of the intra-abdominal esophagus, and effacement of the angle of His (the angle formed by the gastric fundus and the esophagus) all contribute to the reflux (Boix-Ochoa, 1981). The presence of acid reflux is thought to be re-

sponsible, at least in part, for the frequently observed stricture of the anastomosis. An antireflux operation is often indicated to prevent progressive peptic damage (Fonkalsrud, Berquist, Vargas, Ament, & Foglia, 1987). Medical management of gastroesophageal reflux can be very effective in minimizing the damage. The mainstays of treatment include: decreased volume of feedings; neutralization of stomach acid with various antacids or with H_2 blockers (cimetidine, ranitidine); and a prokinetic agent such as metoclopramide (Reglan), domperidone, or cisapride (still experimental in the United States) (McCallum, 1985).

Strictures, even in the absence of documented reflux, are very common, and as many as 50% of patients will need dilatations. Balloon dilatation of the strictures can be safely done with endoscopic equipment presently available (Hoffer, Winter, Fellows, & Folkman, 1987), and results are very satisfactory. The clinical presentation of esophageal stricture is usually the inability to advance the diet with solid foods; choking and dysphagia with solids; and, when more severe, accumulation of secretions and failure to thrive from insufficient intake. Feeding difficulties are the norm, and a great deal of patience is needed to overcome the negative aversions developed in the process of resuming swallowing in the presence of esophageal dysmotility and dysphagia due to physical narrowing in the area of the anastomosis (Nakazato, Landing, & Wells, 1986). Recurrent aspiration pneumonia and hyperreactive airway disease often complicate the picture and add to the management challenges.

Duodenal Atresia and Stenosis

The primary symptom of intestinal obstruction is vomiting. Depending on the level of obstruction, abdominal distention may or may not be present. If the level of involvement is preampullary, the vomiting will be nonbilious; however, most often the atresia is just below the ampulla of Vater and the typical bile-colored secretions will be brought up. Multiple atresias are rare in children with Down syndrome, with anal atresia being more common.

The diagnosis of duodenal atresia will be quite straightforward, as the radiologic examination will confirm the presence of a "double bubble." Air fluid levels may be present, and strong peristaltic gastric waves can sometimes be seen. The treatment is surgical. Because of the chronic obstruction, the prestenotic duodenum might remain distended after surgery and abnormal motility can be discerned radiologically. The clinical implications are sometimes considerable, as advancement of feedings might be difficult and duodenogastric bilious reflux might result in alkali gastritis. These complications tend to abate with time, and reoperation is seldom necessary.

Hirschsprung Disease

Hirschsprung disease, also termed aganglionosis or megacolon, is characterized by a lack of ganglion cells in the myenteric and submucosal plexus of the intestine. It affects the large intestine primarily, although cases of total intestinal involvement have been described. Histologically, the nerve fibers in the myenteric plexus stain intensely for acetylcholinesterase. The absence of ganglion cells results in a state of constant contraction and failure of relaxation of the

segment involved, and this in turn may cause intestinal obstruction. According to Ehrenpreis (1970), Down syndrome is the second most common association of Hirschsprung disease (5%–9%). Urogenital defects are frequently observed in persons with Hirschsprung disease, although at times this is a direct consequence of colonic dilatation and stool impaction and is thus reversible.

The classic presentation in the newborn period is that of an infant who fails to pass meconium in the first 24 hours of life; has abdominal distention; and, if untreated, will usually develop vomiting and all the signs of low intestinal obstruction. In other cases, the presentation includes bloody diarrhea and sepsis (enterocolitis) or the meconium plug syndrome. Diagnosis is made by radiologic demonstration of a "transition zone" (an area that fails to expand with the flow of barium) in the rectosigmoid area and by intestinal biopsies obtained rectally with a suction biopsy or forceps. A venting colostomy is the indicated initial management with a pull-through operation in its various forms planned after the first birthday. Results of the pull-through operations are generally very favorable, although a period of adaptation is the rule, and stooling difficulties are very common for years following correction.

A recent review of 13 children with Down syndrome by a group at Ohio State University College of Medicine and Children's Hospital in Columbus, Ohio (Caniano, Teitelbaum, & Qualman, 1990) who received various pull-through operations documented satisfactory continence in all but 1 child (only 54% of patients came to definitive surgery). Associated congenital anomalies were encountered in 77% of the children (cardiac, duodenal stenosis, and the VATER complex [vertebral defects, anal atresia, tracheoesophageal fistula with esophageal atresia, and radial and renal anomalies]) (Caniano et al., 1990). However, complications were more common and more serious in this group of children. Of particular note was the high incidence of enterocolitis. This is a fulminant complication with a high mortality rate and it can occur at any time before or even after corrective surgery. Management of enterocolitis consists of vigorous colonic irrigations, rectal decompression, intravenous antibiotics, and total parenteral nutrition when indicated. Fecal impaction and "overflow" diarrhea resulting in incontinence can be difficult to manage and will require patience and consistent intervention in the form of irrigations, rectal dilatations, and dietary manipulations. Eventually, the child will develop the sensation of fullness, will sense the need to move the bowels, and will be able to discriminate between flatus and stool. In the Ohio series, most children required regular enemas before bedtime in order to control nocturnal soiling (Caniano et al., 1990). In some individuals, the presence of neuronal intestinal dysplasia (Achem, Owyang, Schuffler, & Dobbins, 1987) has helped explain the frustrating results after pull-through surgery. In these individuals, even though ganglion cells are found in the area of the anastomosis, the bowel continues to behave erratically in its propulsion, resulting in "pseudo-obstructive" symptoms.

Malabsorption Syndrome and Nutritional Issues

The association of Down syndrome and celiac disease has been a matter of some interest in recent years (Simila & Kokkonen, 1990). Celiac disease is characterized by a lifelong intolerance to wheat and rye gluten. Exposure to gluten results in subtotal villus atrophy, with increased intraepithelial lymphocytes and crypt hyperplasia. Onset of symptoms can be insidious, and will result in failure to thrive, abdominal distention, steatorrhea (fat malabsorption), and irritability. The personality changes can be striking, with the child becoming miserable and listless. Conversely, the response to a gluten-free diet can result in dramatic improvement in behavior, even before full gastrointestinal recovery. An increased familial and ethnic incidence of celiac disease has long been recognized (Kelly, Phillips, Elliott, Dias, & Walker-Smith, 1989), and can be as high a 1 in 300 births in certain areas of Ireland. Increased representation of HLA phenotypes B8 and DR3 has been reported, but the pattern of inheritance is seemingly multifactorial, as instances of identical twins being spared have been recorded (Kosnai, Karpati,

Torok, Bucsky, & Gyodi, 1985). The mechanism of damage to the intestinal villi remains to be elucidated. Proposed theories have ranged from an enzymatic defect (Cornell & Rolles, 1978) to an immunologically mediated process (Weiser & Douglas, 1976).

The diagnosis of celiac disease cannot be made without a jejunal biopsy. Documentation of recovery after institution of a strict gluten-free diet and damage induced by re-exposure are the official recommendations of the European Society for Pediatric Gastroenterology published in 1970 (Neeuwisse, 1970). More recently, high sensitivity and specificity have been claimed for serologic tests measuring IgA antibodies against the endomysium of cultured monkey intestinal cell lines, as well as circulating antigliadin antibodies (Kapuscinska et al., 1987). Gliadin is the alcohol-soluble fraction of gluten thought to play the major role in villus damage. Although the serologic screening might be useful in following response to treatment, diagnosis still depends on obtaining morphologic evidence of villus atrophy. Children with Down syndrome are to some degree immunologically compromised (Levin, 1987), but whether the association with celiac disease is coincidental or not remains an open question.

Reports of suspected protein and fat-soluble vitamin malabsorption have appeared sporadically in the literature (Abalan et al., 1990). Recently, a study of vitamin A status and vitamin A absorption in children with Down syndrome and controls failed to document significant differences (Pueschel et al., 1990). In the absence of an underlying gastrointestinal problem, which precludes normal food intake (e.g., tracheo-esophageal fistula or gastroesophageal reflux) or has resulted in compromised bowel length (multiple atresias) or bacterial overgrowth (blind loop syndrome), children with Down syndrome will gain weight appropriately and will not manifest signs or symptoms of malabsorption. It should be kept in mind that the expected growth curves for children with Down syndrome are markedly different from those drawn for children without chromosome disorders; growth monitoring must be done with the appropriate references (Cronk et al., 1988).

CONCLUSION

Congenital gastrointestinal anomalies are an important aspect of the dysmorphology seen in persons with Down syndrome. The impact on the quality of life has been minimized by dependable surgical techniques and attention to postoperative complications. The conflicts and ethical discussions generated in the past about the advisability of performing surgery on the infant with Down syndrome can now be viewed more realistically in the perspective provided by the effective surgical and pediatric involvement seen since the early 1970s. Great progress has been made by surgeons, pediatricians, physical therapists, oral and feeding specialists, and all the other members of the team caring for children with Down syndrome and their special needs.

The prognosis of the child with Down syndrome with a gastrointestinal anomaly such as tracheoesophageal fistula or intestinal atresia seems in many ways comparable to that of a similarly affected child who does not have Down syndrome. Great strides have also been made in the areas of rehabilitation and ultimate function, giving a much brighter overall outlook. This information should have an impact on the way pediatricians feel and act when confronted with gastrointestinal problems. In short, children with Down syndrome who have gastrointestinal anomalies should be treated no differently than "normal" children.

REFERENCES

Abalan, F., Jouan, A., Weerts, M.T., Solles, C., Brus, J., & Sauneron, M.F. (1990). A study of digestive absorption in four cases of Down syndrome. Down syndrome, malnutrition, malabsorption, and Alzheimer's disease. *Medical Hypotheses, 31,* 35–38.

Achem, S.R., Owyang, C., Schuffler, M.D., & Dobbins, W.O., III. (1987). Neuronal dysplasia and chronic intestinal pseudoobstruction: Rectal biopsy as a possible aid to diagnosis. *Gastroenterology, 92,* 805–809.

Barss, V.A., Benacerraf, B.R., & Frigoletto, F.D. (1985). Antenatal sonographic diagnosis of fetal GI malformations. *Pediatrics, 76,* 445.

Biller, J.A., Allen, J.L., Schuster, S.R., Treves, S.T., & Winter, H.S. (1987). Long-term evaluation of esophageal and pulmonary function in patients with repaired esophageal atresia and tracheoesophageal fistula. *Digestive Diseases and Sciences, 32,* 985–990.

Boix-Ochoa, J. (1981). Diagnosis and management of gastroesophageal reflux in children. *Surgery Annals, 13,* 123.

Boyden, E., Cope, J., & Bill, A. (1967). Anatomy and embryology of congenital obstruction of the duodenum. *American Journal of Surgery, 114,* 190–202.

Buchin, P., Levy, J., & Schullinger, J. (1986). Down syndrome and the gastrointestinal tract. *Journal of Clinical Gastroenterology, 8,* 111–114.

Caniano, D.A., Teitelbaum, D.H., & Qualman, S.J. (1990). Management of Hirschsprung's disease in children with trisomy 21. *American Journal of Surgery, 159,* 402–404.

Carter, C. (1958). A life table for mongols with the cause of death. *Journal of Mental Deficiency Research, 2,* 64–74.

Cornell, H.J., & Rolles, C.J. (1978). Further evidence of a primary mucosal defect in celiac disease: In vitro mucosal digestion studies in celiac patients in remission, their relatives, and control subjects. *Gut, 19,* 253–259.

Cronk, C., Crocker, A.C., Pueschel, S.M., Shea, A.M., Zackai, E., Pickens, G., & Reed, R.B. (1988). Growth charts for children with Down syndrome: 1 month to 18 years of age. *Pediatrics, 81,* 102–110.

Ehrenpreis, T.H. (1970). *Hirschsprung's disease.* Chicago: Year Book Medical Publishers.

Fabia, J., & Drolette, M. (1970). Malformations and leukemia in children with Down's syndrome. *Pediatrics, 45,* 60–70.

Fonkalsrud, E.W., Berquist, W., Vargas, J., Ament, M.E., & Foglia, R.P. (1987). Surgical treatment of the gastroesophageal reflux syndrome in infants and children. *American Journal of Surgery, 154,* 11–18.

Franken, E.A., Jr. (1975). *Gastrointestinal radiology in pediatrics.* Hagerstown, MD: Harper & Row, Medical Department.

Gross, R.E. (1953). *Surgery of infancy and childhood.* Philadelphia: W.B. Saunders.

Hoffer, F.A., Winter, H.S., Fellows, K.E., & Folkman, J. (1987). The treatment of postoperative and peptic esophageal strictures after esophageal atresia repair. A program including dilatation with balloon catheters. *Pediatric Radiology, 17,* 454–458.

Holder, T.M., Ashcraft, K.W., Sharp, R.J., & Amoury, R.A. (1987). Care of infants with esophageal atresia, tracheoesophageal fistula, and associated anomalies. *Journal of Thoracic and Cardiovascular Surgery, 94,* 828–835.

Holder, T.M., Cloud, D.T., Lewis, J.E., Jr., & Pilling, G.P. (1964). Esophageal atresia and tracheoesophageal fistula: A survey of its members by the surgical section of the American Academy of Pediatrics. *Pediatrics, 34,* 542–549.

Kapuscinska, A., Zalewski, T., Chorzelski, T.P., Sulej, J., Beutner, E.H., Kumar, V., & Rossi, T. (1987). Disease specificity and dynamics of changes in IgA class anti-endomysial antibodies in celiac disease. *Journal of Pediatric Gastroenterology and Nutrition, 6,* 535–537.

Kelly, D.A., Phillips, A.D., Elliott, E.J., Dias, J.A., & Walker-Smith, J.A. (1989). Rise and fall of coeliac disease 1960–85. *Archives of Disease in Childhood, 64,* 1157–1160.

Knox, G., & Ten Bensel, R. (1972). Gastrointestinal malformations in Down's syndrome. *Minnesota Medicine, 55,* 542–544.

Kosnai, I., Karpati, S., Torok, E., Bucsky, P., & Gyodi, E. (1985). Dermatitis herpetiformis in monozygous twins: Discordance for dermatitis herpetiformis and concordance for gluten-sensitive enteropathy. *European Journal of Pediatrics, 144,* 404–405.

Levin, S. (1987). The immune system and susceptibility to infections in Down syndrome. In E.E. McCoy & C.J. Epstein (Eds.), *Oncology and immunology in Down syndrome* (pp. 143–162). New York: Alan R. Liss.

McCallum, R.W. (1985). Review of the current status of prokinetic agents in gastroenterology. *American Journal of Gastroenterology, 80,* 1008–1016.

Nakazato, Y., Landing, B.H., & Wells, T.R. (1986). Abnormal Auerbach plexus in the esophagus and stomach of patients with esophageal atresia and tracheoesophageal fistula. *Journal of Pediatric Surgery, 21,* 831–837.

Neeuwisse, G.W. (1970). Diagnostic criteria in coeliac disease. *Acta Paediatrica Scandinavica, 59,* 461–463.

Pueschel, S.M., Hillemeier, C., Caldwell, M., Senft, K., Mevs, C., & Pezzullo, J.C. (1990). Vitamin A gastrointestinal absorption in persons with Down syndrome. *Journal of Mental Deficiency Research, 34,* 146–149.

Rothman, T.P., Tennyson, V.M., & Gershon, M.D. (1986). Colonization of the bowel by the precursors of enteric glia: Studies of normal and congenitally aganglionic mutant mice. *Journal of Comprehensive Neurology, 252,* 493–506.

Rowe, R., & Uchida, I. (1961). Cardiac malformation in mongolism. *American Journal of Medicine, 31,* 726–735.

Simila, S., & Kokkonen, J. (1990). Coexistence of celiac disease and Down syndrome. *American Journal of Mental Retardation, 95,* 120–122.

Weiser, M.M., & Douglas, A.P. (1976). An alternative mechanism for gluten toxicity in celiac disease. *Lancet, i,* 567–569.

Wright, T., Orkin, R., Destrempes, M., & Kurnit, D. (1984). Increased adhesiveness of Down syndrome fetal fibroblasts in vitro. *Proceedings of the National Academy of Sciences of the United States of America, 81,* 2426–2430.

CHAPTER 12

Disorders of the Liver

Patricia S. Scola

The major area of investigation regarding liver function in individuals with Down syndrome has been related to hepatitis. Hepatitis, an inflammation of the liver, may result from numerous causes and may be acute or chronic in nature. Of particular interest in persons with Down syndrome is infectious hepatitis of viral etiology, especially that due to hepatitis A virus (HAV) and hepatitis B virus (HBV). Persons with Down syndrome seem to contract HAV at a similar rate as the general population. In contrast, when compared to individuals with other types of retardation, institutionalization of persons with Down syndrome is known to increase the risk of acquiring hepatitis due to HBV. Prevalence of infection with HBV in persons with Down syndrome who have remained in the community is much lower than those living in institutions.

HEPATITIS A

A member of the picornavirus group, HAV is an RNA virus. Transmission is person-to-person by the fecal–oral route. Infection with HAV is common in underdeveloped countries, whereas epidemics in the United States are most likely in households and day-care centers. Jaundice, nausea, anorexia, and fatigue are symptoms that may be associated with acute febrile illness. Asymptomatic infections frequently occur in infants and young children (Committee on Infectious Diseases American Academy of Pediatrics, 1991).

Institutions for persons with mental retardation may be hyperendemic for HAV, as demonstrated by Szmuness, Purcell, Dienstag, and Stevens (1977). In that study, 75.1% of residents exhib-ited antibody to hepatitis A (anti-HAV) antigen. The rate of positivity for anti-HAV was related to length of stay, with residents institutionalized for more than 3 years being significantly more often positive for anti-HAV. Residents with Down syndrome had a rate of anti-HAV that was very similar to the 76.5% positivity rate found in residents with other types of mental retardation. The prevalence of anti-HAV also did not differ between males and females or by age.

Poor hygienic standards are considered contributory to the high prevalence of hepatitis infections in institutions. Renner, Andrle, Horak, and Rett (1985) studied an outpatient population and observed that anti-HAV was not more common in outpatients with mental retardation. Persons with Down syndrome had an anti-HAV rate of 5.6%, persons with mental retardation of other etiologies 9.4%, and "normal" controls 16.7%. The higher rate in controls was attributed to a higher mean age.

HEPATITIS B

Hepatitis B virus is a hepadnavirus that is DNA containing. Antigens include hepatitis B surface antigen (HBsAg), hepatitis B core antigen (HBcAg), and hepatitis B e antigen (HBeAg). The presence of HBsAg is consistent with a current infection with serum antibodies to the hepatitis B antigens providing further diagnostic information. The result of infection ranges from asymptomatic seroconversion; to an illness associated with jaundice, nausea, and anorexia; to an occasionally fatal form of hepatitis. The presence of HBsAg for more than 6 months is indicative of chronic carrier status. A chronic carrier can transmit infection to others and also is at greater risk for developing cirrhosis and hepatocellular carcinoma (Committee on Infectious Diseases American Academy of Pediatrics, 1991).

Transmission by chronic carriers in institutions for persons with mental retardation appears to occur from skin or mucous membrane exposure to blood or other infected body fluids. Residents who are aggressive with biting or scratching behaviors present the greatest risk to other residents and staff.

The combination of large institutional size, host susceptibility of residents with Down syndrome, and the prevalence of hepatitis suggested an infectious etiology to Sutnick, London, Gerstley, Cronlund, and Blumberg (1968). The 1970s provided numerous studies regarding the epidemiology of HBV and Down syndrome and the original term "Australian antigen" was replaced by the current nomenclature of HBsAg. The prevalence of HBsAg in institutionalized residents with Down syndrome was found to range from 23% to 36% although individuals with other forms of retardation in the same institutions had rates from 5% to 17% (Boughton, Hawkes, Schroeter, & Harlor, 1976; Hollinger et al., 1972; Szmuness et al., 1977). These investigators also found that the residents with Down syndrome had antibody to hepatitis B surface antigen (anti-HBs) ranging from 18% to 62% as compared to 45%–52% in residents with other forms of mental retardation.

As more sensitive tests for HBV infection were developed, more information became available about the chronic carrier status of HBV. Hawkes, Boughton, Schroeter, Decker, and Overby (1980) found that all 26 carriers of HBsAg were positive for core antibody with 73% positive for HBeAg, which was recognized as having a high correlation with infectivity. They also determined that of residents who were initially seronegative, 33% of those with Down syndrome became chronic carriers of HBsAg as compared to 10% carrier status in those without Down syndrome who had seroconversion. Those residents with Down syndrome who did develop anti-HBs had significantly lower anti-HBs, but significantly higher antibody to HBcAg (anti-HBc) and antibody to HBeAg (anti-HBe).

With awareness that the carriers of HBsAg who were also HBeAg positive are more infectious than those with anti-HBe, it was possible to define further the carrier rates in institutions for persons with mental retardation. Clarke, Caul, Jancar, and Gordon-Russell (1984) surveyed 7 such institutions with a total population of 2,239 patients and found a HBsAg carrier rate of 5.5%, a third of whom were negative for anti-HBe and thus considered infectious. The residents with Down syndrome were 18 times more likely to be infectious, with the males 6 times more likely to be infectious than females. The higher chronic carrier rate and greater degree of infectivity in males with Down syndrome have been confirmed in several subsequent smaller studies including those by Ditzhuijsen, Kleijnen, Rijntjes, Loon, and Yap (1988); Holt, Goodall, Lees, and Hambling (1986); and Lohiya, Lohiya, Ngo, and Crinella (1986).

As residents of institutions became integrated into community settings, concern arose about the impact of HBV carriers from institutions upon individuals who had never been in institutions. Perrillo, Storch, Bodicky, Campbell, and Sanders (1984) published a report where subtyping suggested that a nonresidential public school student acquired HBV from such a carrier.

The impact of remaining in a home environment upon the prevalence of HBsAg and anti-HBs in persons with Down syndrome has also been studied. Renner et al. (1985) determined that HBsAg was positive in 12.8% and anti-HBs was present in 4.8% of outpatients with Down syndrome, compared to rates of 2.8% for HBsAg and 6.6% anti-HBs in outpatients with mental retardation of other etiologies; controls had rates of 0% for HBsAg and 0.9% for anti-HBs. In contrast, Dicks and Dennis (1987) found HBsAg in only 1 of 37 persons with Down syndrome who had never resided in an institution. A larger study by Pueschel, Bodenheimer, and Dean (1991) of 180 persons with Down syndrome who had never been institutionalized detected 1 patient positive for HBsAg and 1 for anti-HBs. Both of these individuals had received multiple units of blood in the early 1980s during open heart surgery. A nonmatched comparison group of 155 outpatients contained 2 individuals positive for HBsAg, including 1 with a history of numerous transfusions and 1 of Southeast Asian heritage.

Concern about previously institutionalized patients who were carriers for HBV infecting students and staff in public school settings was partially alleviated by the introduction of hepatitis B vaccine, but also provoked discussion as to an immunization policy (Mann, Kane, & Hull, 1983). Heijtink, DeJong, Schalm, and Masurel (1984); Troisi, Heiberg, and Hollinger (1985); and Van Damme, Vranckx, and Meheus (1990) determined that individuals with Down syndrome did have an immune response to vaccination. Troisi et al. concluded that persons with Down syndrome did not represent a special group requiring different guidelines for immunization.

The necessity of vaccination for institutionalized residents with mental disabilities with a low heptatitis carrier rate provoked recent controversy in the United Kingdom (French, Tinsley, Tam, Chan, & Murray, 1989; Green, 1989; McGregor, Cowie, Wassef, Veasey, & Munro, 1988; Tyrer, Codd, Thomson, Rawlins, & James, 1989; Van Damme & Meheus, 1989). In the United States, vaccination is recommended for staff and residents of institutions for persons with developmental disabilities. Vaccination is also recommended for the staff of nonresidential day-care and school programs for children with developmental disabilities. Individuals attending such programs may be at less risk than staff, but vaccination should be encouraged when an HBV carrier classmate is aggressive or may otherwise expose others to blood or bodily secretions. Upon entrance to day or school programs, residents of institutions should be screened for HBsAg to determine their carrier status (Committee on Infectious Diseases American Academy of Pediatrics, 1991).

AUTOIMMUNE CHRONIC ACTIVE HEPATITIS

There have been two reports of persons with Down syndrome who had autoimmune chronic hepatitis (McCulloch, Ince, & Kendall-Taylor, 1982; O'Mahony, Whelton, & Hogan, 1990). These reports underscore the need for awareness that not all persons with chronic active hepatitis have an infectious etiology. The individual described by McCulloch et al. also exhibited other immune disturbances including Hashimoto's thyroiditis, alopecia areata, and elevated antinuclear antibody titres.

LIVER PHYSIOLOGY

The dose effect of trisomy for the 21 chromosome on various enzymes and other cellular functions has long been of interest. Gene mapping has further stimulated such research. Epstein et al. (1985) used mouse trisomy 16 as an animal model for Down syndrome and found fetal liver B cells and pre-B cells were moderately decreased, whereas the transformation by Abelson murine leukemia virus of the fetal liver cells was markedly diminished. The latter finding was unexpected, given the increased susceptibility for developing leukemia in individuals with Down syndrome.

Proteins from human trisomy 21 fetal liver tissue were analyzed by Reichert (1986), who was able to establish three differences in protein patterns when compared to "normal" controls. Control liver tissue synthesized the proteins at a higher level than the trisomic 21 liver tissue. Probing with four chromosome 21–specific genomic sequences of liver and brain from trisomic 21 fetuses and matched controls determined that differences for sequences 21.3, 26c, JG77, and JG90 were significantly different in the brain, but normal in the liver for 21.3, 26C, whereas JG77 and JG90 were normal or decreased (Stefani et al., 1988). Human liver RNA encodes for the trifunctional protein glycinamide ribonucleotide synthetase-aminoimidazole ribonucleotide synthetase-glycinamide ribonucleotide transformylase. A recent study by Aimi, Qiu, Williams, Zalkin, and Dixon (1990) concluded that the levels of RNA are similar in a Down syndrome cell line and a normal fibroblast cell line.

CONCLUSION

Proper hygiene and immunization provide appropriate control measures to decrease the incidence of HBV infection in individuals with Down syndrome. Measures that limit HBV infection decrease the risk for those individuals becoming chronic carriers and thus decrease their risk of developing cirrhosis and hepatocellular carcinoma. Prevention of chronic carriers who may infect others also has important public health benefits. The issue of why individuals with Down syndrome respond differently to HBV infection remains unresolved and suggests intrinsic immunologic and biochemical differences. Continued basic research will help to delineate further the similarities and differences of liver function in individuals with Down syndrome as compared to euploid controls.

REFERENCES

Aimi, J., Qiu, H., Williams, J., Zalkin, H., & Dixon, J.E. (1990). De novo purine nucleotide biosynthesis: Cloning of human and avian cDNAs encoding the trifunctional glycinamide ribonucleotide synthetase-aminoimidazole ribonucleotide synthetase-glycinamide ribonucleotide transformylase by functional complementation in *E. coli*. *Nucleic Acid Research, 18*, 6665–6672.

Boughton, C.R., Hawkes, R.A., Schroeter, D.R., & Harlor, J.A. (1976). The epidemiology of hepatitis B in a residential institution for the mentally retarded. *Australian and New Zealand Journal of Medicine, 6*, 521–529.

Clarke, S.K.R., Caul, E.O., Jancar, J., & Gordon-Russell, J.B. (1984). Hepatitis B in seven hospitals for the mentally handicapped. *Journal of Infection, 8*, 34–43.

Committee on Infectious Diseases American Academy of Pediatrics. (1991). *Report of the Committee on Infectious Diseases*. Elk Grove Village, IL: American Academy of Pediatrics.

Dicks, J.L., & Dennis, E.S. (1987). Down's syndrome and hepatitis: An evaluation of carrier status. *Journal of the American Dental Association, 114*, 637–639.

Ditzhuijsen, T.J.M., Kleijnen, F.M., Rijntjes, P.J.M., Loon, A.M., & Yap, S.H. (1988). The prevalence of serological markers, hepatitis B virus DNA and elevated serum amino transferase values in institutionalized mentally handicapped males and females: An epidemiological study of HBV infections in residents with Down's syndrome or other forms of mental deficiency. *European Journal of Epidemiology, 4*, 349–356.

Epstein, C.J., Hofmeister, B.G., Yee, D., Smith, S.A., Philip, R., Cox, D.R., & Epstein, L.B. (1985). Stem cell deficiencies and thymic abnormalities in fetal mouse trisomy 16. *Journal of Experimental Medicine, 162*, 695–712.

French, G.L., Tinsley, H., Tam, J.S., Chan, R.C.K., & Murray, H.G.S. (1989). Hepatitis B in mental handicap hospitals. *Lancet, ii*, 841.

Green, J. (1989). Hepatitis B in mental handicap hospitals. *Lancet, ii*, 840.

Hawkes, R.A., Boughton, C.R., Schroeter, D.R., Decker, R.H., & Overby, L. (1980). Hepatitis B infection in institutionalized Down's syndrome inmates: A longitudinal study with five hepatitis B virus markers. *Clinical and Experimental Immunology, 40*, 478–486.

Heijtink, R.A., DeJong, P., Schalm, S.W., & Masurel, N. (1984). Hepatitis B vaccination in Down's syndrome and other mentally retarded patients. *Hepatology, 4*, 611–614.

Hollinger, F.B., Goyal, R.K., Hersh, T., Powell, H.C., Schulman, R.J., & Melnick, J.L. (1972). Immune response to hepatitis virus type B in Down's syndrome and other mentally retarded patients. *American Journal of Epidemiology, 95*, 356–362.

Holt, P.A., Goodall, B., Lees, E.M., & Hambling, M.H. (1986). Prevalence of hepatitis B markers in patients and staff in a hospital for the mentally handicapped. *Journal of Hospital Infection, 76*, 799–802.

Lohiya, G., Lohiya, S., Ngo, V.T., & Crinella, R. (1986). Epidemiology of hepatitis B e antigen and antibody in mentally retarded HBsAg carriers. *Hepatology, 6*, 163–166.

Mann, J.M., Kane, M.A., & Hull, H.F. (1983). Hepatitis B, hepatitis B vaccine and education for the handicapped. *Pediatric Infectious Disease Journal, 2*, 273–275.

McCulloch, A.S., Ince, P.G., & Kendall-Taylor, P. (1982). Autoimmune chronic active hepatitis in Down's syndrome. *Journal of Medical Genetics, 3*, 232–234.

McGregor, M.A., Cowie, V.A., Wassef, K., Veasey, D., & Munro, J. (1988). Hepatitis B in a hospital for the mentally subnormal in South Wales. *Journal of Mental Deficiency Research, 32*, 75–77.

O'Mahony, D., Whelton, M.J., & Hogan, J. (1990). Down syndrome and autoimmune chronic active hepatitis: Satisfactory outcome with therapy. *Irish Journal of Medical Science, 159*, 21–22.

Perrillo, R.P., Storch, G.A., Bodicky, C.J., Campbell, C.R., & Sanders, G.E. (1984). Survey of hepatitis B viral markers at a public day school and a residential institution sharing mentally handicapped students. *Journal of Infectious Diseases, 149*, 796–800.

Pueschel, S.M., Bodenheimer, H.C., & Dean, M.K. (1991). The prevalence of hepatitis B surface antigen and antibody in home-reared individuals with Down syndrome. *Research in Developmental Disabilities, 12*, 243–249.

Reichert, G.H. (1986). Two dimensional gel analysis

of proteins from human trisomy 21 fetal liver tissue after DEAE-Sepharose chromotography. *Human Genetics, 73,* 250–253.

Renner, F., Andrle, M., Horak, W., & Rett, A. (1985). Hepatitis A and B in institutionalized mentally retarded patients. *Hepato-gastroenterology, 32,* 175–177.

Stefani, L., Galt, J., Palmer, A., Affara, N., Ferguson-Smith, M., & Nevin, N.C. (1988). Expression of chromosome 21 specific sequences in normal and Down's syndrome tissues. *Nucleic Acids Research, 16,* 2885–2896.

Sutnick, A.I., London, W.T., Gerstley, B.J.S., Cronlund, M.M., & Blumberg, B.S. (1968). Anicteric hepatitis associated with Australian antigen. *Journal of the American Medical Association, 205,* 670–674.

Szmuness, W., Purcell, R.H., Dienstag, J.L., &

Stevens, C.E. (1977). Antibody to hepatitis A antigen in institutionalized mentally retarded patients. *Journal of the American Medical Association, 237,* 1702–1705.

Troisi, C.L., Heiberg, D.A., & Hollinger, F.B. (1985). Normal immune response to hepatitis B vaccine in patients with Down's syndrome. *Journal of the American Medical Association, 254,* 3196–3199.

Tyrer, S.P., Codd, A.A., Thomson, R.G., Rawlins, M.D., & James, P.F.W. (1989). Hepatitis B in mental handicap hospitals. *Lancet, ii,* 842.

Van Damme, P., & Meheus, A. (1989). Hepatitis B in mental handicap hospitals. *Lancet, ii,* 840–841.

Van Damme, P., Vranckx, R., & Meheus, A. (1990). Immunogenicity of a recombinant DNA hepatitis B vaccine in institutionalized patients with Down's syndrome. *Vaccine, 8*(Suppl.), S53–S55.

CHAPTER
13

Genitourinary System

Ilana Ariel and Yigal Shvil

Only scanty information relating to changes of the genitourinary system in persons with Down syndrome is available. Some of this information is mentioned briefly in publications dealing with other aspects of Down syndrome or of urinary tract abnormalities.

MACROSCOPIC AND MICROSCOPIC CHANGES IN KIDNEYS

Small kidneys in persons with Down syndrome were described by Benda (1969). Naeye (1967) calculated a reduction of 9% in renal weight of newborns with Down syndrome compared to controls matched for body weight. A mean reduction of about 14% of renal weight for body length was found in older persons with Down syndrome (Ariel, Wells, Landing, & Singer, 1991). In fetuses with trisomy 21, growth retardation of the kidneys as well as other organs is already well established during the second trimester of pregnancy (Fitzsimmons, Droste, Shepard, Pascoe-Mason, & Fantel, 1990). Whereas both body weight and organ weight were found to be decreased in the latter study, the weight of the kidneys was affected to a greater degree.

In a morphometric study of renal tissue of newborns with Down syndrome, the number of glomeruli was calculated as less than 60% of normal (Naeye, 1967). A decreased number of papillary pores, representing ducts of Bellini, was documented by Heuser, Landing, Dixon, and Shankle (1983). This implies a defect in the process of dichotomous division of the ureteric bud at an early embryonic stage. The number

of generations of glomeruli, representing a later stage of intrauterine renal development, was, however, found to be normal by Ariel et al. (1991).

Postnatal renal growth is produced mainly by tubular lengthening (Fetterman, Shuplock, Phillip, & Gregg, 1965). Postnatal retardation of renal growth relative to gain of body weight was postulated by Benda (1969), but no morphometric data concerning the tubuli in individuals with Down syndrome are available.

Renal hypoplasia, defined as less than two thirds of the normal combined weight of the kidneys (Kissane, 1983), was found in 18 of 84 autopsies in the study by Ariel et al. (1991). Renal failure was the major cause of death in only 3.3% of institutionalized persons with Down syndrome in Texas (Deaton, 1973). Nevertheless, the reduced renal mass and resulting reduced functional reserve in persons with Down syndrome may complicate other medical conditions, thereby increasing the morbidity in such situations.

The microscopic changes of the kidneys of individuals with Down syndrome include glomerular microcysts, tubular dilatation, and immature glomeruli deep in the renal cortex (Gilbert & Opitz, 1988). Ariel et al. (1991) found glomerular microcysts in 23 of 97 (23.7%) persons with Down syndrome. They were not associated with obstructive lesions of the urinary tract. In the same study, focal dilatation of tubules was found in 10, immature glomeruli deep in the cortex in 18, and "simple" cysts (grossly recognized cysts with flat epithelial lining) in 7 persons with Down syndrome. The functional implications of these microscopic abnormalities are not known.

OBSTRUCTIVE
ANOMALIES OF URINARY TRACT

Several types of obstructive lesions along the urinary tract have been described. These may give rise to hydronephrosis or dysplastic changes of the kidneys. An increased prevalence of pyelectasis (dilatation of the pelvis of the kidney) in fetuses with Down syndrome was detected by ultrasonic examination during pregnancy (Benacerraf, Mandell, Estroff, Harlow, & Frigoletto, 1990). Of special interest are the anatomic and functional obstructive lesions of the ureters. The outcome of corrective surgery (i.e., ureteric reimplantation) is usually poor, and nonoperative treatment or ureterostomy should be considered (Ahmed, 1990). A list of all the cases described in the literature appears in Table 13.1.

The true prevalence of obstructive uropathy in persons with Down syndrome is difficult to determine at the present state of knowledge. A severe obstructive lesion early in fetal life may lead to bilateral cystic dysplasia of the kidneys and early postnatal death as a result of pulmonary hypoplasia. Such cases of Potter sequence have not always been routinely karyotyped in the past in order to determine the prevalence of underlying chromosome aberrations. The prevalence of obstructive uropathy for older persons with Down syndrome, who do not have a lethal malformation sequence and thus survive the immediate postnatal period, seems to be 3.5%–6.7% (Ariel et al., 1991; Berg, Crome, & France, 1960; Egli & Stalder, 1973).

URIC ACID AND CREATININE CLEARANCE

A significantly higher level of uric acid was found in the serum and sweat of persons with trisomy 21 (Appleton, Haab, Burti, & Orsulak,

Table 13.1.   Summary of gross urinary tract pathology in Down syndrome

Author	Year	Cases	Gross anatomic abnormalities
Berg, Crome, and France	1960	5/141 autopsy cases of Down syndrome	Unilateral renal agenesis; unilateral renal hypoplasia; horseshoe kidney; urethral valve
Naeye	1967	21 newborns with trisomy 21	Hydronephrosis; ureteropelvic junction stenosis; horseshoe kidney
Egli and Stalder	1973	7/103 autopsies of children with Down syndrome	Hydronephrosis; hydroureter; ureteral stenosis; megacystis; renal cysts
Ozer	1974	1 case of Down syndome	Ureteropelvic junction stricture; hydronephrosis; focal dysplasia
Kravtzova, Lazjuk, and Lurie	1975	Autopsy series of Down syndrome	Hydronephrosis; hydroureter; atresia of ureters
Al Saadi et al.	1984	1 case of trisomy 21 of 21 renal dysplasia	Obstructive uropathy with renal dysplasia
Curry, Jensen, Holland, Miller, and Hall	1984	1 case of Down syndrome of 80 cases of Potter sequence	Obstructive uropathy
Zerres, Volpel, and Weib	1984	1 case of trisomy 21	Prune-belly anomaly[a]
Amacker, Grass, Hickey, and Hisley	1986	2 cases of trisomy 21	Prune-belly anomaly[a]
Passerini-Glazel et al.	1988	1 case of trisomy 21 of 8 urethral hypoplasia	Hydronephrosis; patent urachus
Ahmed	1990	Ureteral implantation in Down syndrome	Vesicoureteral reflux (4); ureterovesical obstruction (1); posterior urethral valves (1)
Ariel, Wells, Landing, and Singer	1991	124 autopsies of Down syndrome; 2/18 2nd trimester fetuses; 2/9 neonates and stillborns; 4/97 older	Bladder neck stenosis; ureterovesical stenosis; hydroureter; hydronephrosis; renal cystic dysplasia; double pelvis and ureter; ureterocele

[a]Malformation sequence that includes urethral obstruction, cryptorchidism, and extreme dilatation of abdominal wall with absence of abnormal muscles.

1969; Danton & Nyhan, 1966; Fuller, Luce, & Mertz, 1962; Goodman, Lofland, & Thomas, 1966; Mertz, Fuller, & Concon, 1963; Nishida, Akaoka, Kobayashi, Maruki, & Oshima, 1979; Pant, Moser, & Krane, 1968). A normal rate of uric acid synthesis was observed by assays using radiolabeled substances (Coburn, Sirlin, & Mertz, 1968; Lesch & Nyhan, 1964). According to Coburn, Seidenberg, and Mertz (1967) and Pant et al. (1968), the mechanism for the increased serum uric acid is a decreased urinary clearance of uric acid. The fractional excretion of uric acid was also found to be lower in persons with Down syndrome compared to controls with other types of mental retardation (Coburn et al., 1967), though both groups were within the normal range of Stapleton's standards (Stapleton, Linshaw, Hassanein, & Gruskin, 1978). The decreased fractional excretion of uric acid has a higher significance in the presence of higher uric acid level in the serum. Blood and erythrocyte levels of substances disturbing tubular reabsorption of uric acid (e.g., lactic acid, lactic dehydrogenase and hydroxybutyrate) were found to be normal (Nishida et al., 1979). (See also Pueschel & Annerén, chap. 23, this volume.)

Creatinine clearance was also found to be significantly reduced in persons with Down syndrome (Coburn et al., 1967; Nishida et al., 1979). The specific gravity of the urine was not different from that of the controls (Coburn et al., 1967).

The understanding of the entire spectrum of glomerular and tubular functions in persons with Down syndrome as well as the correlation between the anatomic and functional abnormalities of the kidney in this chromosome aberration are far from being complete. More research needs to be done in order to clarify these points, and better understanding may enable better care of persons with Down syndrome.

GENITALIA

An increased occurrence of distal hypospadias was reported by Lang, Van Dyke, Heide, and Lowe (1987). Five of the 77 males with Down syndrome in their study had dorsal urethral duplications and/or glanular hypospadias. Renal functions and radiographic studies did not dis-

close any additional abnormalities of the urinary tract or kidneys in these persons. One male with Down syndrome and hypospadias was documented by Ahmed (1990). Different observations were made by other investigators. Hsiang, Berkovitz, Bland, Migeon, and Warren (1987) found the prevalence of hypospadias in 53 males with Down syndrome to be similar to that of the general population. There is also no documentation of any case of hypospadias in a study of the genitalia of 46 adolescents and young adults with Down syndrome (Pueschel, Orson, Boylan, & Pezzullo, 1985).

Hypogenitalism has usually been considered an integral phenotypic characteristic of Down syndrome (Smith & Berg, 1976). Benda (1969) described an infantile penis and small testes in the majority of males with Down syndrome. He reported a 50% incidence of cryptorchidism (failure of one or both testes to descend) at birth, and a frequent occurrence of unilateral undescended testis in older males. Careful examination of Benda's own case reports, however, discloses no case of undescended testes in 11 males with Down syndrome over the age of 18, and only 3 of 25 males between ages of 12–17 (Sylvester & Rundle, 1962). A much lower prevalence of cryptorchidism, probably similar or close to that of the general population, was found by other investigators (Hsiang et al., 1987; Sylvester & Rundle, 1962). No incidence of cryptorchidism was recorded in a study of the genital development in 46 male adolescents with Down syndrome by Pueschel et al. (1985). (See also Pueschel & Blaymore Bier, chap. 22, this volume.)

INTERSEX SYNDROMES

Coincidence of trisomy 21 with conditions associated with intersex syndromes have been reported. Of those, the most common are probably XYY and Klinefelter syndrome (XXY), followed by XXX and Turner syndrome (Smith & Berg, 1976). A person with male pseudohermaphroditism and Down syndrome has been documented by Golbus, Beauchamp, and Conte (1973). Gonadal dysgenesis was described in a 46,XY female mosaic for trisomies 8 and 21 (Sulewski, Dang, Ward, & Ladda, 1980). Another unique individual with Down syndrome, due to translocation occurring concomitantly with virilizing salt-losing congenital adrenal hyperplasia, was reported by Srivuthana, Collipp, Sherman, and Zaino (1971).

TESTICULAR MALIGNANCIES

The increased prevalence of malignancy in persons with Down syndrome is well established. There is a markedly greater risk of developing leukemia as well as a possible association with other tumors (e.g., retinoblastoma, central nervous system tumors, testicular tumors) (Kamidono, Takada, Ishigami, Furumoto, & Urano, 1985). Most of the testicular tumors in Down syndrome were seminoma (Braun et al., 1985; Jackson, Turner, Klauber, & Norris, 1968; Kamidono et al., 1985; Matsaniotis, Karpouzas, & Economou-Mavrou, 1967; Sasagawa et al., 1986), but other malignancies, mostly other types of germ cell tumors, have been documented (Dexeus, Logothetis, Chong, Sella, & Ogden, 1988; Sakashita, Koyanagi, Tsuji, Arikado, & Matsuno, 1980). An increased sensitivity of cells to mutagenic agents is a proposed mechanism, but the carcinogenic effect of persistent high levels of gonadotropins in persons with Down syndrome cannot be excluded (Sasagawa et al., 1986). With better care and increased longevity of persons with Down syndrome today, the prevalence of cancers other than leukemia, particularly seminoma, may increase. (See also Lubin, Kahn, & Scott, chap. 21, this volume.)

CONCLUSION

Small kidneys are a feature of Down syndrome, and, when extreme, may give rise to renal insufficiency. Microscopic changes, including glomerular microcysts, tubular dilatation, and irregular glomerular maturation have been described in persons with Down syndrome, but their functional implications are not clear.

There is an association of obstructive uropathy with Down syndrome. The prevalence is not known, but for older individuals it seems to be approximately 5%. A higher level of serum uric acid is found in persons with Down syndrome, and disturbances in renal function tests include reduced clearance of uric acid and creatinine.

Hypogenitalism, hypospadias, and cryptorchidism have been considered characteristic of persons with Down syndrome. This is probably not true for the latter two according to more recent observations. Down syndrome may occur concomitantly with intersex syndromes.

An increasing number of testicular tumors, especially seminoma, in males with Down syndrome has been described in recent years. This may be the result of increased longevity in individuals with susceptibility to developing malignancy, as exists in this chromosome aberration.

REFERENCES

Ahmed, S. (1990). Vesico-ureteric reflux in Down's syndrome: Poor prognosis. *Australian and New Zealand Journal of Surgery, 60,* 113–116.

Al Saadi, A.A., Yoshimoto, M., Bree, R., Farah, J., Chung, C.H., Sahney, S., Shokeir, M.H.K., & Bernstein J. (1984). A family study of renal dysplasia. *American Journal of Medical Genetics, 19,* 669–677.

Amacker, E.A., Grass, F.S., Hickey, D.E., & Hisley, J.C. (1986). Brief clinical report: An association of prune belly anomaly with trisomy 21. *American Journal of Medical Genetics, 23,* 919–923.

Appleton, M.D., Haab, W., Burti, U., & Orsulak, P.J. (1969). Plasma urate levels in mongolism. *American Journal of Mental Retardation, 74,* 196–199.

Ariel, I., Wells, T.R., Landing, B.H., & Singer, D.B. (1991). The urinary system in Down syndrome. A

study of 124 autopsy cases. *Pediatric Pathology, 11,* 879–888.

Benacerraf, B.R., Mandell, J., Estroff, J.A., Harlow, B.L., & Frigoletto, F.D. (1990). Fetal pyelectasis: A possible association with Down syndrome. *Obstetrics & Gynecology, 76,* 58–60.

Benda, C.E. (1969). *Down's syndrome. Mongolism and its management* (rev. ed.). New York: Grune & Stratton.

Berg, J.M., Crome, L., & France, N.E. (1960). Congenital cardiac malformations in mongolism. *British Heart Journal, 22,* 331–346.

Braun, D.L., Green, M.D., Rausen, A.R., David, R., Wolman, S.R., Greco, M.A., & Muggia, F.M. (1985). *American Journal of Pediatric Hematology/Oncology, 7,* 208–211.

Coburn, S.P., Seidenberg, M., & Mertz, E.T. (1967).

Clearance of uric acid, urea and creatinine in Down's syndrome. *Journal of Applied Physiology, 23,* 579–580.

Coburn, S.P., Sirlin, E.M., & Mertz, E.T. (1968). Metabolism of N15 labeled uric acid in Down's syndrome. *Metabolism, 17,* 560–562.

Curry, C.J.R., Jensen, K., Holland, J., Miller, L., & Hall, B.D. (1984). The Potter sequence: A clinical analysis of 80 cases. *American Journal of Medical Genetics, 19,* 679–702.

Danton, R.A., & Nyhan, W.L. (1966). Concentrations of uric acid in the sweat of control and mongoloid children. *Proceedings of the Society for Experimental Biology and Medicine, 121,* 270–271.

Deaton, J.G. (1973). The mortality rate and causes of death among institutionalised mongols in Texas. *Journal of Mental Deficiency Research, 17,* 117–122.

Dexeus, F.H., Logothetis, C.J., Chong, C., Sella, A., & Ogden, S. (1988). Genetic abnormalities in men with germ cell tumors. *Journal of Urology, 140,* 80–84.

Egli, F., & Stalder, G. (1973). Malformations of the kidneys and urinary tract in common chromosomal aberrations: I.Clinical studies. *Humangenetik, 18,* 1–15.

Fetterman, G.H., Shuplock, N.A., Phillip, F.J., & Gregg, H.S. (1965). The growth and maturation of human glomeruli and proximal convolutions from term to adulthood: Studies by microdissection. *Pediatrics, 35,* 601–619.

Fitzsimmons, J., Droste, S., Shepard, T.H., Pascoe-Mason, J., & Fantel, A. (1990). Growth failure in second-trimester fetuses with trisomy 21. *Teratology, 42,* 337–345.

Fuller, R.W., Luce, M.W., & Mertz, E.T. (1962). Serum uric acid in mongolism. *Science, 137,* 868–869.

Gilbert, E.F., & Opitz, J.M. (1988). Developmental and other pathologic changes in syndromes caused by chromosome abnormalities. *Perspectives in Pediatric Pathology, 7,* 1–63.

Golbus, M.S., Beauchamp, C.J., & Conte, F.A. (1973). Male pseudohermaphroditism in a child with Down's syndrome. *Journal of Medical Genetics, 10,* 189–192.

Goodman, H.O., Lofland, H.B., & Thomas, J.J. (1966). Serum uric acid levels in mongolism. *American Journal of Mental Deficiency, 71,* 437–446.

Heuser, E.T., Landing, B.H., Dixon, L.G., & Shankle, W.R. (1983). Papillary pore counts: A method of studying developmental aberrations in diseased juvenile kidneys. *Pediatric Pathology, 1,* 67–79.

Hsiang, Y.H.H., Berkovitz, G.D., Bland, G.L., Migeon, C.J., & Warren, A.C. (1987). Gonadal function in patients with Down syndrome. *American Journal of Medical Genetics, 27,* 449–458.

Jackson, E.W., Turner, J.H., Klauber, M.R., &

Norris, F.D. (1968). Down's syndrome: Variation of leukemia occurrence in institutionalized populations. *Journal of Chronic Diseases, 21,* 247–253.

Kamidono, S., Takada, K., Ishigami, J., Furumoto, M., & Urano, Y. (1985). Giant seminoma of undescended testis in Down syndrome. *Urology, 25,* 637–640.

Kissane, J.M. (1983). Congenital malformations. In R.H. Heptinstall *Pathology of the kidney* (3rd. ed., pp. 83–140). Boston: Little, Brown.

Kravtzova, G.I., Lazjuk, G.I., & Lurie, I.W. (1975). The malformations of the urinary system in autosomal disorders. *Virchows Archiv A. Pathological Anatomy and Histopathology, 368,* 167–178.

Lang, D.J., Van Dyke, D.C., Heide, F., & Lowe, P.L. (1987). Hypospadias and urethral abnormalities in Down syndrome. *Clinical Pediatrics, 26,* 40–42.

Lesch, M., & Nyhan, W.L. (1964). A familial disorder of uric acid metabolism and central nervous function. *American Journal of Medicine, 36,* 561–570.

Matsaniotis, N., Karpouzas, J., & Economou-Mavrou, C. (1967). Hypothyroidism and seminoma in association with Down's syndrome. *Journal of Pediatrics, 70,* 810–812.

Mertz, E.T., Fuller, R.W., & Concon, J.M. (1963). Serum uric acid in young mongoloids. *Science, 134,* 535.

Naeye, R.L. (1967). Prenatal organ and cellular growth with various chromosomal disorders. *Biology of the Neonate, 11,* 248–260.

Nishida, Y., Akaoka, I., Kobayashi, M., Maruki, K., & Oshima, Y. (1979). Renal impairment in urate excretion in patients with Down's syndrome. *Journal of Rheumatology, 6,* 103–107.

Ozer, F.L. (1974). Kidney malformations in mongolism. *Birth Defects: Original Article Series, X*(4), 189.

Pant, S.S., Moser, H.W., & Krane, S.M. (1968). Hyperuricemia in Down's syndrome. *Journal of Clinical Endocrinology, 28,* 472–478.

Passerini-Glazel, G., Araguna, F., Chiozza, L., Artibani, W., Rabinowitz, R., & Firlit, C.F. (1988). The P.A.D.U.A. (progressive augmentation by dilating the urethra anterior) procedure for the treatment of severe urethral hypoplasia. *Journal of Urology, 140,* 1247–1249.

Pueschel, S.M., Orson, J.M., Boylan, J.M., & Pezzullo, J.C. (1985). Adolescent development in males with Down syndrome. *American Journal of Diseases of Children, 139,* 236–238.

Sakashita, S., Koyanagi, T., Tsuji, I., Arikado, K., & Matsuno, T. (1980). Congenital anomalies in children with testicular germ cell tumors. *Journal of Urology, 124,* 889–891.

Sasagawa, I., Kazama, T., Umeda, K., Kohno, T., Katayama, T., & Miwa, A. (1986). Down's syndrome associated with seminoma. *Urologia Internationalis, 41,* 238–240.

Smith, G.F., & Berg, J.M. (1976). *Down's anomaly* (2nd ed.). Edinburgh: Churchill Livingstone.

Srivuthana, S., Collipp, P.J., Sherman, J., & Zaino, E. (1971). Translocation mongolism with virilizing adrenal hyperplasia. *American Journal of Clinical Pathology, 55,* 232–236.

Stapleton, F.B., Linshaw, M.A., Hassanein, K., & Gruskin, A.B. (1978). Uric acid excretion in normal children. *Journal of Pediatrics, 92,* 911–914.

Sulewski, J.M., Dang, T.P., Ward, S., & Ladda, R.L. (1980). Gonadal dysgenesis in a 46,XY female mosaic for double autosomal trisomies 8 and 21. *Journal of Medical Genetics, 17,* 321–323.

Sylvester, P.E., & Rundle, A.T. (1962). Endocrinological aspects of mental deficiency: II. Maturation status of adult males. *Journal of Mental Deficiency Research, 6,* 87–93.

Zerres, K., Volpel, M.C., & Weib, H. (1984). Cystic kidneys. Genetics, pathologic anatomy, clinical picture and prenatal diagnosis. *Human Genetics, 68,* 104–135.

CHAPTER
14

Gynecologic Care

Thomas E. Elkins

Perhaps the last phase of integration into the medical system for females with mental retardation will be the universal attainment of routine gynecologic care. In a recent survey in New England, gynecologic care and home nursing care were notably lacking even in a population that had achieved full access to most medical resources (Minihan & Dean, 1990). The availability and attainment of reproductive health services for females with mental retardation also appears to be related to the level of mental retardation (and, similarly, the level of cooperation for full physical examinations). Since most females with Down syndrome are able to cooperate with full physical examinations, one would expect them to be more like the general population in their attainment of routine reproductive health care. However, recent surveys still show a diminished use of the health care system—in terms of gynecologic care—for females with Down syndrome (Elkins, Spinnato, & Muram, 1987).

One reason for this is that some may think that females with Down syndrome simply do not need routine reproductive or gynecologic health care. However, other reasons have also been noted in regional surveys. Physicians appear unwilling or ill-prepared to provide full gynecologic services in many instances. Reimbursement programs for females with mental retardation often provide adequate physician payment for inpatient (and surgical) care, but minimal reimbursement for routine gynecologic outpatient care. It is not uncommon, therefore, for a female with Down syndrome to come to the gynecology clinic at the University of Michigan Medical Center, Ann Arbor, for example, for her first pelvic examination at age 35 or 45 years.

Since the mid-1960s, marked advancements have been made in our society for persons with Down syndrome. Improved medical treatment, special (and routine) education efforts, and de-institutionalization have led to an increased life expectancy, increased capacity for work and socialization, and increased community interaction. With these advancements have come the realization that persons with Down syndrome, like all others, have normal concerns about sexuality, socialization, peer acceptance, and self-determination to whatever capacity they can achieve, which is in a normal range for many.

With these concepts in mind, a model clinic for reproductive health concerns in persons with mental retardation was developed at the University of Michigan Medical Center in 1985. Over 500 patients have been seen, with approximately 10%–15% being persons with Down syndrome. The clinic has attempted to provide not only acute, surgically oriented care, but also routine gynecologic care for women and socialization/sexuality counseling for persons of both sexes. This chapter reflects the concepts of health care developed in that clinic setting.

ASPECTS OF ROUTINE GYNECOLOGIC CARE

Physical Development in Females with Down Syndrome

Most females with Down syndrome begin menses between age 10–14. This is not inconsistent with the U.S. national average of 11.4 years now reported in adolescent literature (Frisch & Revelle, 1970). Earlier reports of marked developmental delays in the onset of menses for females with

Down syndrome (even when compared to females with mental retardation of other etiologies) have not been confirmed by current small surveys, or by the clinic population at the University of Michigan (Salerno, Park, & Giannini, 1975). It is very likely that such normalcy in the development of secondary sex characteristics has paralleled the emphasis upon improved health care, nutrition, socialization, and education for persons with Down syndrome since the 1960s and 1970s. Although the many factors that determine the onset of menses are still uncertain, most females with Down syndrome appear to undergo menarche within the same age range seen in society at large.

Pelvic Examinations

In general, initial gynecologic examinations are sought by "normal" adolescents or young women when they develop menstrually related problems, such as menorrhagia or hypermenorrhea (prolonged or profuse menses), irregular bleeding, dysmenorrhea (painful menses), premenstrual syndrome behaviors, or menstrual hygiene concerns; when they become sexually active, or that becomes a consideration; or if they have reached age 17–18 and have still not had menses. The same should be true for females with Down syndrome.

In order to accomplish gynecologic pelvic examinations in females with mental retardation in the least forceful and least threatening fashion, several pre-examination techniques are helpful (Elkins, McNeeley, et al., 1988). Nursing education before an examination is very important and, therefore, should be attempted. Visual aids that depict the routine gynecologic examinations and anatomically correct dolls can also be used to prepare the patient. In some instances in which extreme fear of an examination has been noted, a patient will be allowed to take a hospital gown to wear each evening at home, and a pelvic examination will not even be attempted on the first visit. Family members or other care providers will be asked to accompany the patient into the examining room, especially if excess patient anxiety is noted.

A full gynecologic examination requires palpation and visualization of what should be considered "private" body parts (a term described more fully later in this chapter). All clinic staff are urged to wear the appropriate dress of medical professionals (including white coats, etc.). This enforces the "rule" that a person's private body parts are not to be viewed or touched by those other than health care professionals, unless consenting sexual expressions are considered possible and desirable by the individual.

The breasts and upper body should always be examined before the pelvic examination is attempted. Gentleness and trust may be established with patience, and difficult-to-manage patients may become cooperative. The pelvic examination can be accomplished in a variety of positions, besides the classic lithotomy position with both feet in metal stirrups. For the frightened, anxious patient, simply holding the knees apart and the ankles together in the supine position; elevation of one knee for the debilitated patient with multiple physical disabilities; or the knee–chest position for the young adolescent may be very adequate.

Insertion of a metal or plastic gynecologic speculum (even a pediatric speculum, or an otolaryngology nasal speculum) may be impossible, or at least extremely painful for a virginal or anxious patient. Therefore, persistent efforts to use such instruments should not be pursued if notable difficulty has been initially encountered. A single finger insertion into the vaginal introitus with cervical palpation followed by finger-directed Q-tip insertion to obtain a Pap smear may be readily tolerated when speculum examination is impossible.

Bimanual pelvic examinations are considered the most thorough and appropriate method of pelvic organ evaluation in general. However, relaxation and cooperation are essential features in an adequate examination. In many females with mental retardation, such cooperation is not possible without anesthesia. However, in over 100 instances of examinations in which bimanual evaluations were not possible, transabdominal ultrasonography has been accomplished (Elkins, 1991). This can be done without a full bladder, and uterine, cervical, and adnexal structures can be visualized. Therefore, pelvic ultrasound has become a routine part of gynecologic care for females with mental retardation in whom traditional techniques are unsuccessful.

However, there are some females with mental retardation who are so combative that even the above modifications in pelvic examinations are not helpful. Rather than subject them to the medical risks and economic costs of general anesthesia, an outpatient sedation program has been developed at the University of Michigan (Rosen et al., 1990). Initial reports of the sedation program have revealed high success rates using flavored oral solutions of ketamine and midazolam, with no significant morbidity. Only 1 of over 150 patients required admission for excessive sedation.

Persons with Down syndrome are found in all of the above groups of patients mentioned, from those who are very conversant and who tolerate full gynecologic examinations without difficulty, to those who are so combative that outpatient sedation or, rarely, inpatient general anesthesia is required. Major questions remain about the appropriate frequency and extent of gynecologic examinations that will offer reasonable health care without undue physical harm, psychologic stress, or economic cost. Recent evidence has influenced medical policy so much that yearly Pap smears are not mandatory for cancer screening in asymptomatic persons who have had initial smear(s) that are negative, and who are not sexually active (American Cancer Society, 1980). The American College of Obstetricians and Gynecologists (1989) published recommendations to this effect that urged frequent Pap smears, but allowed variation from annual Pap smears at the patient's discretion. With the major risk for cervical cancer being early sexual intercourse with multiple sex partners, it has become reasonable to utilize Canadian and British standards for cancer screening at least in non–sexually active patients (Harris, 1980; Walton et al., 1976). Certainly, annual general anesthesia or even outpatient sedation, simply to obtain a Pap smear (in an asymptomatic virginal patient with prior negative smear[s]) is unwarranted. However, annual pelvic organ assessment (uterine/ovarian size and content, etc.) is a mainstay of preventive health care that Americans expect, and that females with Down syndrome should be offered as

well. Therefore, in those who require outpatient sedation, after an initial, complete examination with a Pap smear, annual pelvic ultrasonography alone may be used for the next 2–3 years before another full examination is attempted under sedation. This provides reasonable and efficient gynecologic care in a medically reasonable fashion to females with mental retardation.

Menstrually Related Health Care Needs

Similar to "normal" females, females with Down syndrome have an array of menstrually related concerns that become more prominent as age increases. Some appear to be more prevalent in females with Down syndrome.

Hypermenorrhea

Hypermenorrhea or menorrhagia may be especially common in females with Down syndrome for two reasons. First, persons with Down syndrome have a relatively high prevalence of hypothyroidism. Up to 40% of adults with Down syndrome have been thought to develop hypothyroidism, which may result in hypermenorrhea (Murdoch, Ratcliff, McLarty, Rodger, & Ratcliff, 1977). Secondary anemia, which may aggravate existing cardiopulmonary problems in some females with Down syndrome, may follow the development of the menorrhagia. This symptom may be very difficult to control medically, unless the thyroid dysfunction is identified and remedied. Second, another problem related to intermittent episodes of menorrhagia is obesity, again seen frequently in persons with Down syndrome (Pueschel, Canning, Murphy, & Zausmer, 1980). Social isolation, lack of exercise, and poor nutritional habits all contribute to obesity. In women with obesity, adipose tissue creates additional problems. Peripheral conversion of androgens produced by the adrenal glands into estrogen (especially estrone) can lead to persistent high levels of circulating estrogens (Fishman, Boyar, & Hellman, 1975). These hormones, in turn, cause anovulation and excessive stimulation of endometrial glandular tissue, as is seen also in females with polycystic ovary syndrome (Judd, 1978). This endometrial tissue stimulation causes irregular, but often very heavy menses, and may lead to the early development of endometrial hyperplasia and even endometrial carcinoma in younger women (below age 45) with significant constitutional obesity and/or polycystic ovary syndrome.

Numerous authors have noted the success of menstrual hygiene training programs for females with mild to moderate mental retardation (Hamilton, Allen, Stephens, & Davall, 1969; Pattulo & Bernard, 1968). Reduction of heavy bleeding to normal levels plays an important role in aiding menstrual hygiene programs.

Significant menorrhagia requires treatment, which may be medical or surgical. Medical therapy may consist of certain nonsteroidal anti-inflammatory agents (e.g., Ponstel or Naprosyn) that have been shown to reduce menstrual flow by inhibition of prostaglandin synthesis (Anderson, Guillebaud, Haynes, & Turnbull, 1976). More commonly, low-dose oral contraceptives have been shown to reduce menses markedly (in both amount and duration of flow) and to minimize the risks of endometrial hyperplasia/cancer in obese females (Ory, 1982). Most females respond very well to these newer, lower dose preparations. However, many times, females with Down syndrome may also have seizure disorders, which may become worse with estrogens (like those in oral contraceptive tablets), or may be unable to take oral contraceptives because of cardiovascular (e.g., heart failure secondary to congenital heart disease or significant blood clotting problems) or ongoing liver disease (as with chronic hepatitis). A third level of hormonal suppression of menses is to attempt total elimination of menses with medications that have been proven to be effective for endometriosis treatment in the general population. This would include synthetic androgens like danazol (or Danocrine), gonadotropic releasing hormone agonists (e.g., Lupron or Synerrel), and different types of progestins (e.g., Provera, Megace, or Depo-Provera). Depo-Provera has been the most useful in this category because it is inexpensive, causes less break-through bleeding, has been used without major side effects for many years, causes less severe bloating and water retention, and results in more persistent, long-term amenorrhea—which may be a desired result in some females with mental retardation and menstrual dysfunction (Nash, 1975).

Surgical therapy for hypermenorrhea is varied. Dilatation and curettage and hysteroscopy are helpful in diagnosing anatomic causes of severe, heavy bleeding such as endometrial polyps, endometrial hyperplasia, submucous uterine leiomyomas (benign tumors), endometrial carcinoma, and so forth. However, dilatation and curettage seldom provide more than very temporary relief from menorrhagia and should be considered for diagnostic reasons mainly (Scommegna & Dmowski, 1973). Newer methods of endometrial ablation (with laser or electrocautery via hysteroscopy) attempt to destroy the entire endometrial lining to a level beneath the basalis layer. Although effective in some older women, many younger women have recurrent bleeding in a relatively short time (Mishell, 1987).

Hysterectomy may be indicated for females with menstrual problems that have been refractory to other reasonable efforts to control menses or who have obvious uterine pathology (Elkins, McNeeley, Punch, Kope, & Heaton, 1990). The difficulties encountered in performing major surgery in persons with mental retardation have been well documented, making this a therapy of last resort in most instances (McNeeley & Elkins, 1989).

Premenstrual Syndrome

Another significant menstrually related problem for females with Down syndrome is premenstrual syndrome. The symptoms of premenstrual syndrome include bloating, irritability, early cramping, headaches, depression, and agitation that cluster for several days prior to each menstrual period. These are well known to some degree to all cyclically menstruating women, regardless of their mental capacity (O'Brien, 1985). However, unlike the general population, some females with Down syndrome are unable to utilize the psychosocial counseling that is the mainstay of any successful premenstrual syndrome program. Expressive aphasia or other speech dysfunctions may make communication difficult for females with Down syndrome. Rather than finding relief and resolution of premenstrual syndrome concerns through counseling and mild adjuvant medications, a female with mental retardation may respond with frustration, anxiety, and fear, all of which may result in a severe behavior disorder.

Increased disciplinary problems, aggressive behavior, social withdrawal, and decreased attention spans all have been noted by parents and teachers of females with Down syndrome just prior to the onset of menses. Often a 1 kg–1½ kg weight gain just prior to each menses is also documented. All patients requesting help with premenstrual syndrome should have a menstrual calendar given to them to help them document the time, type, and severity of symptoms. This often allows more objective counseling with parents and patients who present with the milder types of symptoms mentioned above. In the University of Michigan clinic, these milder symptoms are seen in patients with moderate and severe mental retardation. Milder symptoms are usually managed readily by family or school counseling, mild diuretics 5–7 days before each period (when water retention is significant), nonsteroidal pain medications (e.g., ibuprofen) when cramping and headaches are significant, and low-dose oral contraceptives to suppress cyclic hormonal swings of estrogen and progesterone.

More severe premenstrual syndrome–like reactions include severe self-destructive or violently combative behavior that is exacerbated prior to each menses. This is usually seen only in females with severe to profound mental retardation, which, fortunately, is uncommon in Down syndrome. However, several females with Down syndrome have presented with this degree of premenstrual syndrome (Ghaziuddin, Elkins, & Kope, 1990). Depo-Provera has been used successfully in 3 such patients, in conjunction with behavior therapy. In those patients unaided by the approach, severe behavior problems continue to occur although they are unrelated to menstrual cycles. Psychiatric referrals that result in the use of major tranquilizing drugs have been helpful in some of the most difficult premenstrual syndrome patients.

REPRODUCTIVE HEALTH CONCERNS

Past studies focused on the delay in development of secondary sex characteristics and pubertal milestones in persons with Down syndrome (Mosier, Grossman, & Dingman, 1968). How-

ever, previous hormonal studies have shown that persons with Down syndrome do have a significant reproductive capacity (Tricomi, Valenti, & Hall, 1964). Although pregnancy in a woman with Down syndrome is not a reportable situation, series of such instances have been collected. A review by Bovicelli, Orsini, Rizzo, Montacut, and Bacchetta (1982) showed that 30 pregnancies in women with Down syndrome impregnated by men without trisomy 21 resulted in 10 infants with Down syndrome, 18 who did not have Down syndrome (one set of twins), and 2 spontaneous abortions. In the 18 infants without Down syndrome, a much higher percentage than usual had congenital anomalies (Bovicelli et al., 1982). This rate of offspring without Down syndrome is higher than the 50% rate expected when one parent has trisomy 21 (Kreutner, 1981). A similar report of 31 pregnancies to mothers with Down syndrome was reported recently by Rani, Jyothi, Reddy, and Reddy (1990).

Parental concerns about unwanted pregnancies occurring in females with Down syndrome are legitimate, especially if regular menstrual function has been established. In Pueschel and Scola's (1988) recent survey, over 50% of the parents of 73 adolescents with Down syndrome wanted their children to have contraception or sterilization. In an earlier survey, parents of persons with Down syndrome overwhelmingly expressed the desire to have the right to request and to authorize sterilization for their family members even when they did not think parents should have complete decision-making rights in neonatal intensive care nursery situations (Elkins et al., 1987). Parents often openly discuss concerns that their daughter could face an unwanted pregnancy, even after the parents have died.

Gynecologic counseling must take the above parental concerns into account, as well as known legal guidelines, ethical issues, and medical knowledge, when offering advice to persons with Down syndrome and their families on reproductive issues.

CONTRACEPTION

Advances in contraceptive technology since the early 1960s have greatly reduced the risk of unwanted pregnancies, along with contraceptive side effects. Newer low-dose oral contraceptives have been shown to have a number of beneficial health effects beyond contraception. Reduction as well as regulation of menses, greatly reduced dysmenorrhea, reduced infection rates with bacterial pelvic inflammatory disease, a marked reduction in the risk of endometrial cancer, a reduction of functional ovarian cysts, suppression of endometriosis, and a probable reduction in ovarian cancer risk may all be attributed to the low-dose oral contraceptive (Derman, 1986). These considerations make oral contraception the first choice for pregnancy prevention in most population groups today. Side effects, though much more rare than before, still occur, and the presence of seizures, liver disease, or cardiovascular disease may contraindicate oral contraceptive use.

The intrauterine contraceptive device has been recommended for any woman who does not want to bear children. However, increased hypermenorrhea is commonly seen with intrauterine contraceptive devices as well as increased dysmenorrhea (Sandmire & Cavanaugh, 1985). This can make menstrual hygiene and premenstrual syndrome problems more difficult to manage. Furthermore, increased pelvic infections, intrauterine contraceptive device perforations, and secondary adjacent organ damage are all potential risks of intrauterine device use. Since pain and discomfort are initial symptoms of these serious problems, delay in diagnosis may occur in females with Down syndrome if diminished verbal skills make discussion of early symptoms difficult.

Depo-Provera is not approved for use as a contraceptive in the United States, even though its efficacy is well documented worldwide. Newer long-acting progestational agents are being approved and may become useful for females with Down syndrome in the future (Chamberlain, Rauh, Passer, McGrath, & Burket, 1984).

Barrier methods, such as the use of condoms and diaphragms, are recommended for the reduction of sexually transmitted diseases. However, all require manual dexterity and highly responsible, controlled behaviors that may

be difficult for some persons with mental disabilities.

STERILIZATION

Sterilization often appears to some care providers and families to be the care option of choice for all young women with Down syndrome. However, this is one of the most controversial issues in gynecologic care for females with mental retardation. Although full discussion of this issue is beyond the scope of this chapter, a few concerns should be noted.

Historically, the legal system has expressed alternating extreme views on several occasions. In 1927, the United States Supreme Court followed a "eugenics" theory and authorized the sterilization of persons with mental retardation in the case of *Buck v. Bell*. After years of escalating numbers of operative procedures, the same Supreme Court justices ruled in *Skinner v. Oklahoma,* in 1942, that reproduction was an "inalienable right," thus reversing their opinion completely from its prior decision. Federal regulations were issued in 1974 that denied payment of federal funds for sterilization operations performed on persons with mental incompetence, as a result of the court decision in *Relf v. Weinberger.*

In light of the above array of legal decisions, it is not surprising that numerous states have developed individual laws governing the sterilization issue, and that a number of challenges to these laws are still before the judicial system. The American College of Obstetricians and Gynecologists Committee on Ethics issued a statement in 1988 to give guidance to its physicians concerning the sterilization issue.

The legal controversies find their bases in deeply rooted ethical concerns about individual dignity and value, as well as societal responsibility. If a person exhibits decisional capacity and desires sterilization, then every effort should be made to perform a sterilizing procedure regardless of the type of mental disability present. However, if the person has been adjudicated mentally incompetent on the basis of age or mental status, then forced sterilization becomes a matter of grave concern. The American College of Obstetricians and Gynecologists Committee on Ethics (1988, p. 3) statement urges that a "best interest of the patient" concern be overriding in such situations.

Hysterectomy has been proclaimed as a procedure of choice for females with mental retardation and parental satisfaction with the procedure has been well documented (Kaunitz, Thompson, & Kaunitz, 1986; Wheeless, 1975). However, hysterectomy does nothing to prevent sexual abuse, the fear of which is one of the most common reasons for the request for hysterectomy (Elkins, Gafford, Wilks, Muram, & Golden, 1986). Although obviously curative for menstrual hygiene problems, much less harmful ways of controlling menses clearly exist through hormonal preparations and patient education. Furthermore, careful consideration must be given to the medical risks of performing surgery on persons with mental retardation, who often have a multitude of associated medical problems (McNeeley & Elkins, 1989). For these reasons, sterilizations (even by laparoscopic tubal procedures) are rarely performed at the University of Michigan, where an advocacy-based committee assists physicians in making the decision to perform such operations (Elkins, Hoyle, Darnton, McNeeley, & Heaton, 1988).

CONCLUSION

There are many gynecologic issues that have not been studied thoroughly in females with Down syndrome. Many of these reflect the progressive advances of the population of persons with Down syndrome. For example, how should menopause be managed for women with Down syndrome? Would estrogen replacement therapy improve the mental status of menopausal women with Alzheimer disease? Questions surrounding marriage, childbearing, and parenting arise only rarely—but how commonly will they occur in the decades ahead?

These are only a few of the many issues that await those who are called upon to provide gynecologic care for females with Down syndrome. It is hoped that the next 20 years will mark a new era of advances in gynecologic care for females with Down syndrome.

REFERENCES

American Cancer Society. (1980). Guidelines for the cancer-related checkup: Recommendations and rationale. *Cancer, 30,* 195–230.

American College of Obstetricians and Gynecologists. (1989). *Report of Task Force on Routine Cancer Screening.* Washington, DC: Author.

American College of Obstetricians and Gynecologists Committee on Ethics. (1988, September). *Committee opinion: Sterilization of women who are mentally handicapped* (Number 63). Washington, DC: Author.

Anderson, A.B.M., Guillebaud, J., Haynes, P.J., & Turnbull, A.C. (1976). Reduction of menstrual blood loss by prostaglandin synthetase inhibitors. *Lancet, i,* 774.

Bovicelli, L., Orsini, L.F., Rizzo, N., Montacut, V., & Bacchetta, M. (1982). Reproduction in Down syndrome. *Obstetrics and Gynecology, 59,* 13S–16S.

Buck v. Bell, 274 U.S. 200 (1927).

Chamberlain, A., Rauh, J., Passer, A., McGrath, M., & Burket, R. (1984). Issues in fertility control for mentally retarded female adolescents: I. Sexual activity, sexual abuse, and contraception. *Pediatrics, 73,* 445–449.

Derman, R. (1986). Oral contraceptives: Assessment of benefits. *Journal of Reproductive Medicine, 31,* 879–885.

Elkins, T.E. (1991). Unpublished raw data.

Elkins, T.E., Gafford, L.S., Wilks, C.S., Muram, D., & Golden, G. (1986). A model clinic approach to the reproductive health concerns of the mentally handicapped. *Obstetrics and Gynecology, 68,* 185–189.

Elkins, T.E., Hoyle, D., Darnton, T., McNeeley, S.G., & Heaton, C.S. (1988). The use of a societally based ethics/advisory committee to aid in decisions to sterilize mentally handicapped patients. *Adolescent and Pediatric Gynecology, 1,* 190–194.

Elkins, T.E., McNeeley, S.G., Punch, M., Kope, S., & Heaton, C. (1990). Reproductive health concerns in Down syndrome: A report of eight cases. *Journal of Reproductive Medicine, 35*(7), 745–750.

Elkins, T.E., McNeeley, S.G., Rosen, D.A., Heaton, C., Sorg, C., DeLancey, J.O.L., & Kope, S.

(1988). A clinical observation of a program to accomplish pelvic exams in difficult-to-manage patients with mental retardation. *Adolescent and Pediatric Gynecology, 1,* 195–198.

Elkins, T., Spinnato, J., & Muram, D. (1987). Sexuality and family interaction in Down syndrome: Parental responses. *Journal of Psychosomatic Obstetrics and Gynecology, 6,* 81–85.

Fishman, J., Boyar, R.M., & Hellman, L. (1975). Influence of body weight on estradiol metabolism. *Journal of Clinical Endocrinology and Metabolism, 41,* 989–992.

Frisch, R.E., & Revelle, R. (1970). Height and weight at menarche and a hypothesis of critical body weights and adolescent events. *Science, 169,* 397–399.

Ghaziuddin, M., Elkins, T.E., & Kope, S. (1990, April). *PMS in persons with mental retardation.* Paper presented at the Annual Meeting of the American Society of Psychosomatic Obstetrics and Gynecology, Houston.

Hamilton, J., Allen, P., Stephens, S., & Davall, E. (1969). Training mentally retarded females to use sanitary napkins. *Mental Retardation, 7,* 40–43.

Harris, R.W.C. (1980). Characteristics of women with dysplasia or carcinoma in situe of the cervix uteri. *British Journal of Cancer, 42,* 359–369.

Judd, H.L. (1978). Endocrinology of polycystic ovarian disease. *Clinical Obstetrics and Gynecology, 21,* 98–108.

Kaunitz, A.M., Thompson, R.F., & Kaunitz, K.K. (1986). Mental retardation: A controversial indication for hysterectomy. *Obstetrics and Gynecology, 68,* 436–438.

Kreutner, A.K. (1981). Sexuality, fertility, and the problems of menstruation in mentally retarded adolescents. *Pediatric Clinics of North America, 28,* 475–485.

McNeeley, S.G., & Elkins, T.E. (1989). Gynecologic surgery and surgical morbidity in mentally handicapped women. *Obstetrics and Gynecology, 74,* 155–159.

Minihan, P.M., & Dean, D.H. (1990). Meeting the needs for health services of persons with mental retardation living in the community. *American Journal of Public Health, 80*(9), 1043–1048.

Mishell, D.R. (1987). Abnormal uterine bleeding. In W. Droegmueller, A.L. Herbst, D.R. Mishell, & M.A. Stenchever (Eds.), *Comprehensive gynecology* (pp. 953–964). St. Louis: C.V. Mosby.

Mosier, H.D., Grossman, H.J., & Dingman, H.F. (1968). Secondary sex development in mentally deficient individuals. *Child Development, 33,* 271–286.

Murdoch, J.C., Ratcliff, W.A., McLarty, D.G., Rodger, J.C., & Ratcliff, J.G. (1977). Thyroid function in adults with Down syndrome. *Journal of Clinical Endocrinology and Metabolism, 44,* 453–458.

Nash, H.A. (1975). Depo-Provera: A review. *Contraception, 12,* 377.

O'Brien, P. (1985). PMS: The premenstrual syndrome: A review. *Journal of Reproductive Medicine, 30,* 113–118.

Ory, H.W. (1982). The noncontraceptive health benefits from oral contraceptive use. *Family Planning Perspectives, 14,* 182–187.

Pattulo, A.W., & Bernard, K.E. (1968). Teaching menstrual hygiene to the mentally retarded. *American Journal of Nursing, 68,* 2572–2575.

Pueschel, S.M., Canning, C.D., Murphy, A., & Zausmer, E. (1980). *Down syndrome: Growing and learning.* Kansas City: Andrews & McMeel.

Pueschel, S.M., & Scola, P.S. (1988). Parents' perception of social and sexual functions in adolescents with Down syndrome. *Journal of Mental Deficiency Research, 32,* 215–218.

Rani, A.S., Jyothi, A., Reddy, P.P., & Reddy, O.S. (1990). Reproduction in Down's syndrome. *International Journal of Gynecology and Obstetrics, 31,* 81–86.

Relf v. Weinberger, 372 F. Supp. 1196 (D.D.C. 1974).

Rosen, D.A., Rosen, K.R., Elkins, T.E., McNeeley, S.G., Heaton, C.J., Sorg, C., & Andersen, H.F. (1990). Ketamine clinic: A model clinic for sedation of mentally handicapped patients undergoing routine gynecologic examinations. In E.F. Domino (Ed.), *Status of ketamine in anesthesiology* (pp. 337–342). Ann Arbor, MI: NPP Books.

Salerno, L.J., Park, J.K., & Giannini, M.J. (1975). Reproductive capacity of the mentally retarded. *Journal of Reproductive Medicine, 143,* 123–129.

Sandmire, H.F., & Cavanaugh, R.A. (1985). Long-term use of intrauterine contraceptive devices in a private practice. *American Journal of Obstetrics and Gynecology, 152,* 169–172.

Scommegna, A., & Dmowski, W.P. (1973). Dysfunctional uterine bleeding. *Clinical Obstetrics and Gynecology, 16,* 221–226.

Skinner v. Oklahoma, 316 U.S. 535 (1942).

Tricomi, V., Valenti, C., & Hall, J.E. (1964). Ovulatory patterns in Down syndrome. *American Journal of Obstetrics and Gynecology, 89,* 651–656.

Walton, R.J., Blanchet, M., Boyes, D.A., Carmichael, J.A., Marshall, K.G., Miller, A.B., Thompson, D.W., & Hill, G.B. (1976). Cervical cancer screening programs. *Canadian Medical Association Journal, 114,* 1003–1033.

Wheeless, C.R. (1975). Abdominal hysterectomy for surgical sterilization in the mentally retarded: A review of parental opinion. *American Journal of Obstetrics and Gynecology, 122,* 872–876.

CHAPTER
15

Musculoskeletal Disorders

Siegfried M. Pueschel and Patricia M. Solga

Numerous musculoskeletal abnormalities have been reported in individuals with Down syndrome. Common problems that may cause significant morbidity are subluxation and dislocation of the cervical spine, hip, and patella. Cervical spine instability at the atlanto-occipital and the atlantoaxial region is one of the potentially most serious orthopedic conditions encountered in persons with Down syndrome. Also, severe scoliosis can cause cardiopulmonary failure, and recurrent patella or hip dislocation may result in significant pain and impair ambulation. Moreover, collapsing flat feet and severe bunion deformity may cause marked discomfort. Most of these problems have been attributed to the generalized ligamentous laxity observed in persons with Down syndrome. Joint capsules, tendons, and ligaments are lax because of the aberrant structure of the underlying biologic material, namely collagen.

Several investigators have attempted to provide an explanation for the ligamentous laxity in persons with Down syndrome. Martel and Tishler (1966) suggested that persons with Down syndrome have a congenital weakness of ligaments. Pueschel, Scola, Perry, and Pezzullo (1981) postulated that children with Down syndrome have an intrinsic defect of their connective tissue that is responsible for the observed general ligamentous laxity. Support for this hypothesis is derived from biochemical studies of tendons from children with Down syndrome that revealed significant abnormalities of the collagen structure. More recently it has been shown that fetal heart collagen is encoded by two genes mapped to the "Down syndrome region" of chromosome 21 (Duff, Williamson, & Richards,

1990). These two genes encode for two chains of collagen type VI molecule during human fetal heart development. It is probable that ligamentous collagen of the musculoskeletal system is either encoded for by the same genes or by other gene(s) on chromosome 21, which if present in triple dosage result in ligamentous laxity, a consistent feature in persons with Down syndrome.

SPINE

Atlanto-occipital Instability

Although many reports have been published on atlantoaxial instability, atlanto-occipital instability in persons with Down syndrome has been mentioned less often in the literature (Brooke, Burkus, & Benson, 1987; Collacott, Ellison, Harper, Newland, & Ray-Chaudhurt, 1989; El-Khoury et al., 1986; Holmes & Hall, 1978; Hungerford, Akkaraju, Rawe, & Young, 1981; Rosenbaum, Blumhagen, & King, 1986). Recently, Tredwell, Newman, and Lockitch (1990) studied 64 children with Down syndrome and found that 43 (61.4%) of the children displayed posterior subluxation in extension. In another study, Gabriel, Mason, and Carango (1990) examined the lateral cervical spine radiographs of 73 persons with Down syndrome. Twenty-seven (37%) showed "anterior posterior translation" of 1 mm or less. None of these 27 had evidence of impaired neurologic functions related to cervical spine instability. Powers et al. (in press) examined 1,228 radiographs of 210 persons with Down syndrome and compared them to 196 radiographs in the control group. They found that 8.5% of the persons with Down syndrome had atlanto-occipital instability; these individuals had a Powers ratio (the ratio between the measured distance from the basion to the anterior surface of the posterior arch of C-1 and the measured distance from the opisthion to the posterior surface of the anterior arch of the C-1 [Powers, Miller, Kramer, Martinez, & Gehweiler, 1979]) of less than 0.55, which is indicative of posterior atlanto-occipital instability. If the bisecting line of the odontoid process is used as the criterion for having posterior atlanto-occipital instability, then 16.5% of children with Down syndrome have this condition (Powers et al., in press).

The discrepancy of the different results is due mainly to variation in methodology and the lack of a definition of what constitutes atlanto-occipital instability. Tredwell et al. (1990) measured the atlanto-occipital relationship as the distance between the anterior margin of the condyles at the base of the skull and the sharp contour of the anterior aspect of the concave joint of the atlas. Gabriel et al. (1990) showed the translational anterior-posterior motion on each side of flexion and extension using the method described by Wiesel, Kraus, and Rothman (1978). Powers et al. (in press) used three different approaches: 1) the dens-basion distance, 2) the perpendicular distance between the basion and the bisecting line of the odontoid process, and 3) the Powers ratio. Although standardized radiographic criteria for the evaluation of the atlanto-occipital joint have not been developed, Powers et al. (in press) found the Powers ratio to be the most reliable radiographic parameter for assessment of atlanto-occipital instability. It yields very consistent values in "normal" persons regardless of neck position and, in addition, it is unaffected by radiographic magnifications.

Based on the results obtained by Tredwell et al. (1990), Gabriel et al. (1990), and Powers et al. (in press), we must presume that, in spite of only a few case reports in the literature, instability at the atlanto-occipital joint is not uncommon in persons with Down syndrome. Atlanto-occipital instability, in addition to the well-documented instability at the atlanto-dens level, must be taken into consideration when reviewing cervical spine radiographs.

Atlantoaxial Instability

Atlantoaxial instability is considered to be present when the atlanto-dens interval is ≥ 5 mm (see Figures 15.1 and 15.2). As in atlanto-occipital instability, atlantoaxial instability in individuals with Down syndrome is primarily due to ligamentous laxity. In atlantoaxial instability, the transverse ligaments that ordinarily hold the odontoid process close to the anterior arch of the atlas are primarily involved.

Although the earliest report of atlantoaxial subluxation dates back some 4,500–5,000 years when Edwin Smith Papyrus described a person's displacement of the cervical vertebra (Power D'Arcy, 1933), atlantoaxial instability in persons with Down syndrome was first reported by Spitzer, Rabinowich, and Wybar in 1961. Since then, several epidemiologic studies have been published on the prevalence of atlantoaxial instability in persons with Down syndrome. It has been estimated that the frequency of this disorder is between 9%–30% (Alvarez & Rubin, 1986; Jagjivan, Spencer, & Hosking, 1988; Martel & Tishler, 1966; Miller, Capusten, & Lampard, 1986; Pueschel & Scola, 1987; Pueschel et al., 1981; Semine, Ertel, Goldberg, & Bull, 1978; Spitzer et al., 1961; Tishler & Martel, 1965; Van Dyke & Gahagan, 1988). In addition, numerous case reports have appeared in the medical literature since the early 1960s (Andrews, 1981; Aoki, 1988; Aung, 1973; Beltran, 1970; Braakhekke et al., 1985; Chaudhry, Sturgeon, Gates, & Myers, 1987; Curtis, Blank, & Fisher, 1968; Finerman, Sakai, & Weingarten, 1976; Gerard, Segal, & Bedoucha, 1971; Giblin & Micheli, 1979; Grobovschek & Strohecker, 1985; Herring, 1982; Hreidarsson, Magram, & Singer, 1982; Hungerford et al., 1981; Khoury, Clark, & Wroble, 1985; Kobori, Takahashi, & Mikawa, 1986; Martel, Uyham, & Stimson, 1969; Moore, McNicholas, & Warran, 1987; Nordt & Stauffer, 1981; Powell, Woodcock, & Luscombe, 1990; Sherk & Nicholson, 1969; Shield, Dickens, & Jensen, 1981; Shikata, Yamamuro, Mikawa, Iida, & Kobori, 1989; Storm, 1986; Thalmann, Scholl, & Tonz, 1972; Whayley & Gray, 1980).

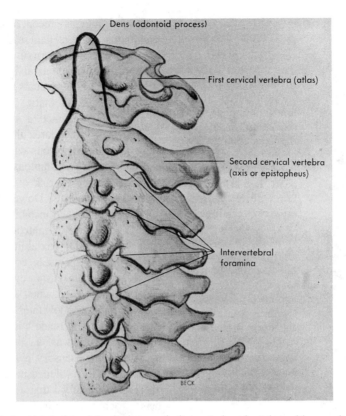

Figure 15.1.   Cervical spine. Note the interrelationship between the first cervical vertebra (atlas) and the second cervical vertebra (axis).

Pueschel and Scola (1987) examined 404 persons with Down syndrome and observed their atlanto-dens intervals and spinal canal widths to be significantly different from children without Down syndrome. Significant differences were also noted between boys and girls with Down syndrome in spinal canal width assessments, but not in atlanto-dens interval measurements. When different neck positions were compared, measurements obtained in flexion were significantly greater than in extension or in neutral position. In addition, more persons had ≥ 5 mm atlanto-dens interval measurements in flexion than in extension or neutral. A total of 59 (14.6%) of 404 persons displayed atlantoaxial instability. Fifty-three (13.1%) persons had asymptomatic atlantoaxial instability, and special precautions will have to be taken with this group of children. Six (1.5%) individuals with symptomatic atlantoaxial instability underwent surgery to prevent further injury to the spinal cord.

Because some of their subjects with symptomatic atlantoaxial instability were remarkably incapacitated and had severe neurologic symptoms, Pueschel et al. (1984) studied the literature and uncovered 42 well-documented cases of symptomatic atlantoaxial subluxation in persons with Down syndrome. Since then, other individuals with symptomatic atlantoaxial instability have been reported and, at this writing, there are more than 70 individuals with Down syndrome and symptomatic atlantoaxial subluxation reported in the literature. Pueschel et al. (1984) observed that there was a preponderance of females; the male-to-female ratio being 1:3.2. The mean age of the onset of symptoms of the 42 individuals was 10.5 years. These persons exhibited a variety of symptoms compatible with spinal cord injury including brisk deep tendon

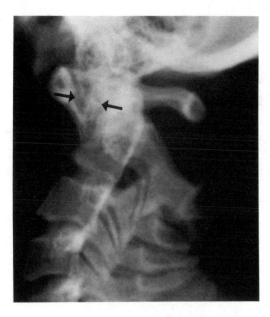

Figure 15.2. X ray of a lateral view of the upper cervical spine indicating with arrows the wide separation between the anterior arch of the atlas and the odontoid process with concurrent narrowing of the spinal canal. This person has significant atlantoaxial instability.

reflexes (64%), extensor plantar responses (52%), ankle clonus (40%), and quadri-, hemi-, or paraplegia (52%). Additional complaints included muscle weakness (52%), gait abnormalities (43%), and difficulties walking (40%). Furthermore, about one third displayed local symptoms with neck pain, limited neck mobility, and head tilt. It is of note that 17% had sustained an injury to the cervical spine, which either had caused atlantoaxial subluxation leading to neurologic symptoms or was a contributing factor augmenting the pre-existing symptoms. All but 7 of the 42 individuals reviewed underwent surgery. The main goal of the surgical procedure is to reduce the atlantoaxial subluxation as much as possible and to stabilize the upper segment of the cervical spine. Using posterior cervical spine fusion by applying wires at the upper cervical vertebra and posterior application of autogenous bone graft, Pueschel et al. (1984) observed that patients with long-standing symptoms and marked neurologic damage showed little or no improvement postoperatively. However,

patients with a more recent onset of this disorder usually made an excellent recovery after surgery.

The primary concern in persons who have asymptomatic atlantoaxial instability is identification of those individuals who are at high risk of becoming symptomatic. Therefore, Pueschel et al. (1987) designed a study to investigate methods and procedures that will identify as early as possible persons with Down syndrome and asymptomatic atlantoaxial instability who are at an increased risk of spinal cord injury. When 27 persons with Down syndrome who did not have atlantoaxial instability were compared with an age- and sex-matched group of 27 persons who had atlantoaxial instability, no significant difference in mean composite neurologic scores and somatosensory evoked responses was observed. However, when a subsample of persons with high and low latencies was formed and comparisons were made with roentgenographic findings, there was a high correspondence between somatosensory evoked potentials and atlanto-dens interval measurements. Pueschel et al. (1987) concluded that a combined approach using roentgenographic, computerized tomographic (CT) scan, neurologic, and neurophysiologic investigations will provide information on the risk status of persons with Down syndrome and atlantoaxial instability.

Recently, Pueschel, Scola, and Pezzullo (in press) enrolled 141 individuals in a longitudinal follow-up study. The results of the atlanto-dens interval measurements of successive radiologic examinations were analyzed using repeated measures of analyses of variance. No significant changes over time were noted. The vast majority of persons had only minor changes of atlanto-dens interval measurements comparing the various examinations. In 11 persons (8%), however, marked changes over time were observed (2 mm–4 mm). Whereas 9 of these persons initially had atlantoaxial instability, in subsequent examinations the atlanto-dens interval was found to be within the normal range; 2 persons who initially had normal measurements were noted to have a marked increase (≥ 5 mm) in follow-up examinations. None of these persons with marked changes of their atlanto-dens interval displayed clinical symptoms on physical examinations and all functioned neurologically within normal limits.

Based on these investigations, Pueschel et al. (in press) proposed that children with Down syndrome should undergo radiologic examination of the cervical spine starting at the age of 2½–3 years and a repeat roentgenographic examination should take place at about the age of 8–9 years, when many children may be entering Special Olympics or other similar sports activities. Those children who have asymptomatic atlantoaxial instability probably should not participate in any sports activities that potentially could injure the neck. Special Olympics Inc., has developed a list of such sport activities that persons with Down syndrome and atlantoaxial instability should avoid (Table 15.1).

It is important that these children be followed closely. The parents should report to the child's physician both local symptoms such as neck discomfort and neuromuscular dysfunction such as gait abnormalities, if they should occur. These children should have annual neurologic examinations and probably biannual radiologic assessments. Persons with atlanto-dens intervals of ≥ 7 mm are at a great risk of developing symptomatic atlantoaxial instability and should be re-examined more often. If symptoms of spinal cord compression are identified either clinically or by a CT scan or magnetic resonance imaging (MRI), then surgical intervention should be considered.

Skeletal Anomalies of the Upper Cervical Spine

Pueschel, Scola, Tupper, and Pezzullo (1990) found that a significant number of children with Down syndrome and atlantoaxial instability have cervical spine anomalies when compared with an age- and sex-matched control group. This suggests that cervical spine anomalies may be a contributing factor in the pathogenesis of atlantoaxial instability. Other investigators also have noted abnormalities of the odontoid process or other skeletal structures of the C1-C2 region in person with Down syndrome (Coria, Quintana, Villalba, Rebollo, & Berciano, 1983; Daw-

Table 15.1. Restriction on participation of sports activities by individuals with Down syndrome with atlantoaxial instability

Training or competition in gymnastics
Diving
Diving start in swimming
Butterfly stroke in swimming
High jump
Pentathlon
Soccer
Alpine skiing
Warm-up exercises placing pressure on head and neck

son & Smith, 1979; Fielding & Griffin, 1974; Finerman et al., 1976; Martel & Tishler, 1966; Roach, Duncan, Wenger, Maravilla, & Maravilla, 1984; Semine et al., 1978).

Other Cervical Spine Abnormalities

Olive, Whitecloud, and Bennett (1988) indicated that, in addition to upper cervical spine problems, attention should also be paid to problems in other parts of the cervical spine. These investigators found an increased prevalence of lower cervical spine spondylosis that significantly correlated with physical findings consistent with cervical myelopathy. Therefore, the authors emphasized the importance of close monitoring of neurologic functions. Flexion and extension lateral radiographs of the cervical spine should be obtained not only to evaluate the C1-C2 area, but also to look for degenerative changes in the lower cervical spine.

Fidone (1986) reported that 16 of 42 persons with Down syndrome had various degrees of degenerative arthritis of the cervical vertebrae and intervertebral disks. The degenerative changes included osteophyte formation, subarticular sclerosis, cystic changes, fusion, and disk narrowing. Although the youngest person with such degenerative changes was only 21 years of age, the majority of degenerative changes were noted with an increased frequency in older persons with Down syndrome. Also, Miller et al. (1986) reported a high prevalence of degenerative changes at the C2-C3 and C3-C4 cervical spine interspaces, especially in persons over the age of 37 years. Four persons demonstrated cervical spine subluxation at interspaces other than C1-C2 and 6 had congenital fusion of either vertebral bodies or facets in the cervical region.

Scoliosis

Poor posture, poor paraspinal muscle tone, and ligamentous laxity may cause scoliosis. There is a wide spectrum in prevalence and severity of scoliosis that is similar to the spectrum of cardiac involvement and mental retardation found in persons with Down syndrome. It has been estimated that over 50% of persons with Down syndrome have thoracic or lumbar scoliosis (Diamond, Lynne, & Sigman, 1981). It should be emphasized that such a high prevalence of scoliosis was observed in persons with Down syndrome residing in an institution. Ordinarily, this musculoskeletal disorder is noted less often in individuals living in the community. For example, only 4.3% of patients with Down syndrome who were admitted to an acute care facility had scoliosis (Diamond et al., 1981).

If scoliosis is present in individuals with Down syndrome, it usually occurs in the thoracolumbar region and is of a mild degree. Bracing is usually not successful in preventing progression of scoliosis. Only rarely will a severe curve develop, necessitating surgical intervention that involves posterior spinal fusion.

HIP

It is uncommon to find congenital dislocation of the hip in the newborn with Down syndrome (Bennet, Rang, Roye, & Aprin, 1982). The acetabulum is usually deep and the acetabular angle is reduced. The child under 2 years of age will usually have equal internal and external rotation of the hips, often up to 90°. Between the ages of 2–10 years, the hip can spontaneously dislocate and reduce without antecedent trauma and with few symptoms. A sudden limp or reluctance to bear weight may be the only sign of hip dislocation. Therefore, a routine examination of the hips should be an essential part of the physical examination, especially in early childhood and adolescence. Approximately 1%–4% of chil-

dren with Down syndrome will have unstable hips (Aprin, Zink, & Hall, 1985).

If hip dislocation has been diagnosed, the hip should be reduced under a general anesthesia. Unfortunately, conservative treatment including closed reduction and immobilization in a spica cast usually will not be successful in preventing redislocation. However, a surgical procedure such as tightening the hip capsule (Gore, 1981) has been shown to prevent future dislocations. If the hip has suffered recurrent dislocations, a bony procedure is usually necessary to correct the architecture of the acetabulum that has been distorted by recurrent dislocations. Acetabular coverage can be improved by performing a pelvic osteotomy. Persistent femoral anteversion may also contribute to the tendency to dislocate. This rotational deformity can be corrected using a varus derotation osteotomy of the proximal femur. A combination of these procedures may be needed to treat the dislocated hip successfully (Aprin et al., 1985; Bennet et al., 1982). Treating a painful hip in the adult with Down syndrome often requires total hip replacement (Skoff & Keggi, 1987).

KNEE

As in the hip, the spectrum of instability of the patellofemoral joint ranges from asymptomatic subluxation to irreducible dislocation (Diamond et al., 1981). However, patella instability is a more common problem than hip instability, affecting close to 20% of individuals with Down syndrome.

Most persons with patellofemoral instability who have full range of motion can walk well. However, some individuals will develop flexion deformities if the chronically dislocated patella causes the quadriceps mechanism to act as a knee flexor. Although moderate to severe patellofemoral instability is usually well tolerated, Dugdale and Renshaw (1986) reported 2 children with Down syndrome with significant functional limitations in walking. A classification of patellofemoral instability was devised in a study of over 350 persons with Down syndrome (Dugdale & Renshaw, 1986): from grade I, no evidence of dislocation, to grade V, the chronically dislocated, irreducible patella. As expected, the largest number of individuals were found to have no instability or mild instability of the patellofemoral joint.

Some controversy exists as to whether individuals who have unstable patellofemoral joints should be treated surgically. Bracing has not been found to be effective. In chronically dislocated joints, subsequent deformities are quite common. However, gait analysis reveals that these persons are able to adapt their gait to walk safely (Dugdale & Renshaw, 1986). Surgical treatment consists of releasing the right lateral retinaculum imbricating the medial capsule of the knee and advancing the vastus medialis. Severe cases necessitate the transfer of part or all of the patellar tendon (Mendez, Keret, & MacEwen, 1988).

FOOT

Flat foot deformity secondary to ligamentous laxity is observed in more than 90% of persons with Down syndrome. The wide-based gait and the tendency to rotate the foot and ankle externally also contribute to the pronation and the collapse of the midfoot (Diamond et al., 1981). Moderately flat feet that are painful may respond to treatment with orthotics. In the very young child who has just started walking, an ankle–foot orthosis may provide stability and assist with ambulation. Shoe inserts or custom foot orthoses with a well-molded heel, such as the University of California at Berkeley Splint, can be used with the older child.

Severely symptomatic flat feet may require surgery. Examination will usually reveal that the person is bearing weight on the pronated talar head. Radiographs may show subtalar arthritis and talar beaking. Since a bony deformity is most often present in these individuals, soft tissue procedures will not correct the problem. A subtalar or triple arthrodesis can stabilize the foot and relieve pain as well as prevent progression of the deformity. The individual should be approaching skeletal maturity when the decision to perform an arthrodesis is made so that the foot will not be left small with no further growth potential. The importance of treatment of this disorder is to ensure independent ambulation. If not treated appropriately, impairment of walking will compromise activities of daily living and will restrict function in the community. In addition, any compromise of mobility may add to the problem of obesity in some persons with Down syndrome.

ARTHROPATHY

There are several reports in the literature describing a juvenile rheumatoid arthritis–like arthropathy in young individuals with Down syndrome. Five case reports of juvenile rheumatoid arthritis in children with Down syndrome have been published in relation to cervical spine abnormalities (Alspaugh & Miller, 1977; Andrews, 1981; Herring, 1982; Sherk, Pasquariello, & Watters, 1982; Thalmann et al., 1972). The arthritic involvement in these children preceded the event of atlantoaxial subluxation, a phenomenon that had been observed previously in individuals with rheumatoid arthritis who did not have Down syndrome. In a recent publication, Olson, Bender, Levinson, Oestreich, and Lovell (1990) discussed ligamentous laxity and joint subluxation in relation to arthritis in children with Down syndrome. The authors indicated that 4 of their 9 patients and 8 of 12 individuals with Down syndrome and arthritis described by other investigators developed various subluxations. Although the most common subluxation occurred in the upper cervical spine, subluxations in other joints such as hands and feet as well as knees and hips were also observed.

Olson et al. (1990) and Yancey, Zmijewski, Athreya, and Doughty (1984) described the rheumatoid arthritis–like arthropathy in persons with Down syndrome in more detail. Their patients displayed polyarthritis existing for over 6 weeks, which was often associated with an elevated erythrocyte sedimentation rate and inflammatory joint fluid. Most of these patients had a progressive course with polyarticular disease complicated by subluxations and a long lag time to diagnosis. The authors were not sure whether the observed arthritis in these individuals with Down syndrome represents a form of juvenile rheumatoid arthritis or whether this is a unique arthropathy only seen in these patients because of the genetic and immunologic abnormalities associated with Down syndrome.

Concerning therapeutic approaches, Olson et al. (1990) mentioned that the arthritis in persons with Down syndrome is often severe and progressive enough to require the use of "second line disease modifying agents" (p. 935). They found that individuals with Down syndrome appear to be more sensitive to some medications as they observed four severe bleeding episodes in 3 of the patients treated with nonsteroidal anti-inflammatory medications.

In 1988, Dacre and Huskisson reported a young man with Down syndrome who had a 10-year history of pain in large joints, particularly in the left elbow, knee, and ankle. The inflammatory polyarthritis resembled juvenile chronic arthritis. However, further investigations noted that his serum uric acid level was significantly increased and that his arthritis was due to gout. The authors emphasized the importance of serum uric acid determination in persons with Down syndrome and coexisting arthritis.

If one compares the chance occurrence of both Down syndrome and chronic juvenile arthritis with the observed data (Yancey et al., 1984), it appears that there is a significantly increased prevalence of arthropathy in persons

with Down syndrome. This may be due to both genetic and immunologic factors.

CONCLUSION

The philosophy of caring for individuals with Down syndrome has evolved into one of promotion of function and independence. When examining persons with Down syndrome, the physician should be aware of the fact that there are various skeletal disorders and orthopedic concerns that need to be taken into consideration. In particular, individuals who have extreme hyperflexibility; those who complain of neck discomfort; those with neurologic involvement and hip, knee, or foot problems; and those with arthritic symptoms resulting in significant disability should be carefully evaluated. It is well known that severe cervical spine pathology may have life-threatening consequences. Likewise, chronic instability of hips, knees, and other joints as well as arthritis may incapacitate the individual's functioning and cause significant morbidity. Persons with Down syndrome who are found to have such musculoskeletal disorders should be provided with optimal medical care and surgical intervention that will ultimately result in a better quality of life. Since most orthopedic concerns in persons with Down syndrome are due to an abnormality of the collagen structure, future molecular genetic studies that will identify genes on chromosome 21 coding for protein(s) involved in the synthesis and production of collagen should result in a better understanding of the underlying pathogenetic mechanisms and may potentially lead to therapeutic interventions.

REFERENCES

Alspaugh, M.A., & Miller, J.J. (1977). A study of specificities of antinuclear antibodies in juvenile rheumatoid arthritis. *Journal of Pediatrics, 90,* 391–395.

Alvarez, N., & Rubin, L. (1986). Atlantoaxial instability in adults with Down syndrome: A clinical and radiological survey. *Applied Research in Mental Retardation, 7,* 67–78.

Andrews, L.G. (1981). Myelopathy due to atlantoaxial dislocation in a patient with Down syndrome and rheumatoid arthritis. *Developmental Medicine and Child Neurology, 23,* 356–360.

Aoki, N. (1988). Atlantoaxial dislocation presenting as sudden onset of quadriplegia in Down's syndrome. *Surgical Neurology, 30,* 153–155.

Aprin, H., Zink, W.P., & Hall, J.E. (1985). Management of dislocation of the hip in Down syndrome. *Journal of Pediatric Orthopedics, 5,* 428–431.

Aung, M.H. (1973). Atlanto-axial dislocation in Down's syndrome: Report of a case with spinal cord compression and review of the literature. *Bulletin of the Los Angeles Neurological Societies, 38,* 197–201.

Beltran, P. (1970). *La dislocation atlanto-axoidienne*

[Atlantoaxial dislocation]. Sandoz de Mexico: Author.

Bennet, G.C., Rang, M., Roye, D.P., & Aprin, H. (1982). Dislocation of the hip in trisomy 21. *Journal of Bone and Joint Surgery, 64*, 289–294.

Braakhekke, J.P., Gabreëls, F.J.M., Renier, W.O., vanRens, T.J.G., Thijssen, H.O.M., & Begeer, J.H. (1985). Craniovertebral pathology in Down syndrome. *Clinical Neurology and Neurosurgery, 87*, 173–179.

Brooke, D.C., Burkus, J.K., & Benson, D.R. (1987). Asymptomatic occipitoatlantal instability in Down syndrome (trisomy 21): Report of two cases in children. *Journal of Bone and Joint Surgery, 69*, 239–295.

Chaudhry, V., Sturgeon, C., Gates, A.J., & Myers, G. (1987). Symptomatic atlantoaxial dislocation in Down's syndrome. *Annals of Neurology, 21*, 606–609.

Collacott, R.A., Ellison, D., Harper, W., Newland, C., & Ray-Chaudhurt, K. (1989). Atlanto-occipital instability in Down's syndrome: Case report. *Journal of Mental Deficiency Research, 33*, 499–505.

Coria, R., Quintana, F., Villalba, M., Rebollo, M., & Berciano, J. (1983). Craniocervical abnormalities in Down's syndrome. *Developmental Medicine and Child Neurology, 25*, 252–255.

Curtis, B.H., Blank, S., & Fisher, R.L. (1968). Atlanto-axial dislocation in Down's syndrome: Report of two patients requiring surgical correction. *Journal of the American Medical Association, 205*, 212–213.

Dacre, J.E., & Huskisson, E.C. (1988). Arthritis in Down's syndrome. *Annals of the Rheumatic Diseases, 47*, 254–255.

Dawson, E.G., & Smith, L. (1979). Atlanto-axial subluxation in children due to vertebral anomalies. *Journal of Bone and Joint Surgery, 61*, 582–587.

Diamond, L.S., Lynne, D., & Sigman, B. (1981). Orthopedic disorders in patients with Down's syndrome. *Orthopedic Clinics of North America, 12*, 57–71.

Duff, K., Williamson, R., & Richards, S.J. (1990). Expression of genes encoding two chains of the collagen type VI molecule during human fetal heart development. *International Journal of Cardiology, 27*, 128–129.

Dugdale, T.W., & Renshaw, T.S. (1986). Instability of the patellofemoral joint in Down syndrome. *Journal of Bone and Joint Surgery, 68*, 405–413.

El-Khoury, G.Y., Clark, C.R., Dietz, F.R., Harre, R.G., Tozzi, J.E., & Kathol, M.H. (1986). Posterior atlantooccipital subluxation in Down syndrome. *Radiology, 15*, 507–509.

Fidone, G.S. (1986). Degenerative cervical arthritis and Down syndrome. *New England Journal of Medicine, 314*, 320.

Fielding, J.W., & Griffin, P.P. (1974). Os odontoideum: An acquired lesion. *Journal of Bone and Joint Surgery, 56*, 187–190.

Finerman, G.A.M., Sakai, D., & Weingarten, S. (1976). Atlanto-axial dislocation with spinal cord compression in a mongoloid child: A case report. *Journal of Bone and Joint Surgery, 58*, 408–409.

Gabriel, K.R., Mason, D.E., & Carango, P. (1990). Occipito-atlantal translation in Down's syndrome. *Spine, 15*, 997–1002.

Gerard, Y., Segal, P., & Bedoucha, J.S. (1971). L'instabilite de l'atlas sur l'axis dans le mongolisme [Instability of the atlantoaxial joint in mongolism]. *La Presse Medicale, 13*, 573–576.

Giblin, P.E., & Micheli, L.J. (1979). The management of atlanto-axial subluxation with neurologic involvement in Down syndrome. *Clinical Orthopedics, 140*, 66–71.

Gore, D.R. (1981). Recurrent dislocation of the hip in a child with Down's syndrome. *Journal of Bone and Joint Surgery, 63*, 823–825.

Grobovschek, M., & Strohecker, J. (1985). Congenital atlanto-axial subluxation in Down's syndrome. *Neuroradiology, 27*, 186–192.

Herring, J.A. (1982). Cervical instability in Down's syndrome and juvenile rheumatoid arthritis. *Journal of Pediatric Orthopedics, 2*, 205–207.

Holmes, J.C., & Hall, J.E. (1978). Fusion for instability and potential instability of the cervical spine in children and adolescents. *Orthopedic Clinics of North America, 9*, 923–943.

Hreidarsson, S., Magram, G., & Singer, H. (1982). Symptomatic atlantoaxial dislocation in Down syndrome. *Pediatrics, 69*, 568–571.

Hungerford, G.D., Akkaraju, V., Rawe, S.E., & Young, G.F. (1981). Atlanto-occipital and atlanto-axial dislocations with spinal cord compression in Down syndrome: A case report and review of the literature. *British Journal of Radiology, 54*, 758–761.

Jagjivan, B., Spencer, P.A.S., & Hosking, G. (1988). Radiological screening for atlanto-axial instability in Down's syndrome. *Clinical Radiology, 39*, 661–663.

Khoury, G.Y., Clark, C.R., & Wroble, R.R. (1985). Fixed atlantoaxial rotary deformity with bilateral facet dislocation. *Skeletal Radiology, 13*, 217–220.

Kobori, M., Takahashi, H., & Mikawa, Y. (1986). Atlanto-axial dislocation in Down's syndrome: Report of two cases requiring surgical correction. *Spine, 11*, 195–200.

Martel, W., & Tishler, J.M. (1966). Observations on the spine in mongolism. *American Journal of Roentgenology, Radium Therapy and Nuclear Medicine, 94*, 630–638.

Martel, W., Uyham, R., & Stimson, C.W. (1969). Subluxation of the atlas causing spinal cord compression in a case of Down's syndrome with a "manifestation of an occipital vertebra." *Radiology, 93*, 839–840.

Mendez, A.A., Keret, D., & MacEwen, G.D. (1988). Treatment of patellofemoral instability in Down's syndrome. *Clinical Orthopedics, 234*, 148–158.

Miller, J.D.R., Capusten, B.M., & Lampard, R. (1986). Changes at the base of skull and cervical spine in Down syndrome. *Journal of the Canadian Association of Radiology, 37,* 85–89.

Moore, R.A., McNicholas, K.W., & Warran, S.P. (1987). Atlantoaxial subluxation with symptomatic spinal cord compression in a child with Down's syndrome. *Anesthesia and Analgesia, 66,* 89–90.

Nordt, J.D., & Stauffer, E.S. (1981). Sequelae of atlanto-axial stabilization in two patients with Down's syndrome. *Spine, 6,* 437–440.

Olive, P.M., Whitecloud, T.S., & Bennett, J.T. (1988). Lower cervical spondylosis and myelopathy in adults with Down syndrome. *Spine, 13,* 781–784.

Olson, J.C., Bender, J.C., Levinson, J.E., Oestreich, A., & Lovell, D.J. (1990). Arthropathy of Down syndrome. *Pediatrics, 86,* 931–936.

Powell, J.F., Woodcock, T., & Luscombe, F.E. (1990). Atlanto-axial subluxation in Down's syndrome. *Anesthesia, 45,* 1049–1051.

Power D'Arcy, L. (1933). Some early surgical cases—The Edwin Smith Papyrus. *British Journal of Surgery, 21,* 1–6.

Powers, B., Miller, M.D., Kramer, R.S., Martinez, S., & Gehweiler, J.A. (1979). Traumatic atlanto-occipital dislocation. *Neurosurgery, 4,* 12–17.

Powers, M., Parfenchuck, B.S., Bertrand, S., Drvaric, D., Lange, N., Pueschel, S.M., & Roberts, J. (in press). Posterior atlanto-occipital instability in Down syndrome: Techniques in evaluation, prevalence and clinical implications. *Journal of Pediatric Orthopedics.*

Pueschel, S.M., Findley, T.W., Furia, J., Gallagher, P.L., Scola, F.H., & Pezzullo, J.C. (1987). Atlantoaxial instability in Down syndrome: Roentgenographic, neurologic, and somatosensory evoked potential studies. *Journal of Pediatrics, 110,* 515–521.

Pueschel, S.M., Herndon, J.H., Gelch, M.M., Senft, K.E., Scola, F.H., & Goldberg, M.J. (1984). Symptomatic atlantoaxial subluxation in persons with Down syndrome. *Journal of Pediatric Orthopedics, 4,* 682–688.

Pueschel, S.M., & Scola, F.H. (1987). Atlantoaxial instability in individuals with Down syndrome: Epidemiologic, radiographic, and clinical studies. *Pediatrics, 80,* 555–560.

Pueschel, S.M., Scola, F.H., Perry, C.D., & Pezzullo, J.C. (1981). Atlantoaxial instability in children with Down syndrome. *Pediatric Radiology, 10,* 129–132.

Pueschel, S.M., Scola, F.H., & Pezzullo, J.C. (in press). A longitudinal study of atlantoaxial instability in individuals with Down syndrome. *Pediatrics.*

Pueschel, S.M., Scola, F.H., Tupper, T.B., & Pezzullo, J.C. (1990). Skeletal anomalies of the upper cervical spine in children with Down syndrome. *Journal of Pediatric Orthopedics, 10,* 607–611.

Roach, J.W., Duncan, D., Wenger, D.R., Maravilla, A., & Maravilla, K. (1984). Atlanto-axial instability and spinal cord compression in children—Diagnosis by computerized tomography. *Journal of Bone and Joint Surgery, 66,* 708–714.

Rosenbaum, D.M., Blumhagen, J.D., & King, H.A. (1986). Atlanto-occipital instability in Down syndrome. *American Journal of Roentgenology, 146,* 1269–1272.

Semine, A.A., Ertel, A.N., Goldberg, M.J., & Bull, M.J. (1978). Cervical spine instability in children with Down syndrome (trisomy 21). *Journal of Bone and Joint Surgery, 60,* 649–652.

Sherk, H.H., & Nicholson, J.T. (1969). Rotatory atlanto-axial dislocation associated with ossiculum terminale and mongolism. *Journal of Bone and Joint Surgery, 51,* 957–964.

Sherk, H.H., Pasquariello, P.S., & Watters, W.C. (1982). Multiple dislocations of the cervical spine in a patient with juvenile rheumatoid arthritis and Down's syndrome. *Clinical Orthopedics, 162,* 37–40.

Shield, L.K., Dickens, D.R.V., & Jensen, F. (1981). Atlanto-axial dislocation with spinal cord compression in Down syndrome. *Australian Paediatrics Journal, 17,* 114–116.

Shikata, J., Yamamuro, T., Mikawa, Y., Iida, H., & Kobori, M. (1989). Atlantoaxial subluxation in Down's syndrome. *International Orthopaedics, 13,* 187–192.

Skoff, H.D., & Keggi, K. (1987). Total hip replacement in Down's syndrome. *Orthopedics, 10,* 485–489.

Spitzer, R., Rabinowich, J.Y., & Wybar, K.C. (1961). A study of abnormalities of the skull, teeth, and lenses in mongolism. *Canadian Medical Association Journal, 84,* 567–572.

Storm, W., (1986). Ventrale Atlasdislokation (Atlanto-axiale Instabilität) bei Kindern mit einer Trisomie 21 (M. Down) [Ventral dislocation of the atlas (atlantoaxial instability) in children with trisomy 21]. *Pädiatrische Praxis, 32,* 149–152.

Thalmann, H., Scholl, H., & Tonz, O. (1972). Spontane Atlas-dislokation bei einem Kind mit Trisomie 21 und rheumatoider Arthritis [Spontaneous dislocation of the atlas of a child with trisomy 21 and rheumatoid arthritis]. *Helvetica Paediatrica Acta, 27,* 391–403.

Tishler, J.M., & Martel, W. (1965). Dislocation of the atlas in mongolism: Preliminary report. *Radiology, 84,* 904–908.

Tredwell, S.J., Newman, D.W., & Lockitch, G. (1990). Instability of the upper cervical spine in Down syndrome. *Journal of Pediatric Orthopedics, 10,* 602–606.

Van Dyke, D.C., & Gahagan, C.A. (1988). Down syndrome cervical spine abnormalities and problems. *Clinical Pediatrics, 27,* 415–418.

Whayley, W.M., & Gray, W.D. (1980). Atlanto-axial

dislocation in Down's syndrome. *Canadian Medical Association Journal, 123,* 35–37.

Wiesel, S., Kraus, D., & Rothman, R.H. (1978). Atlanto-occipital hypermobility. *Orthopedic Clinics of North America, 9,* 969–972.

Yancey, C.L., Zmijewski, C., Athreya, B.H., & Doughty, R.A. (1984). Arthropathy of Down's syndrome. *Arthritis and Rheumatism, 27,* 929–934.

CHAPTER
16

Neurologic Abnormalities

Jesús Flórez

Before discussing the main aspects of brain pathology in Down syndrome, especially as they relate to mental retardation, some points need to be considered in order to prevent a negative impact on the training and education of persons with Down syndrome:

1. It is important to differentiate the brain abnormalities arising during fetal development and the first postnatal years from those observed late in adult life, which are the result of the aging process. Consequently, not all the findings of in vivo and post mortem studies have the same relevance when lesions are to be correlated with neuropsychologic changes and learning difficulties. This chapter focuses primarily on the information obtained during the early years of life.

2. The localization, topographic extension, and severity of the abnormalities of the affected brain areas are determined by the genes coded for on the three #21 chromosomes. Since this genetic expression is a distinct attribute of each individual, it explains in part the extremely wide interindividual variability in the intellectual and cognitive abilities of persons with Down syndrome.

3. In addition to the genetic influences, nutritional and educational environments are important modulators of developmental events in the brain, although the extent and quality of their influence is, as yet, unknown and to some extent, unpredictable.

4. Intelligence is not an "all or nothing" process. Human performance, self-awareness, and other human attributes do not, in fact,

require a high level of intelligence. Consequently, persons with Down syndrome can and should have a high quality of life, as long as the aims and expectations introduced in their lives are not beyond their true capabilities, and match their real basic needs.

BRAIN ABNORMALITIES

The normal development of the brain involves a whole set of processes:

Neuronal formation
Cell movement and migration
Growth of dendrites and axons
Myelination
Formation of synapses
Death and natural elimination of a certain number of neurons and their synapses
Cell differentiation
Functional organization in networks

There is a progressive and selective development that leads to an ordered and programmed organization of the brain networks and circuits composed of neurons and their interconnections. But besides this programmed processing, there are external and internal factors in each individual that, to some extent, influence brain development depending on the plasticity of the neurons. The modification occurring in the physical and electrochemical environments throughout development will determine the final central nervous system function. Of course, the possibilities of change are greater in the early stages of life and are gradually reduced thereafter. However, some degree of neuronal plasticity persists throughout life and allows for input modulation in the central nervous system.

There are widespread alterations in the development of the central nervous system in persons with Down syndrome, and they include several structures and features: 1) there is a reduction in the total number of neurons, which extends to several cortical areas; 2) within the neuron, abnormalities can be observed in subcellular structures, including the synapses; and 3) alterations are found in the functional communication of the interneuronal system.

Morphologic Alterations

Macroscopic Level

Gross neuropathologic abnormalities are usually not observed at birth (Kemper, 1991). Compared to control brains, neuropathologic abnormalities become apparent most often after midinfancy. Several studies have shown that the brain weight of infants with Down syndrome is nearly normal at birth. The brain weight drops below the normal range with increasing age starting after 3–6 months. But in about 20% of children, the brain remains in the lower normal range (Benda, 1971; Kemper, 1988; Wisniewski, 1990). The brain shape of newborns with Down syndrome is normal; however, after 3–5 months, the anterior-posterior diameter becomes shorter due to a reduction of the frontal lobes and a flattening of the occipital lobes. In most instances, the occipitofrontal circumferences are below two standard deviations after midinfancy (Cronk & Pueschel, 1983; Wisniewski, 1990). The superior temporal gyri were found to be narrow in 34 out of 101 brains of individuals with Down syndrome ranging in age from birth to 5 years (Wisniewski, 1990). With increasing age, this finding is observed in approximately one half of the brains (Zellweger, 1977), and may be unilateral or bilateral. According to Kemper (1988), it is twice as likely to occur in the left than in the right cerebral hemisphere. The brainstem and cerebellum are also smaller in children with Down syndrome than in the general population under 5 years (Wisniewski, 1990). Other investigators have found a disproportionate decrease

in the weight of the brainstem and cerebellum compared to that of the cerebrum (Crome, Cowie, & Slater, 1966). The cerebellum often remains hypoplastic throughout due to a reduction in the size of the middle lobes (Zellweger, 1977). Other gross abnormalities found in the brains of some persons with Down syndrome include a decreased development of secondary gyri (Urich, 1976), and hypoplasia of the operculum (Zellweger, 1977), corpus callosum (Gullotta & Rehder, 1974), the anterior commissure, and the hippocampus (Sylvester, 1983, 1986).

Some of these abnormalities have been recently confirmed in vivo by modern brain imaging techniques, such as computerized axial tomography (CAT), and nuclear magnetic resonance imaging (MRI), which can be used to analyze the brain of living humans at a high power of resolution. Both techniques have been applied in individuals with Down syndrome, although their ages have been generally above 25 years.

In CAT studies, young adults with Down syndrome show smaller brains and intracranial volumes than age-matched controls (Schapiro et al., 1989). Magnetic resonance scan gives a higher resolution than computerized axial tomography and allows for a better delineation of grey and white matter as well as of the brain nuclei. By using magnetic resonance and powerful stereologic tools for estimating three-dimensional volumes, Weis (in press) demonstrated in 7 persons with Down syndrome (30–45 years of age) a significant reduction in total brain volume, cerebral cortex, white matter and cerebellum; the brainstem was also smaller, but the difference from that of the control group did not reach statistical significance. Basal ganglia and thalamus were of normal size. In addition, when the normalization procedure was based on cranial cavity rather than on total brain volume, the significant differences between the Down syndrome and the control group persisted.

Kemper (1988) reported that myelination is normal at birth and during early childhood, but a delay of myelin formation was found in 22% of brains from infants and children with Down syndrome (Wisniewski & Schmidt-Sidor, 1989). This delay in myelination affects mainly the associated and intercortical fibers of the fronto-temporal lobes.

Microscopic Level

A reduction in the neuronal density of several areas of the brain cortex has been consistently reported (Kemper, 1988). There is a wide variability between individuals as well as between different areas of the brain in the same individual. It is also important to recognize that a 10%–50% decrease in the number of brain cells can be observed even at birth (Wisniewski, 1990; Wisniewski, Laure-Kamionowska, Connell, & Wen, 1986). In a population of 73 children from birth to 14 years, these authors studied three selected areas; the neocortical 17 (primary visual) and 10 (prefrontal), and the paleocortical 28 (parahippocampal) areas. Although insufficient samples were available for areas 10 and 28, a generalized reduction was evident in all areas studied. All layers of the cortex were affected but primarily layers II and IV, where the small granule cells predominate. A substantial and specific reduction of granular neurons was also found in several cortical areas of the brains of adults with Down syndrome (Ross, Galaburda, & Kemper, 1984). A decreased number of neurons also has been reported in the hippocampus, nucleus basalis, ventral cochlear nucleus, and the cerebellar cortex. This reduction leads to a diffuse loss of the layer cytoarchitecture specific for a given area, thus blurring the boundaries between the cortical areas.

It seems, therefore, that the derangement of granule cells is a distinct feature in Down syndrome even at early developmental stages, thus suggesting the involvement of factors that induce prenatal arrest of neurogenesis. In fact, in the trisomic 16 mouse, which is an animal model of trisomy 21, hypocellularity in the development of the telencephalon has been consistently observed (Oster-Granite, Gearhart, & Reeves, 1986). It will be necessary to determine the molecular link between genetic overexpression and the alterations in neuronal development and maturation. The existence of a genetically determined alteration in neural development does not exclude the influence of additional "toxic" factors, also derived from genetic overexpression, that may accumulate during postnatal life and contribute to a more rapid neural derangement.

Dendritic arborization and synaptic development are severely affected in the cortical neurons of persons with Down syndrome, including the pyramidal cells. At birth, the number of dendritic spines is normal, but during the 1st year of life a marked reduction in the dendritic arborization and development of dendritic spines has been consistently reported, compared to age-matched controls (Becker, Armstrong, & Chan, 1986; Suetsugu & Mehraein, 1980; Takashima, Becker, Armstrong, & Chan, 1981). In addition, the morphology of the spines of individuals with Down syndrome shows abnormal features: The spines may be too long and tortuous in some neurons and extremely short or almost absent in others (Marín-Padilla, 1976; Purpura, 1974). These results indicate that in the brains of persons with Down syndrome the number of spines increases normally during fetal life, but then the increase becomes less and levels off shortly after birth. Although dendritic development in the human brain begins prenatally, it continues for a long time postnatally. Before birth, there are few dendritic spines on dendrites, but after birth they begin to develop and cover the maturing dendrites. This development is genetically programmed to make normal connections, but its full achievement requires the presence of appropriate influences and stimuli, reaching the cortical areas during the early months of life. How much of the reduced development of dendritic branching and spine production in Down syndrome is due to genetic factors during both pre- and postnatal development, and how much is secondary to a failure to respond to environmental stimuli, is difficult to predict. However, both sets of causes may influence each other and contribute to the final outcome.

Ultrastructural studies have also demonstrated that the synaptic density, the pre- and postsynaptic length, and the average surface area per synaptic contact are reduced in the Down syndrome visual cortex, compared to those of the control brain (Scott, Becker, & Petit, 1983; Wisniewski, 1990). Studies in other cortical areas are needed, especially in those that are more severely affected, such as some associational areas.

Neurochemical Alterations

Most reports on the neurochemical activity in Down syndrome are concerned with the brains of elderly people because of the interest in comparing brain aging in persons with Down syndrome with Alzheimer pathology. It is important, however, to know whether individuals with Down syndrome begin life with compromised neurochemical systems.

Cholinergic deficiency in the brains of adults with Down syndrome has been well documented (McCoy & Enns, 1986). However, recent studies in a group of 7 infants with Down syndrome age 1 year or less demonstrated normal or somewhat above-normal activities of choline acetyltransferase, a specific cholinergic marker, in the cerebral and cerebellar cortex, limbic brain, and basal ganglia (Kish et al., 1989). Normal levels of choline acetyltransferase were also found in a fetal trisomy 21 cerebral cortex at midgestation, as compared to controls (Brooksbank, Walker, Balázs, & Jorgensen, 1989). In contrast, relatively low levels of choline acetyltransferase were observed in the cerebral cortex of a 5.5-month-old infant with Down syndrome compared with 2 infants with acquired immunodeficiency syndrome (McGeer et al., 1985). It is of note that these data are confined to cortical and subcortical structures; they do not include the mesencephalic level, nor do they indicate the state of postsynaptic function. A full account of the system would also require the analysis of the cholinergic receptors. A preliminary autoradiographic study of the brains of 2 stillborn infants with Down syndrome (stillbirths at 31 and 39 gestational weeks, respectively) revealed normal densities and distribution patterns of cholinergic muscarinic receptors in the cerebral cortex and striatum, but a marked receptor reduction in the midbrain (superior colliculus and substantia nigra), compared to control age-matched brains (Flórez, del Arco, González, Pascual, & Pazos, 1990). In the fetal brains of mice with trisomy 16, a reduction in muscarinic cholinergic receptors was also found at different levels of the

brain, including the mesencephalon (Kiss, Schlumpf, & Balázs, 1989).

Studies on other neurochemical systems at early ages in Down syndrome are lacking. In the brain of a 5-month-old infant, 5-hydroxytryptamine was decreased in all areas of the brain sampled. Dopamine and noradrenaline concentrations were increased above control values in the putamen and globus pallidus, but decreased in other brain areas (McGeer et al., 1985), which is in partial agreement with data from trisomic mice (Kiss et al., 1989). In young adults, however, a significant elevation of noradrenaline and 5-hydroxyindolacetic acid (a metabolite of 5-hydroxytryptamine) was found in the cerebrospinal fluid, suggesting an increased turnover of monoamines (Schapiro, Kay, et al., 1987). Particular attention has been given to the central nervous system serotonergic function, since it was earlier discovered that plasma 5-hydroxytryptamine was reduced in persons with Down syndrome as a consequence of the limited 5-hydroxytryptamine uptake by platelets (Tukiainen, Tuomisto, Westermareck, & Kupiainen, 1980). Platelets have frequently been considered as a peripheral model of neurons. However, there are marked differences between both types of cells, the most important being the nature of the 5-hydroxytryptamine binding proteins and the inability of the platelet to synthesize 5-hydroxytryptamine in contrast to the serotonergic neuron (Tamir, Bebirian, Muller, & Casper, 1980). Therefore, a reduced uptake of 5-hydroxytryptamine by platelets results in a reduced concentration, but this does not necessarily apply to the neuron. In fact, Ternaux et al. (1979) showed in adults with Down syndrome that, although the serum 5-hydroxytryptamine was markedly decreased, the cerebrospinal fluid levels of 5-hydroxytryptamine and 5-hydroxyindolacetic acid were increased, suggesting an enhanced synthesis and utilization of this amine at the central level.

Many more data are needed to assess the status of the monoaminergic systems during fetal development and early postnatal stages, especially in light of the interesting results obtained by Groner et al. (1990) in a cellular model. These authors reported that rat PC12 cells expressing increased levels of transfected human CuZn superoxide dismutase gene showed impaired uptake of noradrenaline and dopamine. This lesion was localized to the chromaffin granule transport mechanism and was secondary to the failure to maintain the pH gradient across the membrane, which is the main driving force for amine transport. A similar failure was observed in the platelet uptake of 5-hydroxytryptamine. Since monoamine uptake plays a relevant role in the function of the central monoaminergic systems, it is important to determine their functioning in the brain of infants and children with Down syndrome and the role of the CuZn superoxide dismutase gene-dosage in the neurobiologic abnormalities of Down syndrome. However, caution should be exercised in interpreting and correlating these findings because the CuZn superoxide dismutase gene is not essential for the expression of mental retardation in persons with Down syndrome (Kornberg et al., 1990).

In an attempt to clarify whether the pathologic alterations in persons with Down syndrome reflect developmental failures or early degenerative processes, neuronal maturation was assessed by examining the neuronal cell adhesion molecule and some gangliosides in the brain tissue of fetuses with trisomy 21 at 19–24 weeks gestation (Brooksbank et al., 1989). No differences were found in the concentration of the neuronal cell adhesion molecule or in the proportion of its "adult" form, or in the total concentration and composition of gangliosides when compared with the general population. However, derangements in the polyunsaturated fatty acid composition of phosphoglycerides do exist at this stage of brain development in persons with Down syndrome, which have been related to gene-dosage increase of CuZn superoxide dismutase (Balázs & Brooksbank, 1985).

Protein S-100β, a form of the calcium-binding protein S-100, is encoded by a gene mapped to the 21q22 region of chromosome 21 (Allore et al., 1978). Increments in S-100β, but not in S-100α, have been found in the plasma, peripheral T lymphocytes, and nerve cells of individuals with Down syndrome, indicating the existence of a gene-dosage effect (Kato et al., 1990). Several functions have been proposed for S-100β

in the nervous system such as the assembly of microtubules, modulation of phosphorylation of brain proteins, and regulation of glial proliferation and neuronal differentiation. In fact, concentrations of brain S-100β in rats are known to increase sharply during the stages of morphologic differentiation and functional maturation in the central nervous system. However, an increase in the number of S-100β immunoreactive cells and in the total concentration of S-100 has also been found in the brains of persons with Alzheimer disease (Griffin et al., 1989; Jorgensen, Brooksbank, & Balázs, 1990). It is not possible at the present time to conclude whether the excess of S-100β in the brains of individuals with Down syndrome is playing some deleterious role either in the differentiation and development of the brain, or in the aging mechanisms, or in both processes.

Neurophysiologic Alterations

Electrophysiologic alterations have been observed in synaptic transmissions analyzed in cultured dorsal root ganglion neurons taken from human fetuses with Down syndrome. On the one hand, compared with "normal" control human neurons, Scott, Petit, Becker, and Edwards (1982) reported a reduced maximum rate of depolarization of the action potential, elevated specific membrane resistance, reduced hyperpolarizing afterpotential, and a significant increase in specific membrane capacitance and membrane time constant. On the other hand, using dorsal root ganglion neurons cultured with nerve growth factor and examined with a tight-seal whole cell recording technique, Nieminen, Suárez-Isla, and Rapoport (1988) found different results: a shortening of the action potential duration and acceleration of both depolarization and repolarization. The activation rate constants of two outward potassium currents were higher in trisomic than in control neurons, suggesting that acceleration of repolarization of the action potential in trisomic neurons was due to shorter activation time constants of outward potassium currents. Similar results were obtained using cultured murine trisomy 16 dorsal root ganglion neurons (Orozco, Smith, Epstein, & Rapoport, 1987). It is interesting to note that dorsal root ganglion neurons taken from human fetuses with chromosome abnormalities linked to X chromosome did not show electrophysiologic abnormalities. Several differences in procedures used by Scott et al. (1982) and Nieminen et al. (1988) may account for the discrepant results. Both sets of data, however, emphasize the presence of marked alterations in the pattern of synaptic transmission in persons with Down syndrome, which can be explained by the anomalous structure of the synapses demonstrated by morphologic studies.

Further electrophysiologic studies are needed to see whether there are alterations in synaptic transmission at the level of cortical neurons in persons with Down syndrome, similar to those demonstrated in dorsal root ganglion cells. The structural abnormalities of the dendritic spines in the cortical cells would clearly support such findings. If, in addition, there is a marked reduction in the synaptic density and in the number of granular cells in the cortex, it could be anticipated that the input and output functions of the cortical cell columns, which represent the functional unit of the cortical architecture, should be severely compromised. As Courchesne (1988) pointed out, the distortion of integrated neural activity as a result of the dysgenetic process should have a deleterious influence on the capacity to filter, integrate, select, and store information during brain maturation. The presence of neural networks generating abnormal patterns of nervous activity will hinder the subsequent formation of synapses, thereby conditioning a negative influence on the permanent establishment of synaptic connections.

INSTRUMENTAL ANALYSIS OF BRAIN ACTIVITY

Electroencephalographic Patterns

In general, electroencephalographic findings in persons with Down syndrome are rather unspecific and inconsistent. The prevalence of electroencephalographic abnormalities is higher in persons with Down syndrome than in the general population, but lower than in persons with mental retardation due to other etiologies. In a review

of the literature, Ellingson, Menolascino, and Eisen (1970) found that 20%–30% of persons with Down syndrome had electroencephalographic abnormalities. The alterations include delayed maturation, diffuse slow activity, monomorphism, and pathologic slow waves (Ellingson et al., 1970; Laget, 1983; Tangye, 1979). Excessive slowing seems to be more common in older individuals with Down syndrome (over 40 years), which may reflect the neuropathologic characteristics of Alzheimer disease. In a recent study (Devinsky, Sato, Conwit, & Schapiro, 1990), 13 out of 19 young adults with Down syndrome (19–37 years of age) showed normal α background activity, whereas 6 had abnormal α background (either absent or irregular, low-amplitude, mixed frequency). Out of 9 older adults with Down syndrome (42–66 years of age), 5 showed normal and 4 abnormal electroencephalographic activity. Older individuals who had decreased α background also showed dementia and an enlargement of the third ventricle; however, young persons with decreased α background also had enlargement of the third ventricle, but no reduction in cognitive function, compared to the other young persons with normal electroencephalographic activity.

Paroxysmal anomalies (spike and wave activity, polyspike and wave activity, focal sporadic spikes) are rare, and the correlation of these electroencephalographic findings to clinical seizure activity and neurological signs is not evident. This is discussed later in this chapter.

Event-Related Potentials

Event-related potentials have been widely used in persons with Down syndrome to assess the functional activity of the neural systems involved in sensory, cognitive, and motor functions. Significant alterations in timing of the short latency components of the responses to auditory stimuli have been observed (Squires, Ollo, & Jordan, 1986). They reflect the neural activity in the auditory nerve, pons, inferior colliculus, medial geniculate body, and auditory thalamocortical radiations. These abnormalities are independent of the characteristic high frequency of hearing loss often observed in adults with Down syndrome. The cortical sensory-related components of the event-related potentials elicited by auditory, visual, and somatosensory stimuli also show abnormal responses such as increased response amplitudes and response delays (Dustman & Callner, 1979; Lincoln, Courchesne, Kilman, & Galambos, 1985). These abnormalities in the components of the early event-related potentials have been related to deficits in central inhibition or alteration in neuronal excitability in individuals with Down syndrome (Callner, Dustman, Madsen, Schenkenberg, & Beck, 1978). Schafer and Peeke (1982) also observed that P2 and N2 responses in persons with Down syndrome failed to show the normal pattern of short-term habituation that appears after repeated auditory stimuli, indicating a deficiency in modulatory and inhibitory mechanisms.

Longer latency components of the event-related potentials, such as the P300, Sw, and so forth (also called endogenous components), have raised particular interest because they seem to represent neural responses associated with the higher mental processes of stimulus recognition, evaluation, and categorization, and seem to participate in mechanisms related to memory and learning. Several studies have shown increased latencies of P300 in children with Down syndrome as compared to age-matched controls, indicating that visual and auditory information is processed more slowly (Courchesne, 1988; Lincoln et al., 1985; Schantz & Brown, 1990). In addition, abnormalities in amplitude and morphology occur, particularly over the frontal and parietal cortical areas, different from those observed in persons with other developmental disorders.

The Nc component is recorded from frontal cortical areas and is considered as a sign of enhanced selective attention to novel, important, or significant stimuli. With increasing age, "normal" infants display an increased selective enhancement of the Nc response to new information. However, in 12-year-old children with Down syndrome, the Nc responses were as slow as in infants with Down syndrome; and they were as large to non-novel, insignificant information as to novel information (Lincoln et al., 1985). The hippocampus is one of the regions

implicated in the generation of the slow endogenous component of event-related potentials. Since the hippocampal cortex shows gross morphologic as well as microscopic abnormalities in persons with Down syndrome (Sylvester, 1983), event-related potentials studies may serve to validate the behavior impairments involving memory, orienting, and cognition of persons with Down syndrome, and to detect changes during the life course of an individual that may be relevant in follow-up studies.

Positron Emission Tomography (PET)

Modern imaging techniques are being used to characterize brain functions under different physiologic conditions and may serve to identify regions particularly altered in several pathologic conditions. Positron emission tomography provides quantitative images of regional function within the brain and other organs. The emphasis in the application of PET to the brain has been on function, an area in which other imaging methods cannot compete. Although PET, in turn, cannot compete with the exquisite anatomic detail obtained by other techniques (CAT, MRI), progress has been made in the resolution power of PET scanners so that this has became the most favored method to combine the analysis of form and function. Positron emission tomography is being applied in several areas of neuroscience: analysis of degenerative diseases (Parkinson, Alzheimer, etc.), brain tumors, characterization of various neurotransmitter systems (dopamine, opioids, glutamate, γ-aminobutyric acid), and pharmacologic actions of different drugs.

Horwitz, Schapiro, Grady, and Rapoport (1990) have studied regional cerebral metabolic rates for glucose using PET in healthy young adults with Down syndrome, compared with age-matched controls. The correlation analysis between the Down syndrome and the control groups demonstrated especially reduced values in the left hemisphere inferior frontal gyrus of the Down syndrome group, which includes the Broca area. In addition, lower values in the Down syndrome group than in the control were found for many correlations in regions within and between the frontal and parietal lobes. The technique serves to substantiate the central cortical component of the language difficulties, which are so characteristic in persons with Down syndrome (see later section of this chapter). Whether it may have a predictive or prognostic value requires further investigation. Information on frontoparietal correlations is also relevant in view of the reduced size of the frontal lobes in persons with Down syndrome and the cortical abnormalities previously discussed. As Horwitz et al. (1990) pointed out, they may indicate an imbalance between the mutual inhibition of these two cortical areas, the consequences of which will be discussed later in this chapter.

As the age of individuals with Down syndrome increases over 25 years, a significant reduction in the mean hemispheric glucose utilization and in the regional metabolism can be observed in all lobal regions, even in persons with Down syndrome who do not show signs of dementia (Cutler, 1986; Schapiro, Haxby, et al., 1987). This age-related decrement does not appear in age-matched "normal" individuals, indicating that significant age-related neuropsychologic derangements occur in persons with Down syndrome.

BRAIN ACTIVITY AND LEARNING

On the basis of the morphologic and functional data obtained from the brains of individuals with Down syndrome, an attempt is made here to correlate these findings with some of the learning and behavioral difficulties frequently observed in children and young adults with Down syndrome, disregarding any reference to the aging process in Down syndrome. The proposed correlation is summarized in Table 16.1.

A deficiency in cholinergic transmission at the collicular level during the first months of postnatal life, as suggested by the autoradiographic studies (Flórez et al., 1990), may disturb the mechanisms of attention and arousal during such a critical life stage. However, the cerebral cortex is by far the most affected region in the brain of persons with Down syndrome. There is a substantial reduction in the total number of neurons (particularly granule cells), dendritic spines, and synaptic connections as described earlier in this chapter. Neurophysiologic studies have shown deficiencies in synaptic transmission, in the integration of potentials evoked by somatosensory

Table 16.1.   Correlation between brain pathology and cognitive behavior in persons with Down syndrome

Affected structures in the central nervous system	Cognitive behavior
I. Attention, initiative	
Mesencephalus	Distractibility
Thalamocortical interactions	Poor differentiation between old and new stimuli
Frontoparietal cortex interactions	Difficulty in maintaining attention and pursuing a specific task
	Less capacity for self-inhibition
	Less initiative in playing
II. Short-term memory: Penetration and processing of information	
Associative sensory areas	Difficulties in processing specific types of sensory inputs and in
Prefrontal lobes	organizing output responses
III. Long-term memory	
Hippocampus	Reduction in consolidation and retrieval of memory
Corticohippocampal interactions	Reduction in declarative types of memory
IV. Correlation and analysis	
Prefrontal lobes in bidirectional interactions with:	Failure to:
—other cortical and subcortical structures	—integrate and interpret information
—hippocampus	—organize new and deliberate sequential information
	—perform internal conceptualization and programming
	—accomplish serial cognitive operations
	—elaborate abstract thinking and numerical operations

stimuli, and in the intercorrelations between different cortical lobes. Although lesions show a wide distribution throughout the cortex, they seem to affect preferentially some primary sensory and associative areas, some areas of the frontal cortex, the hippocampus, and the cerebellum. Given the role of the granule cells in the function of the cortical columns, the reduction in the number of these cells should severely affect the processing of the input–output information, traveling inside and through the column.

Such widespread and diffuse alteration in several cortical areas and the hippocampus should lead to a severe impairment of the cognitive and learning processes in Down syndrome, because these areas are involved in the mechanisms concerning attention, information processing, integration and correlation, as well as short- and long-term memory (Amaral, 1987; Fuster, 1989; Posner & Petersen, 1990; Squire & Lindenlaub, 1990). In addition, the prefrontal cortex critically intervenes in the initiation and guidance of behaviors. Through the reciprocal interaction with other cortical, hippocampal, and thalamic regions, the prefrontal cortex secures the retention of the information for prospective behavior (Fuster, 1989). Disorders of attention and distractibility, and failures in sustaining attention and maintaining the performance of a task, are common problems in persons with Down syndrome. Visual and auditory information is difficult for individuals to process, retain, and retrieve. This difficulty includes both the receptive and the effector systems, although it has been repeatedly shown that auditory modalities are usually more affected in persons with Down syndrome than are visual modalities; thus, the performance of tasks is always lower after verbal than after visual instruction (Lincoln et al., 1985; Marcell & Armstrong, 1982; Pueschel, Gallagher, Zartler, & Pezzullo, 1987; Rohr & Burr, 1978). According to Elliott, Weeks, and Gray (1990), this difficulty results in a breakdown in the use of verbal information and in the spatial–temporal organization of specific movement programs. This deficiency in information processing may be the result of the dissociation between the functional systems responsible for speech perception (possibly right hemisphere) and the systems involved in the organization of complex movements (left hemisphere). The link between these two systems includes the prefrontal mechanisms, which are involved in programming and sequencing motor behavior, including speech, as well as abstract thinking.

The short-term memory depends heavily upon the function of secondary and tertiary (associative) sensory areas in permanent interaction with the frontal lobes (Dudai, 1989; Squire, 1987). In addition, the hippocampus plays a prominent role in some modalities of long-term memory. Therefore, lesions in these regions as they appear in persons with Down syndrome should be responsible for the impairment of memory and decision-making processes that form essential components of learning and thinking. Individuals with Down syndrome show reduced short-term memory abilities and, contrary to "normal" persons, display greater difficulty in recalling sequences of auditory than visual information (Marcell & Weeks, 1988). This means that they have problems in retaining information and programming sequences behavior, two aspects linked to the frontal lobe activity. It is of no surprise, therefore, that PET metabolic studies in young adults with Down syndrome demonstrated such a low functioning of the frontal cortex in relation to the parietal lobe (Horwitz et al., 1990).

BRAIN ACTIVITY AND LANGUAGE

Language and communication skills are frequently impaired in persons with mental retardation. However, language difficulties in persons with Down syndrome usually exceed those found in persons with mental retardation of other etiologies who have similar cognitive deficiencies. Studies on language development in children with Down syndrome (Miller, 1987, 1988; Rondal, 1986) have demonstrated the following major alterations: 1) an asynchrony in language production relative to language understanding and other cognitive skills, 2) an onset of productive deficits that coincides with word production (vocabulary growth), 3) a slowness in the development of syntactic skills, and 4) a high variation in the profile of language development and production among different individuals.

Although alterations in the auditory function and in the speech structures are common in persons with Down syndrome, the type and intensity of the difficulties observed in language development, processing, and production suggest that the damage to cortical areas involved in language functions is the main factor responsible for this condition. It is a common experience that persons with Down syndrome, quite capable to receive and understand information, present a substantial impairment in their skill to organize the sequence of words, and to combine words syntactically in order to perform long sentences. Indeed, the inadequacy of verbal articulation, the hypotonia of the respiratory and speech muscles (including the tongue), and the congenital abnormalities of the "speech canal" will provide additional impairment to language articulation (Meyers, 1990). Finally, self-awareness of the poor capacity for communication may become a negative reinforcer on the personal initiative to use and improve language skills.

Traditionally, language areas in the brain have been confined to one dominant hemisphere, predominantly the left. They included the anterior prerolandic area in the posterior portion of the inferior frontal gyrus, which is considered important to language production (Broca area), and the posterior postrolandic area in the left angular gyrus of the temporal lobe (Wernicke area), which is important to language understanding. A supplementary area in the posterior part of the superior frontal gyrus is related to the initiation of language output. Connections between the anterior and posterior areas through the arcuate fasciculus would serve as the basis for serial processing of language (Kolb & Whishaw, 1990). However, new studies based on clinical observations from patients with specific brain lesions and from experiments performed during neurosurgical operations have demonstrated that the neural networks on which language depends include structures, both cortical and subcortical, that had not been traditionally considered as language-related areas. For example, the anterior sector of the temporal lobe, which includes the temporal pole (area 38), and the anterior part

of the inferotemporal region (areas 20, 21, 37) have been associated with the ability for naming concrete entities (Damasio & Damasio, 1990). Frontal lesions are also associated with expressive aphasia and some aspects of language understanding.

One emerging concept is that language includes discrete functions, and that specific neural systems, widely distributed in the cortex, are associated with each language function. As Ojemann (1990) has pointed out, each system has essential areas that tend to be highly localized but distributed across several portions of the frontal and/or temporal lobes, in patterns that are highly variable between individuals. In addition, individual neurons in the associative cortex have activity that seems to be specific for each particular language function.

The preceding discussion serves to emphasize that complex language deficiencies existing in persons with Down syndrome cannot be associated with the lesion of one specific area. Indeed, PET studies performed in young adults with Down syndrome showed that there are reduced metabolic patterns in the inferior frontal gyrus that includes the Broca area (Horwitz et al., 1990). Other studies have also suggested the loss of, or at least the reduction in, hemispheric dominance (Giencke & Lewandowski, 1989; Hartley, 1981; Pipe, 1983), due to an early structural and functional deviation in the development and organization of the brain. Nevertheless, what the modern findings and models seem to support is the concept that language deficiencies in persons with Down syndrome are the consequence of the pervasive cellular damage that extends to frontal, temporal, primary, and associative areas, thereby disturbing the cortical interhemispheric organization of language—not so much in the process of understanding as in that involved in the expression and production of words and organized sentences. In this regard, the proposal of Elliott and Weeks (1990) seems particularly appropriate: The specific pattern of language dysfunction in Down syndrome would be related to the dissociation between cerebral areas responsible for speech perception and the production of complex movements including speech. The normal interaction between the right and left hemispheres, each one contributing in its own way to speech perception and movement organization, would be disrupted.

EPILEPSY AND SEIZURE ACTIVITY

Recent reports seem to support some association between seizure activity and Down syndrome. Prevalence figures range widely among different authors: from 1% (Kirman, 1951) to over 13% (Paulson, Son, & Nance, 1969; Romano et al., 1990). As in other issues related to Down syndrome, the age of the population becomes an important factor. Two recent studies reported prevalences of 8.1% (Pueschel, Louis, & McKnight, 1991) and 6.4% (Stafstrom, Patxot, Gilmore, & Wisniewski, 1991), in fair agreement with previous reports (MacGillivray, 1967; Tangye, 1979; Veall, 1974). Pueschel et al. (1991) detected a polymodal distribution in the onset of seizures, as they appeared in a population of 405 individuals with Down syndrome (6 months to 45 years of age). Out of the 25 patients with Down syndrome and seizures, 10 showed seizure activity during the 1st year of life, 6 had infantile spasms, 3 had tonic-clonic seizures with myoclonus, and 1 had febrile seizures. Five patients started the seizure disorder between the age of 1–19 years, whereas another 10 patients developed seizures between 20–30 years of age. These authors suggested that it is possible that a third peak of seizure onset may appear as age increases beyond 40 years when Alzheimer-like changes may appear in the brain.

This age-related increment in seizure prevalence can be considered as a specific feature of Down syndrome because the risk of developing seizures usually decreases with age. The type of seizures most frequently observed during the 1st year of life in Down syndrome is infantile spasms with an hypsarrhythmic electroencephalographic pattern (Le Berre et al., 1986; Pueschel et al., 1991; Romano et al., 1990; Tatsuno, Hayashi, Iwamoto, Suzuki, & Kuroki, 1984), followed by tonic-clonic convulsions. The reasons for this association are not clear. An explanation based on unproven serotonergic deficit is no longer tenable, but some of the morphologic, biochemical, and electrophysiologic alterations, previously described, may account for a loss of balance between excitatory and inhibitory mechanisms in the central nervous system. Stafstrom et al. (1991) have pointed out that seizures in children with Down syndrome are not simply the consequence of abnormal brain development. Complicating factors such as perinatal respiratory distress, hypoxia, cardiac disease, and infections could also contribute to the development of seizures. Le Berre et al. emphasized the deleterious influence of infantile spasms on the psychomotor and educational development of infants with Down syndrome. However, complete control of this seizure disorder can be obtained by adequate therapy with high doses of corticotropin, sodium valproate, or vigabatrin (where available). Therefore, if adequate intervention and educational strategies are maintained in these infants, the prognosis should be much more favorable.

There is disagreement on the prevalence of febrile seizures. Data presented by Romano et al. (1990) (44.4% of patients with seizures had febrile convulsions) are in sharp contrast with data from other surveys (0.04%–1% of all seizures) (Le Berre et al., 1986; Pueschel et al., 1991). This extreme variability may be due to wide differences in diagnostic criteria and the characteristics of the surveys. Other types of epilepsy appearing during childhood, adolescence, and adulthood include tonic-clonic seizures with or without myoclonus, partial simple seizures, and partial complex seizures.

OTHER ABNORMALITIES

Computerized tomography studies have confirmed reports obtained from autopsy that there is a higher incidence of basal ganglia calcification in Down syndrome (10%–30%, depending on age) than in the general population (0.3%–0.6%) (Ieshima, Kisa, Yoshino, Takashima, & Takeshita, 1984; Malamud, 1964; Merikangas, Marasco, & Feczko, 1979; Wisniewski et al., 1982). Although the prevalence and intensity of calcification increase with age, borderline to mild calcium deposition can be observed in children with Down syndrome under 5 years. Basal ganglia calcification is localized predominantly at the medial side of the lateral medullary lamina of globus pallidus, but it also extends to the putamen. Histologic and histochemical examinations have shown that the calcifications occur in the pericapillary and the media of small arteries, but the nerve cells remain unchanged (Takashima & Becker, 1985). This may be related to the amyloid angiopathy that may appear even in young persons with Down syndrome.

CONCLUSION

The genetic inbalance brought about by the trisomy of chromosome 21 seems to be expressed in the central nervous system in a rather specific and consistent manner. As in other organs, however, wide interindividual variations frequently occur. In general, most of the curtailment in brain development appears during the early postnatal months and years, leading to a reduction in the cortical neuronal population and in their synaptic connectivity. Deficiencies in synaptic transmission, integration of event-related potentials, and functional intercorrelation between several cortical lobes are frequently observed. Lesions affect preferentially primary sensory and associative areas, the frontal cortex, the hippocampus, and the cerebellum. Such widespread alterations in the cortical areas seem to account for the specific impairments observed in short- and long-term memory, language skills, and cognitive and learning processes of individuals with Down syndrome. The use of modern brain imaging techniques in conjunction with neurophysiologic and neuropsychologic analysis should serve to further our understanding of the implications of central nervous system lesions, as they appear in Down syndrome, in relation to cognitive and learning difficulties.

Modern and innovative instructional strategies should take into consideration the consequences derived from all these cerebral abnormalities, so that suitable approaches may be applied to the arduous, and yet exciting, task of educating persons with Down syndrome. Consequently, neuropsychologists, neurobiologists, educators, and parents are encouraged to join their efforts in the venture of carrying out longsighted and long-run studies that are directed to overcome, on an individual basis, the learning difficulties derived from the brain anomalies.

REFERENCES

Allore, R., O'Hanlon, D., Price, R., Neilson, K., Willard, H.F., Cox, D.R., Marks, A., & Dunn, R.J. (1978). Gene encoding the β subunit of S-100 protein is on chromosome 21: Implications for Down syndrome. *Science, 239,* 1311–1313.

Amaral, D.G. (1987). Memory: The anatomical organization of candidate brain regions. In F. Plum (Ed.), *Handbook of physiology: Higher functions of the nervous system* (pp. 211–294). Bethesda, MD: American Physiologic Society.

Balázs, R., & Brooksbank, B.W.L. (1985). Neurochemical approaches to the pathogenesis of Down's syndrome. *Journal of Mental Deficiency Research, 29,* 1–14.

Becker, L.E., Armstrong, D.L., & Chan, F. (1986). Dendritic atrophy in children with Down's syndrome. *Annals of Neurology, 20,* 520–526.

Benda, C.E. (1971). Mongolism. In J. Minckler (Ed.), *Pathology of the nervous system* (pp. 1361–1371). New York: McGraw-Hill.

Brooksbank, B.W.L., Walker, D., Balázs, R., & Jorgensen, O.S. (1989). Neuronal maturation in the foetal brain in Down's syndrome. *Early Human Development, 18,* 237–246.

Callner, D.A., Dustman, R.E., Madsen, J.A., Schenkenberg, T., & Beck, E.C. (1978). Life span changes in the averaged evoked responses of Down's syndrome and nonretarded persons. *American Journal of Mental Deficiency, 82,* 398–405.

Courchesne, E. (1988). Physioanatomical considerations in Down syndrome. In L. Nadel (Ed.), *The psychobiology of Down syndrome* (pp. 291–313). Cambridge, MA: MIT Press.

Crome, L., Cowie, V., & Slater, E. (1966). A statistical note on cerebellar and brain stem weight in mongolism. *Journal of Mental Deficiency Research, 10,* 69–72.

Cronk, E., & Pueschel, S.M. (1984). Anthropometric studies. In S.M. Pueschel (Ed.), *A study of the young child with Down syndrome* (pp. 105–141). New York: Human Science Press.

Cutler, N.R. (1986). Cerebral metabolism as measured with positron emission tomography (PET) and [18F]2-deoxy-D-glucose: Healthy aging, Alzheimer's disease and Down syndrome. *Progress in Neuropharmacology & Biological Psychiatry, 10,* 309–321.

Damasio, H., & Damasio, A.R. (1990). The neural

basis of memory, language and behavioral guidance: Advances with the lesion method in humans. *Seminars in the Neurosciences, 2,* 277–286.

Devinsky, O., Sato, S., Conwit, R.A., & Schapiro, M.B. (1990). Relation of EEG alpha background to cognitive function, brain atrophy, and cerebral metabolism in Down's syndrome. *Archives of Neurology, 47,* 58–62.

Dudai, Y. (1989). *The neurobiology of memory.* Oxford: Oxford University Press.

Dustman, R.E., & Callner, D.A. (1979). Cortical evoked responses and response decrement in nonretarded and Down's syndrome individuals. *American Journal of Mental Deficiency, 83,* 391–397.

Ellingson, R.J., Menolascino, F.J., & Eisen, J.D. (1970). Clinical EEG relationships in mongoloids confirmed by karyotype. *American Journal of Mental Deficiency, 74,* 645–650.

Elliott, D., & Weeks, D.J. (1990). Cerebral specialization and the control of oral and limb movements for individuals with Down's syndrome. *Journal of Motor Behavior, 22,* 6–18.

Elliott, D., Weeks, D.J., & Gray, S. (1990). Manual and oral praxis in adults with Down's syndrome. *Neuropsychologia, 28,* 1307–1315.

Flórez, J. (1990). *Brain alterations and learning in Down syndrome.* Paper presented at Il Colloque International sur la Trisomie 21. Université de Lyon.

Flórez, J., del Arco, C., González, A., Pascual, J., & Pazos, A. (1990). Autoradiographic studies of neurotransmitter receptors in the brain of newborn infants with Down syndrome. *American Journal of Medical Genetics, Supplement 7,* 301–305.

Fuster, J.M. (1989). *The prefrontal cortex: Anatomy, physiology, and neuropsychology of the frontal lobe* (2nd ed.). New York: Raven Press.

Giencke, S., & Lewandowski, L. (1989). Anomalous dominance in Down syndrome young adults. *Cortex, 25,* 93–102.

Griffin, W.S., Stanley, L.C., Ling, C., White, L., MacLeod, V., Perrot, L.J., White, C.L., III, & Araoz, C. (1989). Brain interleukin 1 and S-100 immunoreactivity are elevated in Down syndrome and Alzheimer disease. *Proceedings of the National Academy of Sciences of the United States of America, 86,* 7611–7615.

Groner, Y., Elroy-Stein, O., Avraham, K.B., Yarom, R., Schickler, M., Knobler, H., & Rotman, G. (1990). Down syndrome clinical symptoms are manifested in transfected cells and transgenic mice overexpressing the human Cu/Zn-superoxide dismutase gene. *Journal de Physiologie, Paris, 84,* 53–77.

Gullotta, F., & Rehder, H. (1974). Chromosomal anomalies and central nervous system. *Beitrage Pathology, 152,* 74–80.

Hartley, X. (1981). Hemispheric asymmetry in Down's syndrome children. *Canadian Journal of Behavioral Sciences, 13,* 210–217.

Horwitz, B., Schapiro, M.B., Grady, C.L., & Rapoport, S.J. (1990). Cerebral metabolic pattern in young adult Down's syndrome subjects: Altered intercorrelations between regional rates of glucose utilization. *Journal of Mental Deficiency Research, 34,* 237–252.

Ieshima, A., Kisa, T., Yoshino, K., Takashima, S., & Takeshita, K. (1984). A morphometric CT study of Down's syndrome showing small posterior fossa and calcification of basal ganglia. *Neuroradiology, 26,* 493–498.

Jorgensen, O.S., Brooksbank, B.W., & Balázs, R. (1990). Neuronal plasticity and astrocytic reaction in Down syndrome and Alzheimer disease. *Journal of the Neurological Sciences, 98,* 63–79.

Kato, K., Suzuki, F., Kurobe, N., Okajima, K., Ogasawara, N., Nagaya, M., & Yamanaka, T. (1990). Enhancement of S-100β protein in blood of patients with Down's syndrome. *Journal of Molecular Neurosciences, 2,* 109–113.

Kemper, T.L. (1988). Neuropathology of Down syndrome. In L. Nadel (Ed.), *The psychobiology of Down syndrome* (pp. 269–289). Cambridge, MA: MIT Press.

Kemper, T.L. (1991). Down syndrome. In A. Peters & E.G. Jones (Eds.), *Cerebral cortex* (pp. 511–526). New York: Plenum.

Kirman, B.H. (1951). Epilepsy in mongolism. *Archives of Disease in Childhood, 26,* 501–503.

Kish, S., Karlinsky, H., Becker, L., Gilbert, J., Rebbetoy, M., Chang, L-J., DiStéfano, L., & Hornykiewicz, O. (1989). Down's syndrome individuals begin life with normal levels of brain cholinergic markers. *Journal of Neurochemistry, 52,* 1183–1187.

Kiss, J., Schlumpf, M., & Balázs, R. (1989). Selective retardation of the development of the basal forebrain cholinergic and pontine catecholaminergic nuclei in the brain of trisomy 16 mouse, an animal model of Down's syndrome. *Developmental Brain Research, 50,* 251–264.

Kolb, B., & Whishaw, I.R. (1990). *Fundamentals of human neuropsychology* (3rd ed.). New York: W.H. Freeman.

Kornberg, J.R., Kawashima, H., Pulst, S.M., Ikeuchi, T., Ogasawara, N., Yamamoto, K., Schonberg, S.A., West, R., Allen, L., Magenis, E., Ikawa, K., Taginuchi, N., & Epstein, C.J. (1990). Molecular definition of the region of chromosome 21 that causes the Down syndrome phenotype. *American Journal of Human Genetics, 47,* 236–246.

Laget, P. (1983). Electro-neuro-physiological data in Down syndrome. In T. Villa-Elizaga (Ed.), *Síndrome de Down* [Down syndrome] (pp. 71–89). Madrid: Iamer.

Le Berre, C., Journel, C., Lucas, J., Le Mée, F., Betremieux, P., Roussey, M., & Le Marec, B. (1986). L'épilepsie chez le trisomique 21 [Epilepsy in trisomy 21]. *Annales de Pédiatrie, 33,* 579–585.

Lincoln, A.J., Courchesne, E., Kilman, B.A., & Galambos, R. (1985). Neuropsychological correlates of information-processing by children with Down syndrome. *American Journal of Mental Deficiency, 89*, 403–414.

MacGillivray, R.C. (1967). Epilepsy in Down's anomaly. *Journal of Mental Deficiency Research, 11*, 43–48.

Malamud, N. (1964). Neuropathology. In H.A. Stevens & R. Heber (Eds.), *Mental retardation* (pp. 429–452). Chicago: University of Chicago Press.

Marcell, M.M., & Armstrong, V. (1982). Auditory and visual sequential memory of Down syndrome and nonretarded children. *American Journal of Mental Deficiency, 87*, 86–95.

Marcell, M.M., & Weeks, S.L. (1988). Short-term memory difficulties and Down's syndrome. *Journal of Mental Deficiency Research, 32*, 153–162.

Marín-Padilla, M. (1976). Pyramidal cell abnormalities in the motor cortex of a child with Down's syndrome. A Golgi study. *Journal of Comparative Neurology, 167*, 63–82.

McCoy, E.E., & Enns, L. (1986). Current status of neurotransmitter abnormalities in Down syndrome. In C.J. Epstein (Ed.), *The neurobiology of Down syndrome* (pp. 73–87). New York: Raven Press.

McGeer, E.G., Norman, M., Boyes, B., O'Kusky, J., Suzuki, J., & McGeer, P.L. (1985). Acetylcholine and aromatic amine systems in postmortem brain of an infant with Down syndrome. *Experimental Neurology, 87*, 557–570.

Merikangas, J.R., Marasco, J.A., & Feczko, W.A. (1979). Basal ganglia calcification in Down syndrome. *Computerized Tomography, 3*, 111–113.

Meyers, L.F. (1990). Language development and intervention. In D.C. Van Dyke, D.J. Lang, F. Heide, S. van Duyne, & M.J. Soucek (Eds.), *Clinical perspectives in the management of Down syndrome* (pp. 153–164). New York: Springer-Verlag.

Miller, J.F. (1987). Language and communication characteristics of children with Down syndrome. In S.M. Pueschel, C. Tingey, J.E. Rynders, A.C. Crocker, & D.M. Crutcher (Eds.), *New perspectives in Down syndrome* (pp. 233–262). Baltimore: Paul H. Brookes Publishing Co.

Miller, J.F. (1988). The developmental asynchrony of language development in children with Down syndrome. In L. Nadel (Ed.), *The psychobiology of Down syndrome* (pp. 167–198). Cambridge, MA: MIT Press.

Nieminen, K., Suárez-Isla, B.A., & Rapoport, S.I. (1988). Electrical properties of cultured dorsal root ganglion neurons from normal and trisomy 21 human fetal tissue. *Brain Research, 474*, 246–254.

Ojemann, G.A. (1990). Organization of language cortex derived from investigations during neurosurgery. *Seminars in the Neurosciences, 2*, 297–305.

Orozco, C.B., Smith, S.A., Epstein, C.J., & Rapoport, S.I. (1987). Electrophysiological properties of cultured dorsal root ganglion and spinal cord neurons of normal and trisomy 16 fetal mice. *Developmental Brain Research, 32*, 111–122.

Oster-Granite, M.L., Gearhart, J.D., & Reeves, R.H. (1986). Neurobiological consequences of trisomy 16 in mice. In C.J. Epstein (Ed.), *The neurobiology of Down syndrome* (pp. 137–151). New York: Raven Press.

Paulson, G.W., Son, C.D., & Nance, W.E. (1969). Neurological aspects of typical and atypical Down's syndrome. *Diseases of the Nervous System, 30*, 632–636.

Pipe, M.E. (1983). Dichotic listening performance following auditory discrimination training on Down syndrome and developmentally retarded children. *Cortex, 19*, 481–491.

Posner, M.L., & Petersen, S.E. (1990). The attention system of the human brain. *Annual Review of Neurosciences, 13*, 25–42.

Pueschel, S.M., Gallagher, P.L., Zartler, A.S., & Pezzullo, J.C. (1987). Cognitive and learning processes in children with Down syndrome. *Research in Developmental Disabilities, 8*, 21–37.

Pueschel, S.M., Louis, S., & McKnight, P. (1991). Seizure disorders in Down syndrome. *Archives of Neurology, 48*, 318–320.

Purpura, D.P. (1974). Dendritic spine dysgenesis and mental retardation. *Science, 186*, 1126–1128.

Rohr, A., & Burr, D.B. (1978). Etiological differences in patterns of psycholinguistic development of children of IQ 30 to 60. *American Journal of Mental Deficiency, 82*, 549–553.

Romano, C., Tiné, A., Fazio, G., Rizzo, R., Colognola, R.M., & Pavone, L. (1990). Seizures in patients with trisomy 21. *American Journal of Medical Genetics, Supplement 7*, 298–300.

Rondal, J.A. (1986). *Le developpement du langage chez l'énfant trisomique 21*. [The development of language in the child with trisomy 21]. Bruxelles: Pierre Madarga.

Ross, M.H., Galaburda, A.M., & Kemper, T.L. (1984). Down's syndrome: Is there a decreased population of neurons? *Neurology, 34*, 909–915.

Schafer, E.W.P., & Peeke, H.V.S. (1982). Down syndrome individuals fail to habituate cortical evoked potentials. *American Journal of Mental Deficiency, 87*, 332–337.

Schantz, S.L., & Brown, W.S. (1990). P300 latency and cognitive ability. In D.C. Van Dyke, D.J. Lang, F. Heide, S. van Duyne, & M.J. Soucek (Eds.), *Clinical perspectives in the management of Down syndrome* (pp. 139–146). New York: Springer-Verlag.

Schapiro, M.B., Haxby, J.V., Grady, C.L., Duara, R., Schlageter, N.L., White, B., Moore, A., Sundaram, M., Larson, S.M., & Rapoport, S.I. (1987). Decline in cerebral glucose utilisation and cognitive function with aging in Down's syndrome. *Journal of Neurology, Neurosurgery, and Psychiatry, 50*, 766–774.

Schapiro, M.B., Kay, A.D., May, C., Ryker, A.K.,

Haxby, J.V., Kaufman, S., Milstien, S., & Rapoport, S.I. (1987). Cerebrospinal fluid monoamines in Down's syndrome adults at different ages. *Journal of Mental Deficiency Research, 31,* 259–269.

Schapiro, M.B., Luxenberg, J.S., Kaye, J.A., Haxby, J.V., Friedland, R.P., & Rapoport, S.I. (1989). Serial quantitative CT analysis of brain morphometrics in adult Down's syndrome at different ages. *Neurology, 39,* 1349–1353.

Scott, B.S., Becker, L.E., & Petit, T.L. (1983). Neurobiology of Down's syndrome. *Progress in Neurobiology, 21,* 199–237.

Scott, B.S., Petit, T.L., Becker, L.E., & Edwards, B.A.V. (1982). Abnormal electric membrane properties of Down's syndrome DRG neurons in cell culture. *Developmental Brain Research, 2,* 257–270.

Squire, L.R. (1987). *Memory and brain.* New York: Oxford University Press.

Squire, L.R., & Lindenlaub, E. (1990). *The biology of memory.* Stuttgart: F.K. Schattauer Verlag.

Squires, N., Ollo, C., & Jordan, R. (1986). Auditory brainstem responses in the mentally retarded: Audiometric correlates. *Ear and Hearing, 7,* 83–92.

Stafstrom, C.E., Patxot, O.F., Gilmore, H.E., & Wisniewski, K.E. (1991). Seizures in children with Down syndrome. Etiology, characteristics and outcome. *Developmental Medicine and Child Neurology, 33,* 191–200.

Suetsugu, M., & Mehraein, P. (1980). Spine distribution along apical dendrites of the pyramidal neurons in Down's syndrome. *Acta Neuropathologica, 50,* 207–210.

Sylvester, P.E. (1983). The hippocampus in Down's syndrome. *Journal of Mental Deficiency Research, 27,* 227–236.

Sylvester, P.E. (1986). The anterior commissure in Down's syndrome. *Journal of Mental Deficiency Research, 30,* 19–26.

Takashima, S., & Becker, L.E. (1985). Basal ganglia calcification in Down's syndrome. *Journal of Neurology, Neurosurgery, and Psychiatry, 48,* 61–64.

Takashima, S., Becker, L.E., Armstrong, D.L., & Chan, F. (1981). Abnormal neuronal development in the visual cortex of the human fetus and infant with Down's syndrome. *Brain Research, 225,* 1–21.

Tamir, H., Bebirian, R., Muller, F., & Casper, D. (1980). Differences between intracellular platelet and brain proteins that bind serotonin. *Journal of Neurochemistry, 35,* 1033–1044.

Tangye, S.R. (1979). The EEG and incidence of epilepsy in Down's syndrome. *Journal of Mental Deficiency Research, 23,* 17–24.

Tatsuno, M., Hayashi, M., Iwamoto, H., Suzuki, Y., & Kuroki, Y. (1984). Epilepsy in childhood Down syndrome. *Brain Development, 6,* 37–44.

Ternaux, J.P., Mattei, J.F., Faudon, M., Barrit, M.C., Ardissone, J.P., & Giraud, F. (1979). Peripheral and central 5-hydroxytryptamine in trisomy 21. *Life Sciences, 25,* 2017–2022.

Tukiainen, E., Tuomisto, J., Westermarck, T., & Kupiainen, H. (1980). Nature of lowered 5-hydroxytryptamine uptake by blood platelets of patients with Down syndrome. *Acta Pharmacologica et Toxicologica, 47,* 365–370.

Urich, H. (1976). Malformations of the nervous system, perinatal damage and related conditions early in life. In W. Blackwood & J.A.N. Corellis (Eds.), *Greenfield's neuropathology* (pp. 361–496). Chicago: Yearbook Medical Publishers.

Veall, R.M. (1974). The prevalence of epilepsy among mongols related to age. *Journal of Mental Deficiency Research, 18,* 99–106.

Weis, S. (in press). Morphometry and magnetic resonance imaging (MRI) of the human brain in normal controls and Down's syndrome. *Anatomical Record.*

Wisniewski, K.E. (1990). Down syndrome children often have brain with maturation delay, retardation of growth, and cortical dysgenesis. *American Journal of Medical Genetics, Supplement 7,* 274–281.

Wisniewski, K.E., French, J.H., Rosen, J.F., Kozlowski, P.B., Tenner, M., & Wisniewski, H.M. (1982). Basal ganglia calcification (BGC) in Down's syndrome—Another manifestation of premature aging. *Annals of the New York Academy of Sciences, 396,* 179–189.

Wisniewski, K.E., Laure-Kamionowska, M., Connell, F., & Wen, G.Y. (1986). Neuronal density and synaptogenesis in the post-natal stage of brain maturation in Down syndrome. In C.J. Epstein (Ed.), *The neurobiology of Down syndrome* (pp. 29–44). New York: Raven Press.

Wisniewski, K.E., & Schmidt-Sidor, B. (1989). Myelination in Down's syndrome brains (pre- and postnatal maturation) and some clinical-pathological correlations. *Annals of Neurology, 20,* 429–430.

Zellweger, H. (1977). Down syndrome. In P.J. Vinken & G.W. Bruyn (Eds.), *Handbook of clinical neurology* (Vol. 31, Pt. II, pp. 367–469). Amsterdam: North Holland Publishing Co.

CHAPTER
17

Alzheimer Disease

Florence Lai

Alzheimer disease is a primary degenerative disease of the brain that is age related but not a normal part of aging. It is the major cause of dementia, accounting for 50%–60% of all cases. This percentage is even higher when cases coexisting with cerebral infarction are considered (Katzman, 1986). The diagnosis of Alzheimer disease is a neuropathologic one with distinctive features of neuronal cell loss, neurofibrillary tangles, and neuritic plaques, as demonstrated in Figure 17.1. These neuropathologic findings are clustered in specific areas of the central nervous system, namely the nucleus basalis of Meynert in the basal forebrain, the hippocampus of the temporal lobe, and the association areas (temporoparietal) of the neocortex (Braak & Braak, 1990; Kemper, 1984).

Criteria have been established for possible and probable clinical dementia of the Alzheimer type (McKhann et al., 1984). The correlation between clinical diagnosis and definitive neuropathologic diagnosis has varied over the years, but has improved as the criteria for diagnosis have become more specific. A recent work showed an 87% correlation (Joachim, Morris, & Selkoe, 1988). The separation of "Alzheimer disease" (i.e., presenile dementia with onset before 65 years) from "senile dementia of the Alzheimer type" (with onset after 65 years) is a subject of debate. Proponents for separation feel that there are different causations of the Alzheimer neuropathology depending on age at onset, whereas those opposed to separation believe there is a single etiology regardless of age at onset. In this chapter, the term "Alzheimer disease" is used regardless of the age at onset of the disease process.

It is now common knowledge that all persons with Down sydrome over age 35 (with rare exceptions) have the characteristic features of Alzheimer disease in their central nervous system (Malamud, 1966, 1972; Schweber, 1986; Sylvester, 1984; K.E. Wisniewski & Wisniewski, 1983). The localization of a gene for a subgroup of patients with familial early-onset Alzheimer disease (St. George-Hyslop et al., 1987) and a separate gene that encodes beta-amyloid that forms the protein core of neuritic plaques (Tanzi, Gusella, et al., 1987) to chromosome 21 proximal to the locus that delineates Down syndrome made the association between Down syndrome and Alzheimer disease an even closer one.

Despite the neuropathologic evidence of Alzheimer disease in aging persons with Down syndrome, clinical dementia was only reported in a minority of cases (Ropper & Williams, 1980; Williams & Matthysse, 1986; H.M. Wisniewski & Rabe, 1986; K.E. Wisniewski et al., 1985). The retrospective nature of the studies, the presence of mental retardation, and the time lag between neuropathologic and clinical Alzheimer disease may have all contributed to the seemingly low incidence of clinical dementia. Evidence from a prospective study of Alzheimer disease in adults with Down syndrome that the author of this chapter conducted, however,

The author thanks Dr. Miriam Schweber for critiquing several sections of this chapter, Dr. Bradley Hyman for reviewing the neuropathology section, Mr. Daniel Small for photographic work, and Mrs. Sylvia Goldstein for excellent secretarial assistance. The Down Syndrome Memorial Fund for Alzheimer Disease Research at the Shriver Center provided some funding for the production of this chapter.

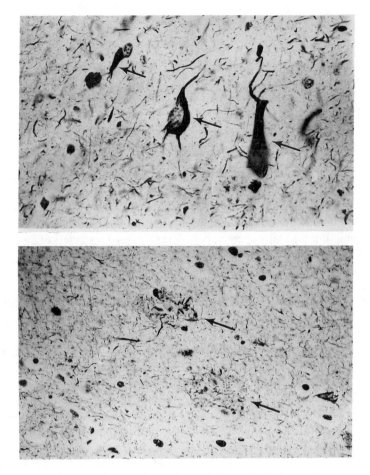

Figure 17.1.   Neurofibrillary tangles (top) and neuritic plaques (bottom) in the neocortex of a person with Alzheimer disease. Bodian stain. 250X. (Photographs courtesy of Thomas L. Kemper, M.D., Boston University School of Medicine.)

seems to indicate that the great majority of these individuals will develop a relentlessly progressive dementia (Lai & Williams, 1989); most likely, this accounts for the sharp decline in survival beyond 44 years of age in these individuals (Baird & Sadovnick, 1988).

The fact that up to 70% of persons with Down syndrome are now living beyond 40 years of age (Baird & Sadovnick, 1987) makes it important that directors of vocational, residential, and institutional programs that include adults with Down syndrome be cognizant of the changing needs of this group as many will become demented with Alzheimer disease. This chapter describes the neuropathologic, neurochemical, neuroradiologic, neurophysiologic, neurogenetic, and clinical features of Alzheimer disease,

particularly as they relate to adults with Down syndrome. In addition, the differential diagnosis, work-up, and management of individuals with Down syndrome and suspected Alzheimer disease are included.

NEUROPATHOLOGIC AND NEUROCHEMICAL CHANGES

The neuropathologic hallmarks of Alzheimer disease are intraneuronal neurofibrillary tangles, extracellular neuritic (senile) plaques, and nerve cell loss (Braak & Braak, 1990; Kemper, 1984). The neurofibrillary tangles are cytoplasmic inclusions of insoluble straight or paired helical filaments, and the neuritic plaques are degenerating neurites (axons and dendrites) surrounding a beta-amyloid core. These same changes in the brains of persons with Down syndrome were first noted in 1929 by Struwe, and it is clear that they appear at much younger ages in persons with Down syndrome than in persons with Alzheimer disease in the general population (Cork, 1990; Jervis, 1948; Mann, 1988a; K.E. Wisniewski, Wisniewski & Wen, 1985). In a large series, Malamud (1972) found Alzheimer disease changes in 30% of the brains from persons with Down syndrome between 31–40 years of age and 100% of those over 41 years of age. Likewise, Sylvester (1984) found Alzheimer changes in 88.9% of all those over 30 years of age. In addition, the numbers of plaques and tangles progressively increased with age in the brains of individuals with Down syndrome (Hyman & Mann, 1991; Motte & Williams, 1989; K.E. Wisniewski et al., 1985).

Although the neuropathology of Alzheimer disease was classified nosologically by the 1970s, its pathogenesis remains unclear. The earliest changes of Alzheimer disease appear to be in the entorhinal cortex and hippocampal formation of the medial temporal lobe (Figure 17.2) (Ball et al., 1985; Hyman & Van Hoesen, 1989; Kemper, 1978). The hippocampus plays a key role in memory function (Damasio, 1984), and it

has been suggested that early pathologic involvement here accounts for the memory disturbance that is prominent in the first stages of Alzheimer dementia. Although a detailed account of the neuroanatomy and connectivity of the hippocampal formation is beyond the scope of this chapter, the schematic diagrams in Figures 17.3, 17.4, and 17.5 of the input to and output from the hippocampal formation may assist the reader in better understanding the topographic pathology in this important region. (The reader is referred to Hyman [1991] and Hyman & Van Hoesen [1989] for detailed discussion.)

The major input to the hippocampus from the cortex (paralimbic, sensory-specific association, and multimodal association areas) and the subcortical regions (anterior thalamus, nucleus basalis of Meynert, and amygdala) is via the entorhinal cortex. Afferents from layer II of the entorhinal cortex form the perforant pathway that projects to the hippocampal formation. (The hippocampal formation consists of the dentate gyrus, CA1-CA4 of the hippocampus proper, and the subicular cortices [see Figure 17.3].) The perforant pathway targets within the hippocampal formation are the granule cells of the dentate gyrus and the pyramids of CA1. The dentate gyrus projects to CA3, which projects to CA1.

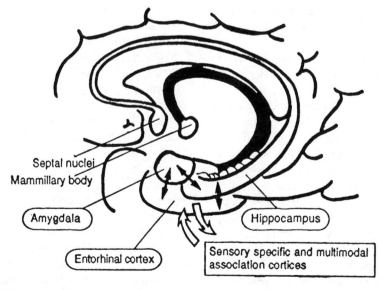

Figure 17.2. Schematic diagram of the medial aspect of the right hemisphere depicting the temporal lobe, and anatomic sites important in the neuropathology of Alzheimer disease. (Courtesy of Bradley T. Hyman, M.D., Ph.D., Massachusetts General Hospital.)

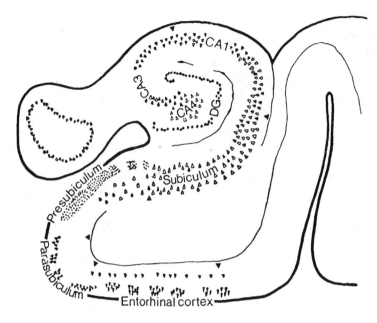

Figure 17.3.   Schematic representation of the organization of the hippocampal formation. DG = dentate gyrus. (Courtesy of Bradley T. Hyman, M.D., Ph.D., Massachusetts General Hospital.)

Other afferents to the hippocampal formation include cholinergic projection from the septal area, serotonergic input from the raphé in the brainstem, and noradrenergic input from the locus ceruleus of the brainstem.

The major transmission of information out of the hippocampal formation is by way of the subiculum to layer IV of the entorhinal cortex. This layer, in turn, projects to widespread areas of the cortex. The subiculum also projects to subcortical regions such as the mammillary bodies, septum, nucleus accumbens, and several of the thalamic nuclei.

In the early stages of Alzheimer disease, pathology in selective areas of the hippocampal formation serves to isolate this structure from the rest of the brain (Hyman, Damasio, Van Hoesen, & Barnes, 1984). Neurofibrillary tangles have a special predilection for neurons in layers II and IV of the entorhinal cortex, which are important in the relay of information to and from the hippocampal formation. The CA1/subicular zones, the origin of hippocampal output, also contain numerous tangles as well as neuritic plaques. The molecular layer of the dentate gyrus, which serves as the endpoint of hippocampal input, is a favored site for plaque formation.

Taking advantage of the inevitable appearance of Alzheimer changes in the brains of persons with Down syndrome, some neuropathologists have studied these brains at various ages using improved histologic and immunocytochemical techniques. This has resulted in an increased understanding of the topography and progressive development of Alzheimer neuropathology (Hyman & Mann, 1991; Mann, Yates, Marcyniuk, & Ravindra, 1986; Motte & Williams, 1989; K.E. Wisniewski et al., 1985). K.E. Wisniewski et al. (1985), studied 100 brains from persons with Down syndrome and showed that plaques and tangles can develop as early as the 3rd decade. This is clearly earlier than in "normal" individuals in which the neurofibrillary tangles make their first appearance in the 4th decade (Matsuyama & Nakamura, 1978) and neuritic plaques in the 5th decade (Jordan, 1971). In addition, the density of the neurofibrillary tangles and neuritic plaques found in the brains of adults with Down syndrome in their 4th decade was comparable to that found in normative brains over age 75 (Kemper, 1988), and the density progressively increased with age in the brains of individuals with Down syndrome. Mann et al. (1986) suggested that the initial focus of plaque and tangle forma-

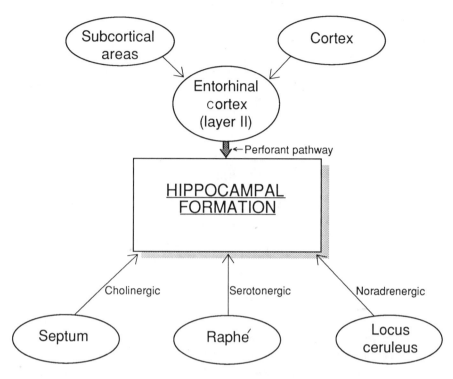

Figure 17.4.   Input to the hippocampal formation.

tion was in the amygdala, entorhinal cortex, and hippocampus, with subsequent spread of pathology to all areas of the cortex, certain subcortical areas, and the olfactory bulbs and tracts. Motte and Williams (1989) found plaques and tangles in 15 brains of persons with Down syndrome ages 25–59 years with a high density of these lesions occurring only after age 40. These changes first appeared in the dentate gyrus, subiculum, and entorhinal and association neocortex. They studied the evolution of neuritic plaque formation in the dentate gyrus and suggested four stages of morphologic development. Their evidence that extracellular amyloid in these brains is present before development into neuritic plaques has also been corroborated by others (Giaccone et al., 1989). Hyman and Mann (1991) showed that the vulnerability to tangle formation in neurons of layers II and IV of the entorhinal cortex, the perforant pathway, and the CA1/subicular zone of the hippocampus of individuals with Down syndrome is identical to the hierarchical patterns of early Alzheimer neuropathology in the general population. There

was steady increase in numbers of tangles in the brains of adults with Down syndrome with age, with mild pathologic changes in the 30s progressing to marked changes after the age of 50 years.

Beta-amyloid protein (or A4) is the major protein component of amyloid deposits in the brain, in blood vessels, and in the amyloid core of mature neuritic plaques. This beta-amyloid protein is identical in persons with Alzheimer disease and in persons with Down syndrome (Glenner & Wong, 1984; Masters et al., 1985). The origin of this protein continues to be the subject of debate, with some favoring a vascular origin (Selkoe, 1989) and others favoring a neuronal one (Masters & Beyreuther, 1987; Neve, 1989). Contributions from the neuropathologic study of individuals with Down syndrome point to a possible different etiology for plaque and vascular amyloid since some investigators have shown that the presence of amyloid plaques precedes that of amyloid angiopathy by a number of years (Mann, 1989; Motte & Williams, 1989). Others view A4 as a developmental protein in the brains of per-

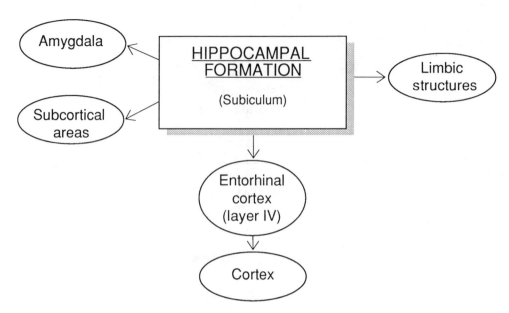

Figure 17.5.   Output from the hippocampal formation.

sons with Down syndrome that reappears as part of the regeneration process when Alzheimer disease supervenes in later life (Takashima et al., 1990).

The identification of Alzheimer disease as a pathologic entity distinct from the effects of normal aging occurred in the 1970s with the identification of neurochemical abnormalities in persons with Alzheimer disease accompanying the neuropathologic changes. Decreases in the neurotransmitters, acetylcholine, norepinephrine, and serotonin reflect the loss of neurons in the nucleus basalis of Meynert in the basal forebrain, the locus ceruleus of the brainstem, and the raphe nucleus in the brainstem, respectively. These same neurotransmitter deficits are evident in middle-age individuals with Down syndrome (Godridge, Reynolds, Czudek, Calcutt, & Benton, 1987; Mann, Yates, Marcyniuk, & Ravindra, 1985) and provide further evidence of the similar (if not identical) process of Alzheimer disease in individuals with Down syndrome. The clinical correlates include deficits in memory and learning due to acetylcholine deficiency and abnormalities in sleep/wake cycles due to norepinephrine deficiency (Aston-Jones, 1986).

Glutamate is the putative neurotransmitter of the hippocampal perforant pathway (delivering information from neocortical and subcortical re-

gions to the hippocampal formation; see Figure 17.4). Depletion of this transmitter has been demonstrated in persons with Alzheimer disease but studies have not yet been carried out in the brains of persons with Down syndrome (Hyman, Van Hoesen, & Damasio, 1987). (The reader is referred to Glenner & Wurtman [1987] and Wurtman, Corkin, Growdon, & Ritter-Walker [1990] for more detailed discussions of the neurochemical and neurotransmitter abnormalities in persons with Alzheimer disease.)

GENETIC LINKAGE
BETWEEN ALZHEIMER
DISEASE AND DOWN SYNDROME

The evidence for a genetic link between Alzheimer disease and Down syndrome has been mixed. Studies that have provided clues include clinical and molecular genetic linkage studies in large family pedigrees with multiple members affected with Alzheimer disease, genetic localization of amyloid precursor protein to chromosome 21, and molecular genetic studies of the gene locus for Down syndrome on chromosome 21.

In the early 1980s, some investigators found an excess of individuals with Down syndrome among relatives of early-onset Alzheimer disease probands in two different sections of the United

States when second- and third-degree relatives were included (Heston, Mastri, Anderson, & White, 1981; Heyman et al., 1983). Other studies showed no increase in the incidence of individuals with Down syndrome, but the number of persons studied was small, and only first-degree relatives were used (Nee et al., 1983; Whalley, Carothers, Collyer, DeMey, & Frackiewicz, 1982). Conversely, when the rate of Alzheimer disease was calculated among relatives of individuals with Down syndrome, the results were again mixed, probably due to inherent limitations in the studies. On the one hand, Yatham, McHale, and Kinsella (1988) found an increased frequency of presenile dementia but not senile dementia in the first- and second-degree relatives of 67 probands with Down syndrome from 8 families. However, neuropathologic confirmation of Alzheimer disease in the 12 relatives with clinical dementia was sparse. On the other hand, when Berr, Borghi, Rethoré, Lejeune, and Alperovitch (1989) surveyed 188 children with Down syndrome and 185 controls for rates of dementia of Alzheimer type among grandparents and great-grandparents, they found no difference between the two groups. However, family members other than direct ancestors were not included in this study.

Among the heterogeneous subgroups of Alzheimer disease (Chui, 1987; Mayeux, Stern, & Spanton, 1985), there is a group that shows a genetic predisposition to develop this condition in a seemingly autosomal dominant pattern (i.e., familial Alzheimer disease). Even within this familial grouping, however, there is heterogeneity. Two groups of investigators have localized a gene for familial early-onset Alzheimer disease to the long arm of chromosome 21, proximal to the gene locus for Down syndrome (Goate et al., 1989; St. George-Hyslop et al., 1987), but two other groups of investigators using family pedigrees with relatively late-onset Alzheimer disease did not show linkage to chromosome 21 (Pericak-Vance et al., 1988; Schellenberg et al., 1988). It should be noted, however, that the families studied by Schellenberg and colleagues were of Volga German ancestry and may represent a founder effect.

After the purification and sequencing of beta-amyloid protein was reported (Glenner & Wong, 1984), several laboratories independently discovered the gene locus of amyloid protein precursor on the long arm of chromosome 21 (Goldgaber, Lerman, McBride, Saffiotti, & Gajdusek, 1987; Kang et al., 1987; Robakis et al., 1987; Tanzi, Gusella, et al., 1987). This discovery seemed to underscore the close association between Alzheimer disease and Down syndrome. However, it was quickly noted that the amyloid protein precursor locus was not close to the gene locus for Down syndrome or familial Alzheimer disease (Tanzi, St. George-Hyslop, et al., 1987) and that this gene was not duplicated in persons with Alzheimer disease (Tanzi, Bird, Latt, & Neve, 1987). Rumble et al. (1989) described a 1.5-fold increase of serum amyloid protein precursor in individuals with Down syndrome not found in "normal" controls or in individuals with Alzheimer disease in the general population; they felt that this increase accounted for the amyloid deposition in the brains of persons with Down syndrome up to 50 years earlier than that in the general population. Since a similar gene-dosage effect was not present in persons with Alzheimer disease without Down syndrome, Rumble et al. postulated that other factors were operative in the brain amyloid deposition of persons with Alzheimer disease without Down syndrome.

Molecular genetic studies of triplicated genes at the locus for Down syndrome (e.g., superoxide dismutase, interferon-α-receptor) do not give convincing evidence of a role in the pathogenesis of Alzheimer disease (Epstein, 1987). The current state of genetic studies in Alzheimer disease has been thoroughly reviewed by Gusella (1991), Martin (1990), Schellenberg, Bird, Wijsman, Moore, and Martin (1989), and St. George-Hyslop et al. (1989).

CLINICAL STUDIES

During the 1980s, a number of review articles on Alzheimer disease in individuals with Down syndrome all mentioned the universality of Alzheimer disease neuropathology in these individuals as they age, but the impression was that only a minority developed clinical dementia (Karlinsky, 1986; Lott, 1982; Oliver & Holland, 1986). This discrepancy is even more notable given the fact that the density of plaques and tangles in the brains of adults with Down syndrome after age 30 exceeds the density criteria for Alzheimer disease neuropathology in the general population (H.M. Wisniewski & Rabe, 1986, Table I, p. 248).

Retrospective and Cross-Sectional Studies

Many reports of the Alzheimer disease association with individuals who have Down syndrome were neuropathologic ones that retrospectively attempted to determine whether there was a concomitant dementia (Burger & Vogel, 1973; Haberland, 1969; Jervis, 1948; Olson & Shaw, 1969; Reid, Maloney & Aungle, 1978; Ropper & Williams, 1980; H.M. Wisniewski & Rabe, 1986). This retrospective study methodology certainly underestimated the incidence of dementia as signs of dementia may not have been recognized in the setting of mental retardation.

When Dalton and Crapper-McLachlan (1986) reviewed all published reports through 1985 that included clinical descriptions of persons with Down syndrome as well as details of their brain pathology, they found that 85% of the 33 patients over age 35 studied had one or more signs suggestive of dementia. The 5 patients who showed Alzheimer disease neuropathology but no recorded signs of dementia were age 35–47 at the time of death. It is possible that these 5 patients had not yet reached the threshold age of dementia onset, which on average is between 51–54 years of age (Evenhuis, 1990; Lai & Williams, 1989; K.E. Wisniewski, Dalton, Crapper-McLachlan, Wen, & Wisniewski, 1985). This threshold effect for clinical dementia, resulting in a seeming discrepancy between the neuropathology of Alzheimer disease and its clinical expression, has also been noted in the general population (Morris & Fulling, 1988).

One of the difficulties in determining dementia in the presence of mental retardation is that there are no standardized criteria for the diagnosis. Cummings and Benson's (1983, p. 1) operational definition for dementia was: "An acquired, persistent impairment of intellectual function with compromise in at least three of the following spheres of mental activity: (1) language, (2) memory, (3) visuospatial skills, (4) emotion or personality, (5) cognition (abstraction, calculation, judgment, etc.)." It is clear that such a definition of dementia for the general population is not appropriate for persons with mental retardation. Thus, studies of aging persons with Down syndrome have used various neuropsychologic, psychometric, functional, and adaptive behavioral assessments to evaluate for the presence of dementia.

Thase, Tigner, Smeltzer, and Liss (1984) showed lower scores for orientation, digit span, visual memory, object naming, and general knowledge in persons with Down syndrome to be especially evident after 50 years of age when compared with controls with mental retardation. Dalton and Crapper-McLachlan (1984) evaluated 49 individuals above the age of 40 years prospectively (1–8 years of follow-up) for memory loss using a visual retention paradigm. They found deficits in 12 patients (24%), but only 6 of these have had subsequent neuropathologic confirmation for Alzheimer disease (K.E. Wisniewski, Dalton, et al., 1985). Schapiro et al. (1987) assessed language, visuospatial ability, attention, and visual recognition memory in 20 persons with Down syndrome and found test scores significantly reduced in 5 of the 6 persons over the age of 47 years concomitant with decreased glucose utilization noted on positron emission tomography, particularly in the temporal and parietal lobes. Only 2 of these 5 older persons were judged to have clinical dementia.

A retrospective longitudinal study assessed changes in scores obtained on the Stanford-Binet Intelligence Scale (Thorndike, Hagen, & Sattler, 1986) in 39 individuals with Down syndrome under 49 years of age (Fenner, Hewitt, & Torpy, 1987) and 23 persons over the age of 50 years (Hewitt, Carter, & Jancar, 1985). The results indicated that 28% of those between 34–49 years and 39% of those over 50 years showed intellectual deterioration with little or no decline in behavioral functioning.

For those aging individuals with Down syndrome who are untestable by standard psychometric batteries, Miniszek (1983) has suggested functional instruments such as Part I of the American Association on Mental Deficiency Adaptive Behavior Scale (AAMD-ABS) (Lambert & Windmiller, 1981). It assesses abilities such as independent function, physical development, economic activity, language development, numbers and time, domestic activity, vocational activity, self-direction, responsibility, and socialization.

Prospective Longitudinal Studies

Retrospective and cross-sectional clinical studies have inherent limitations in defining the natural history of Alzheimer disease in individuals with Down syndrome. Prospective longitudinal studies provide a more accurate description of the clinical dementia that occurs in this group. Only three such reports exist in the current literature (Evenhuis, 1990; Lai & Williams, 1989; K.E. Wisniewski et al., 1985). K.E. Wisniewski et al. (1985) provided neuropathologic confirmation of Alzheimer disease in 7 patients with Down syndrome who had been examined neurologically and cognitively. The average age at dementia onset was 51.0 ± 6.2 years, and the average duration of dementia until death was 5.6 ± 2.2 years. The initial symptoms were visual memory loss, impaired learning ability, and behavioral changes, followed by loss of language, impairment of social–adaptive skills, further personality changes, and loss of personal hygiene. The last phase was marked by mutism, poor sleep, urinary incontinence, seizures, and the inability to walk. Also noted were slow-wave abnormalities in the 5 patients who had electroencephalograms and brain atrophy in the 2 patients who had computerized tomographic scans. The brains of these 7 patients showed widespread neuronal loss and mild gliosis. In decreasing severity, plaques and tangles were seen in the cortical mantle, basal ganglia, thalamus, hypothalamus, and midbrain. Amyloid angiopathy was noted in 5 brains and small infarcts were seen in 4.

In 1989, Lai and Williams reported on a series of 96 individuals with Down syndrome over the age of 35 years who had been followed prospectively for up to 8 years for signs of dementia. When serial assessments were recorded for orientation, memory, verbal and motor skills, and self-care abilities, as well as regular neurologic examinations, a functional decline consistent with dementia was seen in 49 of the 96 individuals, of whom 21 were described previously (Lott & Lai, 1982). The average onset of dementia in these 49 persons was 54.2 ± 6.1 years, and the average duration of dementia was 4.6 ± 3.2 years in the 23 people who died during the course of the study. The prevalence of dementia was calculated for a group of 53 institutionalized individuals with Down syndrome over the age of 35 years, which showed a marked increase with age (8% in those 35–49 years old, 55% in those 50–59 years old, and 75% in those over 60 years old [the figure for those over 60 years has increased to 100% since publication of the study]). Dementia was manifested in the initial stage as memory impairment, temporal disorientation, and reduced verbal output in the higher functioning individuals and as apathy, inattention, and decreased social interaction in the individuals with more severe mental retardation. In the second phase, loss of self-help skills in dressing, toileting, and feeding was seen in addition to slowed gait, deterioration in workshop performance, and the emergence of seizures. In the final phase, the individuals were nonambulatory and incontinent, and exhibited pathologic reflexes.

Seizures, mostly of the generalized tonic–clonic variety, developed in 84% of the 49 persons with Down syndrome who had dementia, usually within 2 years of dementia onset (Lai & Williams, 1989). All 23 persons with dementia who died had seizures. In all those with seizures, 65% also developed myoclonus (Lai & Brodie, 1991). This high frequency of seizures contrasts with the low prevalence in nondemented persons with Down syndrome (Pueschel, Louis, & McKnight, 1991; Romano et al., 1990; Veall, 1974) and the 10%–64% seizure frequency in the later stages of Alzheimer disease in the general population (Hauser, Morris, Heston, & Anderson, 1986; Risse et al., 1990), and probably reflects the neuropathology of Alzheimer disease superimposed on the already developmentally abnormal brain of individuals with Down syndrome (de la Monte & Hedley-Whyte, 1990; Ross, Galaburda, & Kemper, 1984). In addition, a gene for a progressive form of myoclonus epilepsy has been localized to the long arm of chromosome 21 (Lehesjoki et al., 1991) and could perhaps account for the unusually high frequency of seizures and myoclonus in individuals with Down syndrome as they develop dementia. Parkinsonian features (bradykinesia, flexed posture, masked facies, cogwheel rigidity) occurred in one fifth of the study subjects with dementia, which correlated with that seen in Alzheimer disease in the general population (Ditter & Mirra, 1987). It also corroborates a recent study of extrapyramidal features in adults with Down syndrome (Vieregge et al., 1991). Hypothyroidism was present in 59% of the study group with Down syndrome who had dementia, compared with only 33% in the nondemented group with Down syndrome.

Computerized tomographic (CT) scans of 43 of the 49 persons with dementia showed substantial brain tissue loss, especially in the temporal lobes (Lai & Williams, 1989). Neuropathologic confirmation of Alzheimer disease was available for 12 persons with Down syndrome who were demented (this has increased to 21 since publication of the study). The great majority had moderate to marked ventricular enlargement, and all had prominent neurofibrillary tangles and neuritic plaques in the hippocampus, parahippocampal gyrus, amygdala, and neocortex.

In 1990, Evenhuis reported an additional 17 middle-age individuals with Down syndrome who were followed prospectively, 15 of whom had dementia, based on decline in daily functional abilities. The average age of dementia onset in these 15 individuals was 52.5 years and the average duration of dementia until death was 4.9 years. The manifestations and natural course of the dementia were very similar to that described by Lai and Williams (1989). Epileptic seizures or myoclonus occurred in all of the individuals studied and started within 2 years of dementia onset in the group with severe mental retardation and slightly later in the group with moderate mental retardation. Eight of the 15 persons with dementia had autopsy examination, which showed many neurofibrillary tangles and neuritic plaques in widespread areas of the cortex as well as the hippocampus. Amyloid angiopathy was also noted in arachnoidal and cortical vessels. One of these 8 persons also demonstrated several cerebral infarctions and had had a stroke during life. Two persons with Down syndrome, ages 49 and 50 years respectively, were not considered demented during life but already showed the same qualitative neuropathologic changes of Alzheimer disease as in the patients with Down syndrome who had dementia.

The three prospective clinical studies just described demonstrate that dementia can be diagnosed even in individuals with Down syndrome who are severely mentally retarded by using functional and neuropsychologic assessments. The important factor is longitudinal evaluation of the same person using the same assessment parameters. The reported average age of dementia onset between 51–54 years is clearly 15–20 years later than the age of reported neuropathologic changes of Alzheimer disease in individuals with Down syndrome. This latency between neuropathologic and clinical Alzheimer disease may in part account for the low incidence of dementia in many retrospective neuropathologic studies of Alzheimer disease in persons with Down syndrome. Nevertheless, persons with Down syndrome still develop a clinical dementia several decades earlier than those in the general population; perhaps the deposition of amyloid A4 protein in the brains of persons with Down syndrome up to 50 years earlier than that in "normal" aging individuals (Rumble et al., 1989) will play a role in this phenomenon. Of greater interest, however, is that the existence of plaques and tangles, even in numbers that surpass the criteria for Alzheimer disease in the general population, is not sufficient to cause a clinical dementia in persons with Down syndrome. Additional factors must be operative.

NEUROIMAGING STUDIES

Since Alzheimer disease insidiously destroys selected areas of the brain, it is sometimes possible to make the diagnosis with relative certainty during life, employing various neuroimaging tests. These tests must be used in conjunction with careful clinical assessments because brain atrophy and ventricular enlargement can also occur as the result of brain damage from stroke or craniocerebral trauma. They can also occur in normal aging individuals, but the rate of change is more rapid in those with dementia of the Alzheimer type, as noted in several CT studies (de Leon et al., 1989; Luxenberg, Haxby, Creasey, Sundaram, & Rapoport, 1987). Although assessments of brain atrophy and ventricular dilatation are not specific for Alzheimer disease, rating of temporal horn enlargement on computerized tomographic scans can accurately diagnose dementia of the Alzheimer type in 82%–89% of cases (George et al., 1990; LeMay et al., 1986). Similar studies of temporal lobe atrophy in individuals with Down syndrome confirm the high correlation with clinical dementia (LeMay & Alvarez, 1990; Pearlson et al., 1990). Lai and LeMay (1990) found a progressive brain tissue loss in the temporal lobe and temporoparietal areas in individuals with Down syndrome directly related to increasing duration of the dementia process. When comparisons were made with persons with Alzheimer disease from the "normal" population, the more aggressive nature of the disease process was evident in individuals with Down syndrome. Figure 17.6 illustrates the progressive enlargement of the temporal, occipital, and frontal horns of the lateral ventricle in a woman with Down syndrome who had serial scans over a 6-year period of time (i.e., 1 year after dementia onset until 1 year before death).

The selective regional loss of brain tissue as seen on CT scans corresponds to the neuropathologic process of Alzheimer disease in which early destruction occurs in the entorhinal cortex of the temporal lobe. The entorhinal cortex transmits information from the cortical association areas (in the temporoparietal area) to the hippocampus; thus its destruction leads to atrophy of the hippocampus and cortical association areas, which is reflected in temporal horn and occipital horn enlargement, respectively.

Basal ganglia calcification is a frequent finding on CT scans of individuals with Down syndrome, which far exceeds that found in the general population. It is felt to be a manifestation of premature aging and not related to dementia per se (Mann, 1988b; K.E. Wisniewski et al., 1982).

The use of magnetic resonance imaging (MRI) scans does not supply additional information regarding selective brain atrophy. However, in some research centers, the technique may make possible areal and volumetric analysis of select brain areas such as the hippocampus (Naidich et al., 1987; Scheltens et al., 1991).

ELECTROPHYSIOLOGIC STUDIES

In persons with Alzheimer disease who are already exhibiting moderate or severe dementia, electroencephalograms show a decrease and loss of the normal alpha rhythm (8 Hz–13 Hz [cycles per second]), and replacement by more and more theta (4 Hz–7 Hz) and delta activity (1 Hz–3 Hz). Since slowing of background activity can be seen in organic brain conditions other than Alzheimer disease, the usefulness of the electroencephalogram, especially in the early stages of Alzheimer disease, is limited. In addition, normality or abnormality of the electroencephalogram may not distinguish between mild and moderate Alzheimer disease, nor correlate with duration or severity of dementia (Soininen et al., 1989). However, preservation of the alpha background rhythm in persons with Alzheimer disease may correlate with relative intactness of parietal lobe function (Sheridan et al., 1988).

Cortical evoked potential studies in persons with Alzheimer disease show that the P300 response (a long latency response 300 msec after the stimulus) is increased in latency and decreased in amplitude when compared with controls (Blackwood, St. Clair, Muir, Oliver, & Dickens, 1988). However, prolongation of P300 can also occur in normal aging. Blackwood et al. applied this same technique to individuals with Down syndrome and found a marked increase in P300 latency starting at age 37, which coincides with the appearance of Alzheimer disease neuropathology in these individuals. In addition, the majority of those who showed a clinical deterioration when followed longitudinally displayed an increase in P300 latency (Muir et al., 1988). Although these results are interesting, the changes in P300 latency may not be specific enough to predict the onset of a clinical dementia in the

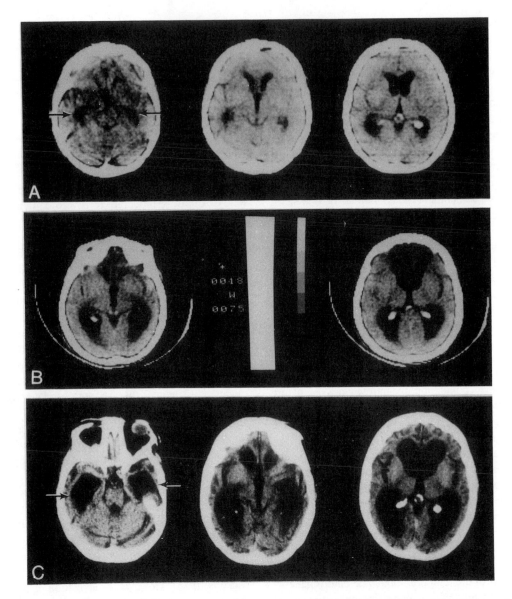

Figure 17.6.   Computerized tomographic scans from a woman with Down syndrome and Alzheimer disease: (A) age 55, 1 year after dementia onset, 7 years before death; (B) age 57, 3 years after dementia onset, 5 years before death; (C) age 61, 7 years after dementia onset, 1 year before death. Note the progressive ventricular enlargement, particularly of the temporal horns (arrows).

presence of the already-existing neuropathology of Alzheimer disease.

WORK-UP AND MANAGEMENT

Differential Diagnosis

In the work-up of individuals with Down syndrome who have symptoms suggestive of de-

mentia, it is important to rule out conditions that mimic dementia and also to rule out any treatable causes of dementia. Since Alzheimer disease is a relentlessly progressive condition without a cure (at least at the present time), there is no advantage in labeling someone with this condition early in the evaluation process before other conditions have been satisfactorily excluded.

Conditions that can present with a dementia-like syndrome were outlined by Cummings and Benson (1983). For persons with mental retardation, the following conditions should be considered in the differential diagnosis of Alzheimer disease: multiple cerebral infarctions; toxic metabolic states such as B_{12} deficiency, folate deficiency, and hypothyroidism; hydrocephalic dementia; and the pseudodementia of depression.

Multi-infarct dementia has an abrupt onset of focal neurologic signs and symptoms with stepwise deterioration often in the context of cardiovascular disease or previous strokes. The personality is preserved and a reactive depression is common. Neuroimaging studies reveal the areas of infarction. It should be noted, however, that Alzheimer disease can occur concomitantly with multiple infarcts and has been reported to occur in persons with Down syndrome (Evenhuis, 1990; Lai & Williams, 1989).

The dementia of B_{12} deficiency (pernicious anemia) may precede the hematologic changes by months or years and manifests as confusion, memory impairment, depression, hallucinations, and delusions. It is treatable with monthly B_{12} injections. Lai (1991) observed the presence of low B_{12} levels in several persons with Down syndrome who had dementia, but despite replacement therapy, these individuals' dementia became progressively worse.

The dementia from folate deficiency is very rare, with manifestations similar to that of B_{12} deficiency. Poor diet, jejunal resection, and decreased absorption of folate from phenytoin or primidone are predisposing factors. Treatment is with daily oral folic acid.

Dementia can occur in 5% of individuals with hypothyroidism in the general population. The hypothyroidism that presents in up to one third of adults with Down syndrome (Dinani & Carpenter, 1990; Mani, 1988) is usually on an autoimmune basis and often is subclinical in nature with elevation of thyroid-stimulating hormones with or without depression of thyroxine levels. It occurs more frequently in individuals with Down syndrome who have manifestations of Alzheimer disease than in those who do not have dementia (Lai & Williams, 1989; Percy et al., 1990).

Adults with spontaneously arrested hydrocephalus may develop dementia even after minor cranial insult. An acquired hydrocephalus can occur after subarachnoid hemorrhage or cranial trauma. The clinical triad of hydrocephalic dementia includes an initial spastic gait disturbance followed by dementia and then incontinence. The CT scan shows ballooned lateral ventricles (frontal and temporal horns greater than occipital horns) that are suggestive of obstruction. Shunting is the procedure of choice, but the dementia may or may not be reversible, depending on the stage at which intervention is carried out.

Depression, which can masquerade as dementia, with apathy and social withdrawal as prominent symptoms, may be difficult to diagnose in persons with mental retardation. Pirodsky et al. (1985) suggested that the clinical symptoms of depression in this group may differ from that in the general population, and may include antisocial behavior, repetitive/stereotypic movements, temper tantrums, and screaming/crying episodes. Because of this, they suggested that the use of the dexamethasone suppression test may be helpful in diagnosing depression in persons with mental retardation. Complicating the differentiation between dementia and depression is that loss of social skills and impaired intellectual functioning can accompany depression in individuals with mental retardation (Helsel & Matson, 1988), and depression can occur with dementia in persons with mental retardation just as it can in the general population (Harper & Wadsworth, 1990). It may be a greater diagnostic challenge when depression occurs in individuals with Down syndrome, but an onset of symptoms before age 35 without clear memory impairment, a fluctuating course of behavioral regression, and prominent change in vegetative function should point to depression rather than Alzheimer disease as the prime consideration (Warren, Holroyd, & Folstein, 1989).

Functional Assessment

Longitudinal follow-up of the individual over several years, preferably by the same examiner, reveals the natural history of the disease process in question and helps to distinguish Alzheimer disease from other conditions. Details of the person's highest level of functioning and subsequent decline should be carefully recorded. In this regard, it is important that the caregiver who accompanies the individual to the evaluation be someone who knows him or her well. Table 17.1 outlines the general areas of functioning in persons with mental retardation that can be used as a check-off list.

Expressive language becomes truncated as the dementia progresses, and comprehension also declines. Notation should be made of the individual's ability to answer open-ended questions and his or her ability to carry out one-step commands and multistep instructions. Information about the person's language abilities in day-to-day situations is helpful since language abilities may appear worse than they really are in the office setting.

In Alzheimer disease, short-term memory is usually affected before long-term memory. The ability to remember details of past and recent events should be recorded, as well as the ability to recognize or remember names of family members and staff. More immediate memory can be tested by having the individual repeat a simple story or repeat the names of three objects after 5 minutes or find an object hidden in the room after several minutes. If the individual begins to misplace or lose personal belongings, this may be a sign of memory impairment. Difficulty learning new skills may be an early manifestation of Alzheimer disease and is especially evident in those who attend a workshop where acquiring new skills is mandatory.

Decreased sociability and attention span are early recognizable signs of dementia in individuals with Down syndrome. Sometimes behavioral changes are manifested as irritability, stubbornness, and agitation.

Activities of daily living such as eating, dressing, toileting, food preparation, housekeeping tasks, travel skills, and money management should be noted according to the level of independence. The onset of incontinence should be recorded. Spatial and temporal orientation can often be assessed in higher functioning individuals, and impairment can be manifested as getting lost going to familiar places outside or inside the home, and confusion about sequence of events, time of day, and so forth. Dyspraxia can be manifested in the loss of ability to put on clothing in the right order, tie shoelaces, or use food utensils or personal care items like combs and toothbrushes properly.

In individuals who are employed, dementia may appear as disinterest in work, increased lethargy, poor quality of work, and decreased productivity. This last feature can be measured as a decline in "normal production average," which is an objective measure of work productivity compared with "normal" individuals in assembly line or piecemeal type of work.

The individual's fund of knowledge and academic skills can be probed as outlined in Table

---

Table 17.1. Functional levels in persons with mental retardation

Language
  Full sentences
  Phrases
  Single words
  Nonverbal
  Sign language (number of signs)
Memory/learning
  Remote and short-term for events, people
  Ability to learn new skills
Sociability/attention span/behavioral changes
Daily living skills
  Independent
  Verbal prompts
  Physical assistance
  Totally dependent
Spatial and temporal orientation
Work performance
  Normal production average
Fund of knowledge/academic skills
  Orientation (date, place, person)
  Days of week
  Months of year
  Birth date/age
  Colors
  Body parts
  Reading and writing
  Arithmetic
  Figure drawing

17.1, and a drop in performance can be readily appreciated with progression of the Alzheimer disease process.

Physical and Neurologic Assessment

In the general physical examination, special attention should be paid to vision and hearing since adults with Down syndrome are prone to develop premature cataracts and presbyacusis. Impairment in these sensory modalities will hamper daily functioning in persons without dementia and will make persons with dementia even more dysfunctional. Any limitation of neck movement should be noted as there is an increased incidence of premature degenerative disc disease as well as atlantoaxial subluxation in persons with Down syndrome. Significant cervical spinal pathology may be manifested as upper extremity motor or sensory impairment in a nerve root distribution or a myelopathy presenting with lower limb spasticity, hyperreflexia, extensor plantar responses, and hesitancy and precipitancy in urination.

During the neurologic examination, the individual's posture and movements should be observed for signs of parkinsonism such as masked facies, hypophonia, bradykinesia, cogwheel rigidity, flexed posture, decreased arm swing, and a small-stepped gait. These parkinsonian features were noted in 20% of adults with Down syndrome who had dementia (Lai & Williams, 1989).

When testing the cranial nerves, intactness of the gag reflex should be noted since diminution or loss of the gag reflex will predispose the individual to aspiration pneumonia. Alternative means of feeding may need to be considered.

With progression of Alzheimer disease, muscle tone assumes a gegenhalten quality (i.e., a variable resistance to passive movement with a seeming inability to relax the muscles on command). The deep tendon reflexes may or may not be increased, and the plantar responses in some persons may be extensor. Pathologic reflexes become prominent as the individual slips into the more advanced stages of the disease. Inability to extinguish eye blinking to tapping the bridge of the nose (Meyerson sign) is characteristically seen in Parkinson disease but is noted with increased frequency in persons with Down syndrome who had dementia, with and without parkinsonian features. The palmomental reflex (scratch of the palm elicits a twitch of the ipsilateral mentalis muscle on the chin) is occasionally seen in normal individuals, but occurs more frequently in persons with Alzheimer disease. The palmar grasp, and snout, suck, and root reflexes, are clearly abnormal and reflect widespread cerebral disease.

Laboratory Tests

Tests to rule out treatable causes of dementia should be done. These include tests for thyroid-stimulating hormone, thyroxine level, B_{12} and folate levels, and a syphilis serology. An unenhanced CT scan will help to rule out infarction and brain tumor. Serial CT scans help to document the progressive nature of the disease. An electroencephalogram may show slowing of background rhythm.

If psychologic services are available, the following tests are suggested: Stanford-Binet Intelligence Scale (4th ed.) (Thorndike et al., 1986), Peabody Picture Vocabulary Test–Revised (Dunn & Dunn, 1981), Vineland Adaptive Behavior Scales (expanded form) (Sparrow, Balla, & Cicchetti, 1984), and Expressive One-Word Vocabulary Test–Revised (Gardner, 1990). The Stanford-Binet can better assess lower functioning individuals than the Wechsler Adult Intelligence Scale–Revised (Wechsler, 1981). Also, by means of the various composite scores, it can be determined whether the dementia is generalized, occurs only in particular areas, or is confined to specific abilities. The Peabody Picture Vocabulary Test–Revised is a nonverbal test of receptive vocabulary available in two forms, which is helpful if a person is tested on multiple occasions. The expanded form of the Vineland Adaptive Behavior Scale provides the best ability to discriminate among individuals in the moderate range of mental retardation. Expressive language skills appear particularly susceptible to decline when persons with Down syndrome become demented, and the Expressive

One-Word Vocabulary Test–Revised may provide an objective measure of this decline.

Management

Unfortunately, there are currently no proven treatments for Alzheimer disease. The best that can be offered is to keep the individual functional and comfortable for as long as possible. Although the average duration of dementia in individuals with Down syndrome is between 4–5 years, some have lived for more than a decade.

If vision is impaired by cataracts or hearing diminished because of presbyacusis or conduction defects, consideration should be given for cataract surgery and the feasibility of hearing aids— particularly if the person is in the early stages of dementia or if the progression appears to be very slow. It should not be attempted if the individual is already unaware of his or her environment.

Adults with Down syndrome who are dementing should be kept in familiar surroundings with a regular schedule as long as they are not in danger of hurting themselves or others. Sudden and radical changes adversely affect their functional capabilities, and they will appear more demented. Any necessary change should be gradual and carefully explained.

Intercurrent illnesses such as pneumonias and urinary tract infections should be promptly treated. When the individual has reached the terminal stages of the disease, opinions vary regarding aggressive treatment, and the decision often depends on the personal philosophy of the family and physician. In the same regard, the decision to put in a gastrostromy tube for feeding will be subject to personal philosophies. In the advanced stages of the disease, the individual's comfort will be dependent on skilled nursing care to prevent decubitus ulcers and to keep the individual well hydrated and as infection free as possible.

If death appears imminent, the family may decide to forego cardiopulmonary resuscitative measures, and the physician in charge should note this in the orders and the patient's chart.

The importance of an autopsy cannot be overstated. The neuropathologic examination of persons with Down syndrome, particularly by investigators at regional Alzheimer Disease Research Centers, may help in the understanding of Alzheimer disease in the general population, and may aid in the search for an eventual cure.

CONCLUSION

For many decades, it has been known that the brains of individuals with Down syndrome past the age of 35–40 years inevitably develop the neuropathology of Alzheimer disease. Recent studies have indicated that the clinical dementia of Alzheimer disease is just as inevitable, albeit with an average age at onset in the mid 50s. It is possible to diagnose dementia even in the setting of mental retardation by demonstrating an objective decline in functional and adaptive behavioral assessment parameters. The main differential diagnostic considerations are depression and hypothyroidism.

The clinical course of Alzheimer disease in individuals with Down syndrome is one of steady decline in memory, language, motor, and sphincteric functions, as well as inexorable deterioration in social skills and personality. The development of seizures is almost universal and some persons also develop parkinsonian features. There are no specific diagnostic tests for Alzheimer disease during life, although the electroencephalogram usually shows generalized slowing, and neuroimaging studies show brain atrophy and ventricular enlargement, particularly of the temporal horns. Management is mainly supportive with medications as indicated for seizures, parkinsonism, and infections.

The long arm of chromosome 21 (21q), which is triplicated in persons with Down syndrome, may play a key role in the development of Alzheimer disease in general. Both the gene for the precursor of beta-amyloid (an important component of the characteristic neuritic plaque of Alzheimer disease) and the gene for some cases of familial early-onset Alzheimer disease have been localized to 21q. The more aggressive nature of Alzheimer disease in persons with Down syndrome compared with the general population is reflected in the greater density of neuritic plaques and neurofibrillary tangles and the more dramatic ventricular enlargement (especially of the temporal horns) in the brains of persons with

Down syndrome. Perhaps the triplication of the gene for beta-amyloid precursor or some other as yet undiscovered factor on 21q causes a more severe expression of Alzheimer disease in adults with Down syndrome.

The pathogenesis of Alzheimer disease is not entirely clear, and at present there is no cure for this degenerative neurologic disease. Since the development of Alzheimer disease appears inevitable in older persons with Down syndrome, careful and systematic evaluation of these individuals during life, and an equally intensive study of their brains after death, may yield answers to the basic understanding of Alzheimer disease that may then lead to rational therapeutic interventions for this devastating condition.

REFERENCES

Aston-Jones, G. (1986). Physiological characteristics of noradrenergic and cholinergic cortical afferent neurons: Functional implications and changes with age. In C.J. Epstein (Ed.), *The neurobiology of Down syndrome* (pp. 219–238). New York: Raven Press.

Baird, P.A., & Sadovnick, A.D. (1987). Life expectancy in Down syndrome. *Journal of Pediatrics, 110,* 849–854.

Baird, P.A., & Sadovnick, A.D. (1988). Life expectancy in Down syndrome adults. *Lancet, ii,* 1354–1356.

Ball, M.J., Fisman, M., Hachinski, V., Blume, W., Fox, A., Kral, V.A., Kirshen, A.J., Fox, H., & Merskey, H. (1985). A new definition of Alzheimer's disease: A hippocampal dementia. *Lancet, i,* 14–16.

Berr, C., Borghi, E., Rethoré, M.O., Lejeune, J., & Alperovitch, A. (1989). Absence of familial association between dementia of Alzheimer type and Down syndrome. *American Journal of Medical Genetics, 33,* 545–550.

Blackwood, D.H.R., St. Clair, D.M., Muir, W.J., Oliver, C.J., & Dickens, P. (1988). The development of Alzheimer's disease in Down's syndrome assessed by auditory event-related potentials. *Journal of Mental Deficiency Research, 32,* 439–453.

Braak, H., & Braak, E. (1990). Morphology of the cerebral cortex in relation to Alzheimer's dementia. In K. Maurer, P. Riederer, & H. Beckmann (Eds.), *Alzheimer's disease: Epidemiology, neuropathology, neurochemistry, and clinics* (pp. 85–91). Wien, Federal Republic of Germany: Springer-Verlag.

Burger, P.C., & Vogel, F.S. (1973). The development of the pathological changes of Alzheimer's disease and senile dementia in patients with Down's syndrome. *American Journal of Pathology, 73,* 457–476.

Chui, H.C. (1987). The significance of clinically defined subgroups of Alzheimer's disease. *Journal of Neural Transmission Supplementum, 24,* 57–68.

Cork, L.C. (1990). Neuropathology of Down syndrome and Alzheimer disease. *American Journal of Medical Genetics Supplement 7,* 282–286.

Cummings, J.L., & Benson, D.F. (1983). *Dementia: A clinical approach.* Boston: Butterworth.

Dalton, A.J., & Crapper-McLachlan, D.R. (1984). Incidence of memory deterioration in aging persons with Down's syndrome. In J.M. Berg (Ed.), *Perspectives and progress in mental retardation: Vol. 2. Biomedical aspects* (pp. 55–62). Baltimore: University Park Press.

Dalton, A.J., & Crapper-McLachlan, D.R. (1986). Clinical expression of Alzheimer's disease in Down's syndrome. *Psychiatric Clinics of North America, 9,* 659–670.

Damasio, A.R. (1984). The anatomic basis of memory disorders. *Seminars in Neurology, 4,* 223–225.

de la Monte, S.M., & Hedley-Whyte, E.T. (1990). Small cerebral hemispheres in adults with Down's syndrome: Contributions of developmental arrest and lesions of Alzheimer's disease. *Journal of Neuropathology and Experimental Neurology, 49,* 509–520.

de Leon, M.J., George, A.E., Reisberg, B., Ferris, S.H., Kluger, A., Stylopoulos, L.A., Miller, J.D., LaRegina, M.E., Chen, C., & Cohen, J. (1989). Alzheimer's disease: Longitudinal CT studies of ventricular change. *American Journal of Roentgenology, 152,* 1257–1262.

Dinani, S., & Carpenter, S. (1990). Down's syndrome and thyroid disorder. *Journal of Mental Deficiency Research, 34,* 187–193.

Ditter, S.M., & Mirra, S.S. (1987). Neuropathologic and clinical features of Parkinson's disease in Alzheimer's disease patients. *Neurology, 37,* 754–760.

Dunn, L.M., & Dunn, L.M. (1981). *Peabody Picture Vocabulary Test–Revised.* Circle Pines, MN: American Guidance Service.

Epstein, C.J. (1987). Down's syndrome and Alzheimer's disease: What is the relation? In G.G. Glenner & R.J. Wurtman (Eds.), *Advancing frontiers in Alzheimer's disease research* (pp. 155–173). Austin: University of Texas Press.

Evenhuis, H.M. (1990). The natural history of dementia in Down's syndrome. *Archives of Neurology, 47,* 263–267.

Fenner, M.E., Hewitt, K.E., & Torpy, D.M. (1987). Down's syndrome: Intellectual and behavioral functioning during adulthood. *Journal of Mental Deficiency Research, 31*, 241–249.

Gardner, M.F. (1990). *Expressive One-Word Picture Vocabulary Test–Revised.* Novato, CA: Academic Therapy Publications.

George, A.E., de Leon, M.J., Stylopoulos, L.A., Miller, J., Kluger, A., Smith, G., & Miller, D.C. (1990). CT diagnostic features of Alzheimer disease: Importance of the choroidal/hippocampal fissure complex. *AJNR—American Journal of Neuroradiology, 11*, 101–107.

Giaccone, G., Tagliavini, F., Linoli, G., Bouras, C., Frigerio, L., Frangione, B., & Bugiani, O. (1989). Down patients: Extracellular preamyloid deposits precede neuritic degeneration and senile plaques. *Neuroscience Letters, 97*, 232–238.

Glenner, G.G., & Wong, C.W. (1984). Alzheimer's disease: Initial report of the purification and characterization of a novel cerebrovascular amyloid protein. *Biochemical and Biophysical Research Communication, 120*, 885–890.

Glenner, G.G., & Wurtman, R.J. (Eds.). (1987). *Advancing frontiers in Alzheimer's disease research.* Austin: University of Texas Press.

Goate, A.M., Haynes, A.R., Owen, M.J., Farrall, M., James, L.A., Lai, L.Y.C., Mullan, M.J., Roques, P., Rossor, M.N., Williamson, R., & Hardy, J.A. (1989). Predisposing locus of Alzheimer's disease on chromosome 21. *Lancet, i*, 352–354.

Godridge, H., Reynolds, G.P., Czudek, C., Calcutt, N.A., & Benton, M. (1987). Alzheimer-like neurotransmitter deficits in adult Down's syndrome brain tissue. *Journal of Neurology, Neurosurgery, and Psychiatry, 50*, 775–778.

Goldgaber, D., Lerman, M.I., McBride, O.W., Saffiotti, U., & Gajdusek, D.C. (1987). Characterization and chromosomal localization of a cDNA encoding brain amyloid of Alzheimer's disease. *Science, 235*, 877–880.

Gusella, J.F. (1991). The search for the genetic defects in Huntington's disease and familial Alzheimer's disease. In P.R. McHugh & V.A. McKusick (Eds.), *Genes, brain, and behavior* (pp. 75–83). New York: Raven Press.

Haberland, C. (1969). Alzheimer's disease in Down syndrome: Cliniconeuropathological observations. *Acta Neurologica Belgica, 69*, 369–380.

Harper, D.C., & Wadsworth, J.S. (1990). Dementia and depression in elders with mental retardation: A pilot study. *Research in Developmental Disabilities, 11*, 177–198.

Hauser, W.A., Morris, M.L., Heston, L.L., & Anderson, V.E. (1986). Seizures and myoclonus in patients with Alzheimer's disease. *Neurology, 36*, 1226–1230.

Helsel, W.J., & Matson, J.L. (1988). The relationship of depression to social skills and intellectual functioning in mentally retarded adults. *Journal of Mental Deficiency Research, 32*, 411–418.

Heston, L.L., Mastri, A.R., Anderson, E., & White, J. (1981). Dementia of the Alzheimer's type. Clinical genetics, natural history and associated conditions. *Archives of General Psychiatry, 38*, 1085–1090.

Hewitt, K.E., Carter, G., & Jancar, J. (1985). Ageing in Down's syndrome. *British Journal of Psychiatry, 147*, 58–62.

Heyman, A., Wilkinson, W.E., Hurwitz, B.J., Schmetchel, D., Sigman, A.H., Weinberg, T., Helms, M.J., & Swift, M. (1983). Alzheimer's disease: Genetic aspects and associated clinical disorders. *Annals of Neurology, 14*, 507–516.

Hyman, B.T. (1991, April). Hippocampal anatomy and Alzheimer's disease. In *Neurochemistry* (Course #340). (Available from American Academy of Neurology, 2221 University Ave., S.E., Suite 335, Minneapolis, MN 55414.)

Hyman, B.T., Damasio, A.R., Van Hoesen, G.W., & Barnes, C.L. (1984). Alzheimer's disease: Cell specific pathology isolates the hippocampal formation. *Science, 298*, 83–95.

Hyman, B.T., & Mann, D.M.A. (1991). Alzheimer-type pathological changes in Down's syndrome individuals at various ages. In K. Iqbal, D.R.C. McLachlan, B. Winblad, & H.M. Wisniewski (Eds.), *Alzheimer's disease: Basic mechanisms, diagnosis and therapeutic strategies* (pp. 105–113). New York: John Wiley & Sons.

Hyman, B.T., & Van Hoesen, G.W. (1989). Hippocampal and entorhinal cortex cellular pathology in Alzheimer's disease. In V. Chan-Palay & C. Köhler (Eds.), *The hippocampus—new vistas* (pp. 499–512). New York: Alan R. Liss.

Hyman, B.T., Van Hoesen, G.W., & Damasio, A.R. (1987). Alzheimer's disease: Glutamate depletion in the hippocampal perforant pathway zone. *Annals of Neurology, 22*, 37–40.

Jervis, G. (1948). Early senile dementia in mongoloid idiocy. *American Journal of Psychiatry, 105*, 102–106.

Joachim, C.L., Morris, J.H., & Selkoe, D.J. (1988). Clinically diagnosed Alzheimer's disease: Autopsy results in 150 cases. *Annals of Neurology, 24*, 50–56.

Jordan, S.W. (1971). Central nervous system. *Human Pathology, 2*, 561.

Kang, J., Lemaire, H.G., Unterbeck, A., Salbaum, J.M., Masters, C.L., Gzreschik, K.H., Multaup, G., Beyreuther, K., & Muller-Hill, B. (1987). The precursor of Alzheimer's disease amyloid A4 protein resembles a cell-surface receptor. *Nature, 325*, 733–736.

Karlinsky, H. (1986). Alzheimer's disease in Down's syndrome: A review. *Journal of the American Geriatrics Society, 34*, 728–734.

Katzman, R. (1986). Alzheimer's disease. *New England Journal of Medicine, 314*, 964–973.

Kemper, T.L. (1978). Senile dementia: A focal disease in the temporal lobe. In K. Nandy (Ed.), *Senile dementia: A biomedical approach* (pp. 105–113). Amsterdam: Elsevier, North Holland.

Kemper, T.L. (1984). Neuroanatomical and neuropathological changes in normal aging and in dementia. In M. Albert (Ed.), *Clinical neurology of aging* (pp. 9–52). London: Oxford University Press.

Kemper, T.L. (1988). Neuropathology of Down syndrome. In L. Nadel (Ed.), *The psychobiology of Down syndrome* (pp. 269–289). Cambridge, MA: MIT Press.

Lai, F. (1991). Early versus late onset of Alzheimer disease in Down syndrome individuals. *Neurology, 41* (Suppl. 1), 215.

Lai, F., & Brodie, J.S. (1991, November). *The myoclonus of Alzheimer disease in Down syndrome.* Presented at Massachusetts Alzheimer's Disease Research Center, Sixth Annual Scientific Poster Session, Boston. (Available from Massachusetts Alzheimer's Disease Research Center, Massachusetts General Hospital, Boston, MA 02114.)

Lai, F., & LeMay, M. (1990, November). *Changes in regional lateral ventricular size in Alzheimer disease with and without Down syndrome.* Massachusetts Alzheimer's Disease Research Center, Fifth Annual Scientific Poster Session. (Available from Massachusetts Alzheimer's Disease Research Center, Massachusetts General Hospital, Boston, MA 02114.)

Lai, F., & Williams, R.S. (1989). A prospective study of Alzheimer disease in Down syndrome. *Archives of Neurology, 46*, 849–853.

Lambert, N., & Windmiller, M. (1981). *AAMD Adaptive Behavior Scale, School Edition.* Monterey, CA: CTR/McGraw-Hill.

Lehesjoki, A-E., Koskiniemi, M., Sistonen, P., Miao, J., Hästbacka, J., Norio, R., & de la Chapelle, A. (1991). Localization of a gene for progressive myoclonus epilepsy to chromosome 21q22. *Proceedings of the National Academy of Sciences of the United States of America, 88*, 3696–3699.

LeMay, M., & Alvarez, N. (1990). The relationship between enlargement of the temporal horns of the lateral ventricles and dementia in aging patients with Down syndrome. *Neuroradiology, 32*, 104–107.

LeMay, M., Stafford, J.L., Sandor, T., Albert, M., Haykal, H., & Zamani, A. (1986). Statistical assessment of perceptual CT-scan ratings in patients with Alzheimer type dementia. *Journal of Computerized Assisted Tomography, 10*, 802–809.

Lott, I.T. (1982). Down's syndrome, aging, and Alzheimer's disease: A clinical review. *Annals of the New York Academy of Sciences, 396*, 15–27.

Lott, I.T., & Lai, F. (1982). Dementia in Down's syndrome: Observations from a neurology clinic. *Applied Research in Mental Retardation, 3*, 233–239.

Luxenberg, J.S., Haxby, J.V., Creasey, H., Sundaram, M., & Rapoport, S.I. (1987). Rate of ventricular enlargement in dementia of the Alzheimer type correlates with rate of neuropsychological deterioration. *Neurology, 37*, 1135–1140.

Malamud, N. (1966). The neuropathology of mental retardation. In I. Philips (Ed.), *Prevention and treatment of mental retardation* (pp. 24–32). New York: Basic Books.

Malamud, N. (1972). Neuropathology of organic brain syndromes associated with aging. In C.M. Gaitz (Ed.), *Aging and the brain* (3rd ed., pp. 63–87). New York: Plenum.

Mani, C. (1988). Hypothyroidism in Down's syndrome. *British Journal of Psychiatry, 153*, 102–104.

Mann, D.M.A. (1988a). Alzheimer's disease and Down's syndrome. *Histopathology, 13*, 125–137.

Mann, D.M.A. (1988b). Calcification of the basal ganglia in Down's syndrome and Alzheimer's disease. *Acta Neuropathologica, 76*, 595–598.

Mann, D.M.A. (1989). Cerebral amyloidosis. ageing and Alzheimer's diesase; a contribution from studies on Down's syndrome. *Neurobiology of Aging, 10*, 397–399.

Mann, D.M.A., Yates, P.O., Marcyniuk, B., & Ravindra, C.R. (1985). Pathological evidence for neurotransmitter deficits in Down's syndrome of middle age. *Journal of Mental Deficiency Research, 29*, 125–135.

Mann, D.M.A., Yates, P.O., Marcyniuk, B., & Ravindra, C.R. (1986). The topography of plaques and tangles in Down's syndrome patients of different ages. *Neuropathology and Applied Neurobiology, 12*, 447–457.

Martin, R.L. (1990). The genetics of Alzheimer disease: Identification of persons at high risk. In R.E. Becker & E. Giacobini (Eds.), *Alzheimer disease: Current research in early diagnosis* (pp. 31–48). New York: Taylor & Francis.

Masters, C.L., & Beyreuther, K. (1987). Neuronal origin of cerebral amyloidogenic proteins: Their role in Alzheimer's disease and unconventional virus disease of the nervous system. In G. Bock & M. O'Connor (Eds.), *Selective neuronal death, CIBA Foundation Symposium* (Vol. 126, pp. 49–64). Chicester, UK: John Wiley & Sons.

Masters, C.L., Simms, G., Weinman, N.A., Multhaup, G., McDonald, B.L., & Beyreuther, K. (1985). Amyloid plaque core protein in Alzheimer disease and Down syndrome. *Proceedings of the National Academy of Sciences of the United States of America, 82*, 4245–4249.

Matsuyama, H., & Nakamura, S. (1978). Senile changes in the brain in the Japanese: Incidence of Alzheimer's neurofibrillary change and senile plaque. In R. Katzman, R.D. Terry, & K.L. Blick

(Eds.), *Alzheimer's disease: Senile dementia and related disorders* (pp. 287–297). New York: Raven Press.

Mayeux, R., Stern, Y., & Spanton, S. (1985). Heterogeneity in dementia of the Alzheimer type: Evidence of subgroups. *Neurology, 35*, 453–461.

McKhann, G., Drachman, D., Folstein, M., Katzman, R., Price, D., & Stadlan, E.M. (1984). Clinical diagnosis of Alzheimer's disease: Report of the NINCDS-ADRDA work group under the auspices of Department of Health and Human Services Task Force on Alzheimer's disease. *Neurology, 34*, 939–944.

Miniszek, N.A. (1983). Development of Alzheimer disease in Down syndrome individuals. *American Journal of Mental Deficiency, 87*, 377–385.

Morris, J.C., & Fulling, K. (1988). Early Alzheimer's disease: Diagnostic considerations. *Archives of Neurology, 45*, 345–349.

Motte, J., & Williams, R.S. (1989). Age related changes in density and morphology of plaques and neurofibrillary tangles in Down syndrome brain. *Acta Neuropathologica, 77*, 535–546.

Muir, W.J., Squire, I., Blackwood, D.H.R., Speight, M.D., St. Clair, D.M., Oliver, C., & Dickens, P. (1988). Auditory P300 response to the assessment of Alzheimer's disease in Down's syndrome: A 2-year-follow-up study. *Journal of Mental Deficiency Research, 32*, 455–463.

Naidich, T.P., Daniels, D.L., Haughton, V.M., Williams, A., Pojunas, K., & Palacios, E. (1987). Hippocampal formation and related structures of the limbic lobe: Anatomic-MR correlation. Part I: Surface features and coronal sections; Part II: Sagittal sections. *Radiology, 162*, 747–761.

Nee, L.E., Polinsky, R.J., Eldridge, R., Weingartner, H., Smallberg, S., & Ebert, M. (1983). A family with histologically confirmed Alzheimer's disease. *Archives of Neurology, 40*, 203–208.

Neve, R.L. (1989). Genetic studies support a neuronal origin for the beta amyloid polypeptide. *Neurobiology of Aging, 10*, 400–402.

Oliver, C., & Holland, A.J. (1986). Down's syndrome and Alzheimer's disease: A review. *Psychological Medicine, 16*, 307–322.

Olson, M.I., & Shaw, C.M. (1969). Presenile dementia and Alzheimer's disease in mongolism. *Brain, 92*, 147–156.

Pearlson, G.D., Warren, A.C., Starkstein, S.E., Aylward, E.H., Kumar, A.J., Chase, G.A., & Folstein, M.F. (1990). Brain atrophy in 18 patients with Down syndrome: A CT study. *AJNR—American Journal of Neuroradiology, 11*, 811–816.

Percy, M.E., Dalton, A.J., Markovic, V.D., Crapper-McLachlan, D.R., Gera, E., Hummel, J.T., Rusk, A.C.M., Somerville, M.J., Andrews, D.F., & Walfish, P.G. (1990). Autoimmune thyroiditis associated with mild "subclinical" hypothyroidism in adults with Down syndrome: A comparison of patients with and without manifestations of Alzheimer disease. *American Journal of Medical Genetics, 36*, 148–154.

Pericak-Vance, M.A., Yamaoka, L.H., Haynes, C.S., Speer, M.C., Haines, J.L., Gaskell, P.C., Hung, W-Y., Clark, C.M., Heyman, A.L., Trofatter, J.A., Eisenmenger, J.P., Gilbert, J.R., Lee, J.E., Alberts, M.J., Dawson, D.V., Bartlett, R.J., Earl, N.L., Siddique, T., Vance, J.M., Conneally, P.M., & Roses, A.D. (1988). Genetic linkage studies in Alzheimer's disease families. *Experimental Neurology, 102*, 271–279.

Pirodsky, D.M., Gibbs, J.W., Hesse, R.A., Hsieh, M.C., Krause, R.B., & Rodriguez, W.H. (1985). Use of the dexamethasone suppression test to detect depressive disorders of mentally retarded individuals. *American Journal of Mental Deficiency, 90*, 245–252.

Pueschel, J.M., Louis, S., & McKnight, P. (1991). Seizure disorders in Down syndrome. *Archives of Neurology, 48*, 318–320.

Reid, A.H., Maloney, A.F.J., & Aungle, P.G. (1978). Dementia in aging mental defectives: A clinical and neuropathological study. *Journal of Mental Deficiency Research, 22*, 223–241.

Risse, S.C., Lampe, T.H., Bird, T.D., Nochlin, D., Sumi, S.M., Keenan, T., Cubberley, L., Peskind, E., & Raskind, M.A. (1990). Myoclonus, seizures, and paratonia in Alzheimer disease. *Alzheimer Disease & Associated Disorders, 4*, 217–225.

Robakis, N.K., Wisniewski, H.M., Jenkins, E.C., Devine-Gage, E.A., Houck, G.E., Yao, X-L., Ramakrishna, N., Wolfe, G., Silverman, W.P., & Brown, W.T. (1987). Chromosome 21q21 sublocalization of gene encoding beta amyloid peptide in cerebral vessels and neuritic (senile) plaques of people with Alzheimer disease and Down syndrome. *Lancet, i*, 384–385.

Romano, C., Tiné, A., Fazio, G., Rizzo, R., Colognola, R.M., Sorge, G., Bergonzi, R., & Pavone, L. (1990). Seizures in patients with trisomy 21. *American Journal of Medical Genetics Supplement, 7*, 298–300.

Ropper, A.H., & Williams, R.S. (1980). Relationship between plaques, tangles, and dementia in Down syndrome. *Neurology, 30*, 639–644.

Ross, M.H., Galaburda, A.M., & Kemper, T.L. (1984). Down's syndrome: Is there a decreased population of neurons? *Neurology, 34*, 909–916.

Rumble, B., Retallack, R., Hilbich, C., Simms, G., Multhaup, G., Martins, R., Hockey, A., Montgomery, P., Beyreuther, K., & Masters, C. (1989). Amyloid A4 protein and its precursor in Down's syndrome and Alzheimer's disease. *New England Journal of Medicine, 320*, 1446–1452.

Schapiro, M.B., Haxby, J.V., Grady, C.L., Duara, R., Schlageter, N.L., White, B., Moore, A., Sundaram, M., Larson, S.M., & Rapoport, S.I. (1987). Decline in cerebral glucose utilisation and cognitive function with aging in Down's syndrome. *Journal of Neurology, Neurosurgery, and Psychiatry*, *50*, 766–774.

Schellenberg, G.D., Bird, T.D., Wijsman, E.M., Moore, D.K., Boehnke, M., Bryant, E.M., Lampe, T.H., Sumi, S.M., Deeb, S.M., Beyreuther, K., & Martin, G.M. (1988). Absence of linkage of chromosome 21q21 markers to familial Alzheimer's disease in autopsy-documented pedigrees. *Science*, *241*, 1507–1510.

Schellenberg, G.D., Bird, T.D., Wijsman, E.M., Moore, D.K., & Martin, G.M. (1989). The genetics of Alzheimer's disease. *Biomedicine and Pharmacotherapy*, *43*, 463–468.

Scheltens, P., Leys, D., Barkhof, F., Huglo, D., Weinstein, H., Vermersch, P., Steinling, M., Wolters, E.C., & Valk, J. (1991). Hippocampal atrophy on magnetic resonance imaging in Alzheimer's disease and normal aging. *Neurology*, *41* (Suppl. 1), 341–342.

Schweber, M. (1986). Interrelation of Alzheimer disease and Down syndrome. In S.M. Pueschel, C. Tingey, J.E. Rynders, A.C. Crocker, & D.M. Crutcher (Eds.), *New perspectives on Down syndrome* (pp. 135–144). Baltimore: Paul H. Brookes Publishing Co.

Selkoe, D.J. (1989). Molecular pathology of amyloidogenic proteins and the role of vascular amyloidosis in Alzheimer's disease. *Neurobiology of Aging*, *10*, 387–395.

Sheridan, P.H., Sato, S., Foster, N., Bruno, G., Cox, C., Fedio, P., & Chase, T.N. (1988). Relation of EEG alpha background to parietal lobe function in Alzheimer's disease as measured by positron emission tomography and psychometry. *Neurology*, *38*, 747–750.

Soininen, H., Partanen, J., Laulumaa, V., Helkala, E.L., Laakso, M., & Riekkinen, P.J. (1989). Longitudinal EEG spectral analysis in early stage of Alzheimer's disease. *Electroencephalography and Clinical Neurophysiology*, *72*, 290–297.

Sparrow, S.S., Balla, D.A., & Cicchetti, D.V. (1984). *Vineland Adaptive Behavior Scales (Expanded Form)*. Circle Pines, MN: American Guidance Service.

St. George-Hyslop, P.H., Myers, R.H., Haines, J.L., Farrer, L.A., Tanzi, R.E., Abe, K., James, M.F., Conneally, P.M., Polinsky, R.J., & Gusella, J.F. (1989). Familial Alzheimer's disease: Progress and problems. *Neurobiology of Aging*, *10*, 417–425.

St. George-Hyslop, P.H., Tanzi, R.E., Polinsky, R.J., Haines, J.L., Nee, L., Watkins, P.C., Myers, R.H., Feldman, R.G., Pollen, D., Drachman, D., Growdon, J., Bruni, A., Foncini, J-F., Salmon, D., Frommelt, P., Amaducci, L., Sorbi, S., Piacentini, S., Stewartt, G.C., Hobbs, W.J., Conneally, P.M., & Gusella, J.F. (1987). The genetic defect causing familial Alzheimer's disease maps on chromosome 21. *Science*, *135*, 885–890.

Struwe, F. (1929). Histopathologische untersuchungen über Entstehung und Wesen der senilen Plaques [Histopathologic investigation of the origin and form of senile plaques]. *Zeitschrift für die Gesamte Neurologie und Psychiatrie*, *122*, 291–307.

Sylvester, P.E. (1984). Ageing in the mentally retarded. In J. Dobbing, A.D.B. Clarke, J.A. Corbett, J. Hogg, & R.O. Robinson (Eds.), *Scientific studies in mental retardation* (pp. 259–277). London: Royal Society of Medicine/MacMillan Press.

Takashima, S., Kuruta, H., Mito, T., Nishizawa, M., Kunishita, T., & Tabira, T. (1990). Developmental and aging changes in the expression patterns of beta-amyloid in the brains of normal and Down syndrome cases. *Brain Development*, *12*, 367–371.

Tanzi, R.E., Bird, E.D., Latt, S.A., & Neve, R.L. (1987). The amyloid β protein gene is not duplicated in brains from patients with Alzheimer's disease. *Science*, *238*, 666–669.

Tanzi, R.E., Gusella, J.F., Watkins, P.C., Bruns, G.A.P., St. George-Hyslop, P., Van Keuren, M.L., Patterson, D., Pagan, S., Kurnit, D.M., & Neve, R.L. (1987). Amyloid β protein gene: cDNA, mRNA distribution, and genetic linkage near the Alzheimer locus. *Science*, *235*, 880–884.

Tanzi, R.E., St. George-Hyslop, P.H., Haines, J.L., Polinsky, R.J., Nee, L., Foncin, J-F., Neve, R.L., McClatchey, A.I., Conneally, P.M., & Gusella, J.F. (1987). The genetic defect in familial Alzheimer's disease is not tightly linked to the amyloid β-protein gene. *Nature*, *329*, 156–157.

Thase, M.E., Tigner, R., Smeltzer, D.J., & Liss, L. (1984). Age-related neuropsychological deficits in Down's syndrome. *Biological Psychiatry*, *19*, 571–585.

Thorndike, R.L., Hagen, E.P., & Sattler, J.M. (1986). *Stanford-Binet Intelligence Scale* (4th ed.). Chicago: Riverside.

Veall, R.M. (1974). The prevalence of epilepsy among mongols related to age. *Journal of Mental Deficiency Research*, *18*, 99–106.

Vieregge, P., Ziemens, G., Freudenberg, M., Piosinski, A., Muysers, A., & Schulz, B. (1991). Extrapyramidal features in advanced Down's syndrome: Clinical evaluation and family history. *Journal of Neurology, Neurosurgery, and Psychiatry*, *54*, 34–38.

Warren, A.C., Holroyd, S., & Folstein, M.F. (1989). Major depression in Down's syndrome. *British Journal of Psychiatry*, *155*, 202–205.

Wechsler, D. (1981). *Wechsler Adult Intelligence Scale–Revised*. New York: Psychological Corporation.

Whalley, L.J., Carothers, A.D., Collyer, S., DeMey, R., & Frackiewicz, A. (1982). A study of familial factors in Alzheimer's disease. *British Journal of Psychiatry*, *140*, 249–256.

Williams, R.S., & Matthysse, S. (1986). Age-related

changes in Down syndrome brain and the cellular pathology of Alzheimer disease. In D.F. Swaab, E. Fliers, M. Mirmiran, W.A. Van Gool, & F. Van Haaren (Eds.), *Progress in brain research* (Vol. 70, pp. 49–67). New York: Elsevier.

Wisniewski, H.M., & Rabe, A. (1986). Discrepancy between Alzheimer-type neuropathology and dementia in persons with Down's syndrome. *Annals of the New York Academy of Sciences*, 477, 247–259.

Wisniewski, K.E., Dalton, A.J., Crapper-McLachlan, D.R., Wen, G.Y., & Wisniewski, H.M. (1985). Alzheimer's disease in Down's syndrome: Clinico-pathological studies. *Neurology*, 35, 957–961.

Wisniewski, K.E., French, J.H., Rosen, J.F., Koz-lowski, P.B., Tenner, M., & Wisniewski, H.M. (1982). Basal ganglia calcification (BGC) in Down's syndrome (DS)—Another manifestation of premature aging. *Annals of the New York Academy of Sciences*, 396, 179–189.

Wisniewski, K.E., & Wisniewski, H.M. (1983). Age-associated changes and dementia in Down's syndrome. In R. Reisberg (Ed.), *Alzheimer's disease: The standard reference* (pp. 319–326). New York: Free Press.

Wisniewski, K.E., Wisniewski, H.M., & Wen, G.Y. (1985). Occurrence of neuropathological changes and dementia of Alzheimer's disease in Down's syndrome. *Annals of Neurology*, 17, 278–282.

Wurtman, R.J., Corkin, S., Growdon, J.H., & Ritter-Walker, E. (1990). *Alzheimer's disease: Vol. 51. Advances in neurology*. New York: Raven Press.

Yatham, L.N., McHale, P.A., & Kinsella, A. (1988). Down's syndrome and its association with Alzheimer's disease. *Acta Psychiatrica Scandinavica*, 77, 38–41.

CHAPTER 18

Psychiatric Disorders

Beverly A. Myers

In order to examine the relationship of psychiatric disorders to Down syndrome, one must ask questions as to whether the psychiatric condition is related to the presence of the extra chromosome, to mental retardation per se, to the impact of psychosocial attitudes and environmental conditions, or to the same influences as in the general population. To obtain accurate answers to these questions, one must conduct careful epidemiologic studies, comparing persons with Down syndrome, individuals with other forms of mental retardation, and those in the general population. One then looks for discrepancies between persons with Down syndrome and the other two populations.

The coexistence of two relatively infrequent conditions raises the question of an interrelationship between the two disorders. An increased frequency of a psychiatric disorder in persons with Down syndrome compared to other forms of mental retardation and the general population would suggest such an interrelationship. Alzheimer disease, noted in increased frequency in persons with Down syndrome, is apparently one such condition. Its mechanism probably relates to beta-amyloid protein precursors whose gene is located on chromosome 21 (St. Clair, 1987). Whether the extra genetic material due to the supernumerary chromosome leads to any other increase or decrease in psychopathology remains to be evaluated. (For an in-depth discussion of Alzheimer disease and Down syndrome, the reader is referred to Lai, chap. 17, this volume.)

This chapter reviews what is known about the psychiatric conditions in individuals with Down syndrome. In the context of this review, information on the relative frequencies of psychiatric disorders in people who have mental retardation of other etiologies and in the general population is presented in order to see relationships, where possible. The review is conducted with an awareness that it is possible only to raise hypotheses rather than to draw any conclusions from the limited information available regarding psychiatric disorders in persons with Down syndrome.

EPIDEMIOLOGY

There are only a few surveys of psychopathology in individuals with Down syndrome; three studies explored the frequency and nature of psychiatric disorders in children, and one study focused on adults. In children, Menolascino (1965) observed 11 of 86 (13%) outpatients with Down syndrome under 12 years of age to have psychiatric disorders. In an institutionalized sample, Menolascino (1970) found 35 of 95 (37%) children and adolescents with Down syndrome to have psychiatric disorders. A controlled study by Gath and Gumley (1986) revealed that 73 of 193 (38%) children and adolescents with Down syndrome had psychiatric disorders. In comparison, 49% of age-, sex-, and physical and mental disability–matched controls with mental retardation and 4% of siblings were found to have psychiatric disorders.

In a recent study, Myers and Pueschel (1991b) surveyed 497 children and adults with Down syndrome. Four hundred twenty-five were followed as outpatients of the Child Development Center of Rhode Island Hospital. There were 261 individuals below 20 years of age and 164 patients 20 years and older. In addition, 72 adults with Down syndrome who resided at a nearby state institution were included in the sample. As shown in Table 18.1, the overall frequency of psychiatric disorders was 110 of 497 (22.1%). There were 46 of 261 (17.6%) Child Development Center outpatients below 20 years, 42 of 164 (25.6%) Child Development Center outpatients 20 years and older, and 22 of 72 (30.6%) state institution residents (28.1% of all adults) identified to have psychiatric disorders.

The frequency of 17.6% psychiatric disorders in children with Down syndrome in this study is markedly lower than the 30% prevalence of psychiatric disorders in children with mental retardation in the Isle of Wight study, but higher than

Table 18.1. Psychiatric disorders

Disorders	Child Development Center[a] outpatients < 20 years (n = 261)		Child Development Center[a] outpatients ≥ 20 years (n = 164)		State institution[b] residents (n = 72)		Total (n = 497)	
	No.	%	No.	%	No.	%	No.	%
Disruptive disorders								
Attention deficit hyperactivity disorder	16	6.1	4	2.4	1	1.3	21	4.2
Conduct/oppositional disorder	14	5.4	3	1.8	1	1.3	18	3.6
Aggressive behavior	17	6.5	10	6.1	9	1.2	36	7.2
Anxiety disorders								
Phobias	4	1.5	1	0.6			5	1
Obsessive-compulsive behavior			1	0.6	3	4.1	4	0.8
Conversion disorder			1	0.6				
Gastrointestinal disorders								
Eating problems	2	0.8	3	1.8	1	1.3	6	1.2
Elimination difficulties	4	1.5	1	0.6	3	4.1	8	1.6
Repetitive behaviors								
Tourette syndrome	1	0.4	2	1.2			3	0.6
Stereotypic behavior	7	2.7	7	4.3			14	2.8
Self-injurious behavior	2	0.8	2	1.2	4	5.5	8	1.6
Affective disorders								
Major depressive disorders			10	6.1			10	2
Manic-depressive disorders			1	0.6			1	0.2
Organic affective syndromes					1	1.3	1	0.2
Others								
Dementias			1	0.6	5	6.1	6	1.1
Paraphilias			3	1.2			3	0.6
Psychoses			1	0.6			1	0.2
Schizophrenia			0	0	0	0	0	0
Autism	3	1.2	2	1.2			5	1
Total[c]	46	17.6	42	25.6[d]	22	30.6[d]	110	22.1

[a]Child Development Center is located in Providence, Rhode Island.
[b]State institution is located in Massachusetts.
[c]Some patients have more than one psychiatric disorder.
[d]Of these adults, 28.1% have psychiatric disorders.

the 6.6% prevalence in the general population (Rutter, Graham, & Yule, 1970). It is probably lower than other epidemiologic studies of children with mental retardation, which have shown prevalence figures in the range of 30%–50% (Birch, Richardson, Baird, Horobin, & Ilsey, 1970; Chazen, 1964; Corbett, 1977; Gillberg, Persson, Grafman, & Themner, 1986; Hagberg, Hagberg, Lewerth, & Lindberg, 1981; Koller, Richardson, Katz, & McLaren, 1983). Stein and Susser (1975) and Groden, Dominique, Pueschel, and Deignan (1982) found prevalences of 20% and 25%, respectively.

Thus, there is evidence in the literature that children and adolescents with Down syndrome are likely at lower risk for psychiatric disorders than are children and adolescents with mental retardation of other etiologies. However, children and adolescents with Down syndrome are probably at higher risk than those in the general population.

In adults, only two psychiatric surveys of individuals with Down syndrome have been completed. Lund's studies (1985, 1988) of 324 adults with mental retardation, including 44 with Down syndrome, living in a community found that 11 of 44 (25%) persons with Down syndrome had psychiatric disorders as compared to 27.1% of the remaining individuals with mental retardation. Myers and Pueschel's (1991b) study found 27.1% of adults with Down syndrome to have psychiatric disorders (see Table 18.1; 42 of 164 adult outpatients and 22 of 72 state institution residents equals 27.1%). From these studies, it appears that the prevalence of psychiatric disorders in adults with Down syndrome may be similar to those with other forms of mental retardation.

Several epidemiologic studies of psychiatric disorders in persons with mental retardation reveal prevalence ranges of 30%–50% (Ballenger & Reid, 1977; Corbett, 1979; Department of Health and Social Security [DHSS], 1972; Gostason, 1985; Jacobson, 1982; Leck, Gordon, & McKeown, 1967; Lund, 1985; Penrose, 1938; Primrose, 1971; Williams, 1971). Moreover, four other studies of mental retardation showed prevalence figures of 10%–14% (Borthwick-Duffy & Eyman, 1991; Eaton & Menolascino, 1982;

Reiss, 1982, 1990). Some reasons for the wide variation in prevalence figures of psychiatric disorders include the variety of facilities or programs studied (individuals in residential settings have a higher prevalence of psychiatric disorders), level of retardation (individuals with mild mental retardation have higher prevalences of psychiatric disorders), type of data obtained (questionnaires reveal a higher prevalence of psychiatric disorders than chart reviews), and type of problem (aggressive behavior is more often identified) (Benson, 1985; Borthwick-Duffy & Eyman, 1991; Reiss, 1990).

TYPES OF PSYCHIATRIC DISORDERS

Adjustment Disorders

A maladaptive reaction to an identifiable psychosocial stressor that occurs within 3 months and lasts no more than 6 months constitutes an adjustment reaction. Impairment in school, occupational, or social functioning is invariably seen in persons with adjustment disorders. Types of reactions include disturbances of mood (anxious or depressed) or conduct; physical complaints; social withdrawal; or work inhibition. People with mental retardation are probably as vulnerable to stressors, if not more so, as people of average intelligence. One may observe responses to stress that are dramatically intense and might suggest grave severity and prognosis. Prompt resolution of the reaction is common, giving a better prognosis than expected (B.A. Myers, personal observation).

Whether people with Down syndrome have a different vulnerability to stress than persons with mental retardation of other etiologies or the general population is not known. Different diagnostic nomenclatures over time and place, the often short duration of an adjustment reaction, and the different manifestations of adjustment reactions make comparisons impossible. Menolascino noted 4.6% of children with Down syndrome had adjustment reactions in his 1965 study, and 8% in his 1970 study, whereas none was observed in studies by Gath and Gumley (1986), Lund (1988), and Myers and Pueschel (1991b).

Affective Disorders

Serious affective disorders include major depressive disorder and mania. Major depressive disorder is characterized by a depressed mood or loss of interest or pleasure and at least four of the following seven symptoms: weight loss or gain, poor or excessive sleep, psychomotor agitation or retardation, fatigue or loss of energy, feelings of worthlessness or excessive guilt, poor concentration or indecisiveness, and thoughts of death or suicide. Mania is characterized by an elevated or irritable mood and at least four of the following eight symptoms: inflated self-esteem, short sleeping, excessive talking, flight of ideas, distractibility, increased activity or agitation, buying sprees, or sexual indiscretions.

There are no case reports or epidemiologic studies of depression in children with Down syndrome, but there are such reports in the adult population. Several case reports of depression in persons with Down syndrome have been published (Jakab, 1978; Keegan, Pettigrew, & Parker, 1974; Roith, 1961; Sovner & Hurley, 1983; Szymanski, 1984; Warren, Holroyd, & Folstein, 1990). Mania has been reported (Cook & Leventhal, 1987; McLaughlin, 1987), although it was previously doubted to exist in persons with Down syndrome (Sovner, Hurley, & Labrie, 1985).

In epidemiologic studies in adults with Down syndrome, Lund (1988) found no depression, but Myers and Pueschel (1991b) noted major depressive disorders in 10 of 164 (6.1%) outpatient adults with Down syndrome (see Table 18.1). The prevalence of major affective disorders in the general population has been estimated at 1.8%–2.6% (Regier & Burke, 1985). The prevalence of major affective disorders in persons with mental retardation of other etiologies has been estimated at 1%–3.5% (Corbett, 1979; Forrest & Ogunremi, 1974; Heaton-Ward, 1976; Leck et al., 1967; Lund, 1988; Penrose, 1938; Reid, 1972; Wright, 1982). Thus, it seems that adults with Down syndrome may be at a greater risk for major depressions than other adults with mental retardation and adults of average intelligence. This leads to a hypothesis that, as in Alzheimer disease, people with Down syndrome

are at increased risk of depression because of the extra 21 chromosome. Much more research needs to be conducted to confirm or deny this hypothesis.

Depression in persons with Down syndrome is difficult to treat. Serotonergic antidepressants may be more effective than other medications (B.A. Myers, personal observation). Sometimes neuroleptics may be required. Although there may be difficulties in identifying depression in individuals with Down syndrome, particularly in persons with Alzheimer disease, it is important to diagnose this condition correctly. The quality of life of a depressed person with Down syndrome is impaired, yet remediable (Storm, 1990).

Anorexia Nervosa and Other Eating Disorders

Anorexia nervosa is defined as intense fear of gaining weight or becoming fat, weight loss to below 15% expected body weight, distorted perception of body as fat, and amenorrhea. There have been five reports in the literature describing people with Down syndrome and eating disorders (Cottrell & Crisp, 1984; Fox, Karan, & Ratatori, 1981; Holt, 1988; Hurley & Sovner, 1979; Morgan, 1989; Szymanski, 1984). As is common in people with average intelligence (Halmi, 1985), grief or depression was noted in 3 of these 5 individuals with Down syndrome and eating disorders.

Although there were no observations of eating disorders by Gath and Gumley (1986), Lund (1988), and Menolascino (1965, 1970), there were 2 persons who presented with self-induced vomiting and 1 individual with anorexia nervosa in Myers and Pueschel's (1991b) study. One of the 2 who presented with self-induced vomiting subsequently developed a major depressive disorder.

Anxiety Disorders

Characterized by anxiety and avoidance behavior, these disorders include panic disorder with and without agoraphobia, social and simple phobias, obsessive-compulsive disorder, and post-traumatic stress disorder.

Observations of anxiety in Down syndrome have been difficult to discern. Menolascino (1970) noted 3 children with psychoneurotic reactions (chronic anxiety and conversion reactions). Gath and Gumley (1986) found 6 of 194 (3%) children with Down syndrome and 4 of 153 (2.6%) controls with mental retardation of other etiologies to exhibit anxiety and fearfulness. Myers and Pueschel (1991b) described 4 children with simple phobias, which are fears of specific objects that do not pervasively interfere with daily functioning.

In adults with Down syndrome, Lund (1988) did not note anxiety disorders. Myers and Pueschel (1991b) described 1 of 236 adults (0.4%) to have simple phobias. The prevalence of phobias in the general population has been noted recently to be 4%–5% (Regier & Burke, 1985). In adults with mental retardation, anxiety and phobic behavior has been noted to occur at lower rates than the general population (Hurley & Sovner, 1982; Jacobson, 1991).

Obsessions, defined as repetitive thoughts, may be difficult to recognize in a nonverbal person with mental retardation. However, compulsions, signified by repetitive, purposeful, and intentional behavior performed in a ritualistic manner according to certain rules and causing impairment in a person's life, can be recognized. Myers and Pueschel (1991a) described obsessive-compulsive disorder in 4 of 236 (1.7%) people with Down syndrome. This prevalence of 1.7% is in the range of the general population of 1.6% to 2.5% (Rasmussen, 1990), but is lower than the 3.5% in adults with mental retardation in Vitiello, Spreat, and Behar's (1989) study. This suggests no greater vulnerability of obsessive-compulsive disorder in adults with Down syndrome.

Thus, anxiety disorders of several varieties exist in persons with Down syndrome. At the present time, it seems that the prevalence of such disorders is not significantly increased in persons with Down syndrome.

Autistic Disorders

Infantile autism, as it is often called, includes impairments in reciprocal social interaction and in verbal and nonverbal communication; a restricted repertoire of activities and interests, along with stereotypies; intolerance of change; and insistence on a rigid routine.

There have been only two reports of a child with Down syndrome and autistic disorder (Bregman & Volkmar, 1988; Wakabayashi, 1979). In addition, Gath and Gumley (1986) found no difference in the frequency of children with Down syndrome and infantile autism (1%) as compared with controls with mental retardation of other etiologies (2%). Myers and Pueschel (1991b) noted 3 of 261 (1.2%) children with Down syndrome (see Table 18.1) as compared to a prevalence of autistic disorder in the general population of 0.02%–0.05% (Volkmar, 1991).

Concerning adults with Down syndrome, Lund (1988) found 5 of 44 (11.4%) to have infantile autism, as compared to 6.9% of 258 adults with mental retardation of other etiologies. Myers and Pueschel's (1991b) observation of 2 of 236 (0.8%) adults with autism may be higher than the general population.

Thus, it appears that children and adults with Down syndrome, as those with mental retardation of other etiologies, are at a greater risk for autism than the general population.

Dementia

Dementia includes impairments in short-term and long-term memory, abstract thinking, judgment, and other higher cortical functioning, and changes in personality. People with Down syndrome show a clearly increased risk of Alzheimer disease (one form of dementia), both clinically and neuropathologically (Oliver & Holland, 1986; Zigman, Schupf, Lubin, & Silverman, 1987). (This topic is discussed in detail in Lai, chap. 17, this volume.)

Lund's 1988 study reflects this significantly increased risk for Alzheimer disease in persons with Down syndrome (9.1%) as opposed to 2% in persons with mental retardation of other etiologies. Myers and Pueschel's (1991b) study of two groups of adults with Down syndrome reflects the age-related development of Alzheimer disease. The mean age of the outpatient population was 27 years; 1 in 164 (0.6%) had clinical evidence of dementia. The mean age of the state institution population was 40.7 years; 5 of 72 (6.1%) patients had dementia.

Disruptive Behavior Disorders

Disruptive behavior disorders include attention deficit hyperactivity disorder, conduct disorder, and oppositional disorder. These disorders constitute a large proportion of the psychopathology seen in children with Down syndrome.

Attention Deficit Hyperactivity Disorder

The symptoms of attention deficit hyperactivity disorder include: fidgetiness, out-of-seat behavior, distractibility, impatience, speaking out of turn, inattentiveness, incompletion of activities, poor following of instructions, rowdy play, excessive talking, poor listening, frequent loss of things, and poor regard of danger. It is identifiable in children with mental retardation and is often responsive to psychostimulant medications (Handen, Breaux, Gosling, Ploof, & Feldman, 1990).

There have been major positive changes in the classification of child psychiatric disorders with the publication of the American Psychiatric Association's *Diagnostic and Statistical Manual of Mental Disorders* in 1980 (*DSM-III*) and 1987 (*DSM-III-R*). Thus, it is not possible to discuss any studies done prior to 1980, when this disorder was labeled differently (e.g., minimal cerebral dysfunction, brain-damaged syndrome).

A controlled study of attention deficit hyperactivity disorder in a small group of children with Down syndrome was carried out by Green, Dennis, and Bennets (1989). They noted 4 of 13 children ages 2–4 years to have attention deficit hyperactivity disorder. Their study suggests that attention deficit hyperactivity disorder is probably a separate condition from Down syndrome. It is not present in the majority of individuals with Down syndrome.

In one epidemiologic survey of children with Down syndrome, Gath and Gumley (1986) found attention deficit hyperactivity disorder in only 2 of 194 (1%) children with Down syndrome. They also had a category of hyperkinetic conduct disorder, which was identified in 7.5% of the children. In comparison, 6% of the controls with mental retardation had attention deficit hyperac-

tivity disorder plus 1.3% had hyperkinetic conduct disorder. Myers and Pueschel (1991b) found attention deficit hyperactivity disorder in 16 of 261 (6.1%) children with Down syndrome. It is said to occur in 3%–5% of children in the general population (Brunstetter & Silver, 1985). Thus, if both of Gath and Gumley's categories are included, no marked differences are observed when children with Down syndrome are compared with those with mental retardation of other etiologies, but both are probably greater than the general population.

In adults with Down syndrome, Lund (1988) did not note any persons with attention deficit hyperactivity disorder. However, Myers and Pueschel (1991b) observed 5 of 236 (2%) adults to have attention deficit hyperactivity disorder.

Conduct and Oppositional Behavior Disorders

Conduct disorder consists of a wide variety of antisocial behavior including fighting, temper tantrums, destructiveness, stealing, running away, and firesetting. Oppositional disorder primarily involves uncooperative behavior within the family. Both are very common problems in childhood and adolescence, with a prevalence of 5%–10%.

In Menolascino's 1965 study of children with Down syndrome, 6 of 86 (7%) outpatients had conduct disorders, then called "chronic brain syndrome with behavior reactions"; in his 1970 study, 17 of 95 (17%) were so diagnosed. Gath and Gumley (1986) found conduct disorders in 40 of 193 (20%) children with Down syndrome, compared to 29 of 153 (20%) controls with mental retardation. In Myers and Pueschel's (1991b) population of children with Down syndrome, 31 of 264 (12%) exhibited conduct or oppositional disorders or aggressive behaviors. With the prevalence of conduct disorders in the general population of 5%–10%, it is likely that children with Down syndrome and those with mental retardation of other etiologies (12%–20%) are both at increased risk for conduct disorders.

Lund (1985, 1988) found that 2 of 44 (4.5%) adults with Down syndrome displayed behavior disorders as compared to 12% of 258 adults with mental retardation of other etiologies. Myers and Pueschel (1991b) observed 23 of 236 (10%)

adults with Down syndrome to have conduct disorders, many exhibiting aggressive behaviors. In comparison, a study by Corbett (1979) noted that 25% of persons with mental retardation of other etiologies had behavior disorders. This suggests that adults with Down syndrome have a lower rate of conduct disorders than do other persons with mental retardation.

Elimination Disorders

Encopresis is involuntary passage of feces in the presence of adequate neurologic and intellectual function. Encopresis was not reported in the three studies involving children with Down syndrome (Gath & Gumley, 1986; Menolascino, 1965, 1970), or in Lund's (1988) study of adults with Down syndrome. Myers and Pueschel (1991b) noted encopresis in 4 children and 4 adults; 4 of these 8 persons had associated conduct disorders.

Paraphilias

Paraphilias consist of intense sexual urges and fantasies and sexual behavior involving nonhuman objects, children, and other nonconsenting persons; or suffering or humiliation of oneself or one's partner. Three outpatient adolescents with Down syndrome who exposed themselves or masturbated in inappropriate situations were reported by Myers and Pueschel (1991b). Sadistic behavior was noted in 1 state institution resident, but his partners were consenting. Medroxyprogesterone suspension can be used to treat these disorders when behavioral and psychotherapeutic measures are unsuccessful (Myers, 1991).

Repetitive Behaviors

Repetitive behaviors can be differentiated in people with mental retardation into stereotypic behaviors such as banging, rocking, flipping, or swinging; pleasurable nonstereotypic behaviors such as verbal perseveration, humming, demanding attention, stealing, pacing, masturbation, and compulsive eating, drinking, or smoking; self-injurious behaviors; and tic disorders, including Tourette syndrome. Compulsive behaviors, described earlier, can be distinguished from these repetitive behaviors (Vitiello et al., 1989). Because there are specific treatments available for most of these behaviors, it is important to distinguish between them. These treatments include clomipramine for obsessive-compulsive disorder; haloperidol for Tourette syndrome; and antidepressants, naloxone, lithium, propranolol, and benzodiazepines for self-injurious behavior (Myers, 1990).

Tourette Syndrome and Other Tic Disorders

Tourette syndrome consists of multiple motor and vocal tics. The presence of Tourette syndrome in individuals with Down syndrome has been reported in 5 individuals by Barabas, Wardell, Sapiro, and Matthews (1986); Collacott and Ismail (1988); Karlinsky, Sandor, Berg, Moldofsky, and Crawford (1986); and Sachs (1982). With only these 5 individuals and Myers and Pueschel's (1991b) observation of 3 patients in 497 (0.6%) who had both Down syndrome and Tourette syndrome, it is unlikely that there is an interrelationship between these two disorders, although both may involve disturbances of similar neurotransmitters (serotonin) (Collacott & Ismail, 1988). Tourette syndrome may be overlooked in persons with Down syndrome and in those with other forms of mental retardation due to the failure to differentiate various types of repetitive behaviors. The dramatic response to a small dose of haloperidol makes skillful diagnosis essential.

Stereotypic Disorders

The essential features of stereotypic disorders are intentional and repetitive behaviors that are nonfunctional and serve no constructive or socially acceptable purpose. Included are both self-injurious behavior such as head banging, hitting or biting parts of one's own body, face slapping, and hand biting; and non-self-injurious behavior such as teeth grinding, bodily manipulations, vocalizations, breath holding, hyperventilation, and air swallowing.

Stereotypic behavior probably progressively develops during childhood and adolescence. The prevalence of stereotypic behavior in Myers and Pueschel's (1991b) study was 7 of 261 (2.7%) children and adolescents with Down syndrome and 7 of 164 (4.3%) adults followed as outpatients.

Self-Injurious Behavior

In a number of studies involving people with mental retardation, 8%–15% of those living in institutions exhibit self-injurious behavior (Oliver, Murphy, & Corbett, 1987). This contrasts with 3% living in the community. People with Down syndrome have been noted for their low rate of self-injurious behavior as compared to de Lange, Riley-Day, and other syndromes (Oliver et al., 1987). Myers and Pueschel (1991b) observed 6 of 236 (2.5%) adults with Down syndrome with self-injurious behavior, which includes 1.2% followed as outpatients and 5.5% who were state institution residents.

The treatment of self-abusive behavior includes a variety of behavior modification approaches and, when needed, psychotropic medications such as antidepressants, lithium, naloxone, benzodiazepines, propranolol, and, sometimes, neuroleptic medications.

Schizophrenia and Other Psychoses

Schizophrenia is a chronic disorder lasting at least 6 months that is manifested by personality change, hallucinations, delusions, incoherence of thought, flat or inappropriate affect, catatonic behavior, social isolation, and impairment in self-care and role functioning. Menolascino (1970) noted 2 adolescents with "propfschizophrenia," whereas Gath and Gumley (1986) and Myers and Pueschel (1991b) found no schizophrenia in children and adolescents with Down syndrome. The frequency of schizophrenia in children in the general population is less than 0.05% (Kolvin et al., 1971).

In adults with Down syndrome, Lund (1988) and Myers and Pueschel (1991b) did not find schizophrenia. It was observed in 1.3%–6.2% of people with mental retardation due to other etiologies (Corbett, 1979; Eaton & Menolascino, 1982; Heaton-Ward, 1976; Leck et al., 1967; Lund, 1985; Penrose, 1938; Reid, 1972; Wright, 1982) and in 0.5%–0.8% of the general population (Regier & Burke, 1985).

There are a wide variety of other acute psychoses (gross impairment in reality testing) that include delirium, toxic or organic psychoses, reactive psychoses, and acute schizophreniform

reaction, which potentially can occur in persons with Down syndrome as well as persons with mental retardation of other etiologies.

Menolascino noted chronic psychotic reactions in 1 of 86 (1.2%) children with Down syndrome in 1965 and 4 in 95 children and adolescents in 1970. Myers and Pueschel (1991b) observed none in children, but noted chronic psychoses in 1 of 236 adults with Down syndrome.

PSYCHIATRIC DISORDERS NOT OBSERVED

Personality Disorders

There have been several studies relating to the personality traits in people with Down syndrome, both supporting and failing to support their agreeable, affectionate, happy, cheerful, and good-natured temperament (Blacketer-Simmonds, 1953; Domino, 1965; Domino, Goldschmid, & Kaplan, 1964; Moore, Thuline, & Capes, 1968; Tredgold & Soddy, 1956). However, there have not been any reports on specific personality disorders.

Psychoactive Substance Abuse Organic Mental Disorders

The general absence of mental disorders related to alcoholism and substance abuse, such as alcohol withdrawal and toxic psychosis, in people with Down syndrome is probably related to their living and working in supervised conditions.

CONCLUSION

The preceding review of psychiatric disorders in persons with Down syndrome suggests that, in addition to the well-recognized increased prevalence of Alzheimer disease in persons with Down syndrome, major depressive disorders are also observed more frequently. Autistic disorders, attention deficit hyperactivity disorders, and conduct disorders may be observed at an increased frequency in persons with Down syndrome, as in persons with mental retardation of other etiologies. Obsessive-compulsive disorder and Tourette syndrome occur no more frequently than in the general population.

In view of the limited number of carefully executed epidemiologic studies of psychiatric disorders in people with Down syndrome, further investigations need to be done to clarify the question of the relative risk of psychiatric disorders in persons with Down syndrome and their relationship to the extra chromosomal material.

Therapeutically, it is important to make specific diagnoses, since a number of interventions are available. Medications are available for affective disorders (lithium, antidepressants, and neuroleptics), anxiety (antidepressants, benzodiazepines), obsessive-compulsive disorder (serotonergic antidepressants), attention deficit hyperactivity disorder (psychostimulants), par-

aphilias (medroxyprogesterone), schizophrenia (neuroleptics), Tourette syndrome (haloperidol), and aggressive and self-injurious behavior (lithium, neuroleptics, beta-blockers, and anticonvulsants [carbamazepine and valproic acid]). In addition, behavioral and psychotherapeutic interventions can be used in adjustment, eating, anxiety, autistic, conduct, self-injurious, elimination, and paraphilia disorders. The two general approaches are not mutually exclusive but frequently need to be skillfully combined. The need to discover further knowledge and interventions is great.

REFERENCES

American Psychiatric Association. (1980). *Diagnostic and statistical manual of mental disorders* (3rd ed.). Washington, DC: Author.

American Psychiatric Association. (1987). *Diagnostic and statistical manual of mental disorders* (3rd ed., rev.). Washington, DC: Author.

Ballenger, B.R., & Reid, A.H. (1977). Psychiatric disorders in an adult training centre and a hospital for the mentally handicapped. *Psychological Medicine, 7,* 525–528.

Barabas, G., Wardell, B., Sapiro, M., & Matthews, W.S. (1986). Coincident Down's and Tourette syndrome: Three case reports. *Journal of Child Neurology, 1,* 358–360.

Benson, B.A. (1985). Behavior disorders and mental retardation: Associations with age, sex, and level of functioning in an outpatient clinic sample. *Applied Research in Mental Retardation, 6,* 79–85.

Birch, H.G., Richardson, S.A., Baird, D., Horobin, G., & Ilsey, R. (1970). *Mental subnormality in the community: A clinical and epidemiologic study.* Baltimore: Williams & Wilkins.

Blacketer-Simmonds, D.A. (1953). An investigation into the supposed differences existing between mongols and other mentally defective subjects with regard to certain psychological traits. *Journal of Mental Science, 90,* 702–719.

Borthwick-Duffy, S.A., & Eyman, O. (1991). Who are the dually diagnosed? *American Journal on Mental Retardation, 94,* 586–595.

Bregman, J.D., & Volkmar, F.R. (1988). Autistic social dysfunction and Down syndrome. *American Academy of Child and Adolescent Psychiatry, 27,* 440–441.

Brunstetter, R.W., & Silver, L.B. (1985). Attention deficit disorder. In H.I. Kaplan & B.J. Sadock (Eds.), *Comprehensive textbook of psychiatry* (4th ed., pp. 1684–1690). Baltimore: Williams & Wilkins.

Chazen, M. (1964). The incidence and nature of maladjustment among children in schools for the educationally subnormal. *British Journal of Educational Psychology, 34,* 292–304.

Collacott, R.A., & Ismail, I.A. (1988). Tourettism in a patient with Down's syndrome. *Journal of Mental Deficiency Research, 32,* 163–166.

Cook, E.H., & Leventhal, B.L. (1987). Down's syndrome with mania. *British Journal of Psychiatry, 150,* 249–250.

Corbett, J.A. (1977). Studies of mental retardation. In P.J. Graham (Ed.), *Epidemiologic approaches in child psychiatry.* London: Academic Press.

Corbett, J.A. (1979). Psychiatric morbidity and mental retardation. In F.E. James & R.P. Snaith (Eds.), *Psychiatric illness and mental handicap* (pp. 11–25). London: Gaskell Press.

Cottrell, D.J., & Crisp. A.H. (1984). Anorexia nervosa in Down's syndrome—A case report. *British Journal of Psychiatry, 145,* 195–196.

Department of Health and Social Security. (1972). *Census of mentally handicapped patients in England and Wales at the end of 1970.* London: Her Majesty's Stationery Office.

Domino, G. (1965). Personality traits in institutionalized mongoloids. *American Journal of Mental Deficiency, 69,* 568–570.

Domino, G., Goldschmid, M., & Kaplan, M. (1964). Personality traits of institutionalized mongoloid girls. *American Journal of Mental Deficiency, 68,* 498–502.

Eaton, L.F., & Menolascino, F.J. (1982). Psychiatric disorders in the mentally retarded: Types, problems and challenges. *American Journal of Psychiatry, 139,* 1297–1303.

Forrest, A.D., & Ogunremi, O.O. (1974). The prevalence of psychiatric illness in a hospital for the mentally handicapped. *Health Bulletin, 32,* 199–202.

Fox, R., Karan, O.C., & Ratatori, A.F. (1981). Regression including anorexia nervosa in a Down's syndrome adult: A seven year follow up. *Journal of Behavior Therapy and Experimental Psychiatry, 12,* 351–354.

Gath, A., & Gumley, D. (1986). Behaviour problems in retarded children with special reference to Down's syndrome. *British Journal of Psychiatry, 149,* 156–161.

Gillberg, C., Persson, E., Grafman, M., & Themner, U. (1986). Psychiatric disorders in mildly and severely mentally retarded urban children and adolescents: Epidemiological aspects. *British Journal of Psychiatry, 149,* 68–74.

Gostason, R. (1985). Psychiatric illness among the mentally retarded: A Swedish population study. *Acta Psychiatrica Scandinavica, 71,* 1–113.

Green, J.M., Dennis, J., & Bennets, L.A. (1989). Attention disorder in a group of young Down's syndrome children. *Journal of Mental Deficiency Research, 33,* 105–122.

Groden, G., Dominique, D., Pueschel, S.M., & Deignan, L. (1982). Behavioral and emotional problems in mentally retarded children and youth. *Psychological Reports, 51,* 143–146.

Hagberg, B., Hagberg, G., Lewerth, A., & Lindberg, V. (1981). Mild mental retardation in Swedish school children: II. Etiologic and pathogenetic aspects. *Acta Paediatrica Scandinavica, 70,* 445–452.

Halmi, K.A. (1985). Anorexia nervosa. In H.I. Kaplan & B.J. Sadock (Eds.), *Comprehensive textbook of psychiatry* (4th ed., pp. 1143–1148). Baltimore: Williams & Wilkins.

Handen, B.L., Breaux, A.M., Gosling, A., Ploof, D.L., & Feldman, H. (1990). Efficacy of methylphenidate among mentally retarded children with attention deficit hyperactivity disorder. *Pediatrics, 86,* 922–930.

Heaton-Ward, W.A. (1976). Psychosis in mental handicap. *British Journal of Psychiatry, 130,* 525–533.

Holt, G.M. (1988). Down syndrome and eating disorders. *British Journal of Psychiatry, 152,* 847–848.

Hurley, A.D., & Sovner, R. (1979). Anorexia nervosa and mental retardation: A case report. *Journal of Clinical Psychiatry, 40,* 480–482.

Hurley, A.D., & Sovner, R. (1982). Phobic behavior and mentally retarded persons. *Psychiatric Aspects of Mental Retardation, 1,* 41–44.

Jacobson, J.W. (1982). Problem behavior and psychiatric impairment within a developmentally disabled population: Behavior severity. *Applied Research in Mental Retardation, 3,* 121–139.

Jacobson, J.W. (1991). Do some mental disorders occur less frequently among persons with mental retardation? *American Journal on Mental Retardation, 94,* 596–602.

Jakab, I. (1978). Basal ganglia calcification and psy-

chosis in mongolism. *European Neurology, 17,* 300–314.

Karlinsky, H., Sandor, P., Berg, J.M., Moldofsky, H., & Crawford, E. (1986). Gilles de la Tourette's syndrome in Down's syndrome—A case report. *British Journal of Psychiatry, 148,* 601–604.

Keegan, D.L., Pettigrew, A., & Parker, Z. (1974). Psychosis in Down's syndrome treated with amitriptyline. *Canadian Medical Association Journal, 110,* 1128–1133.

Koller, H., Richardson, S., Katz, M., & McLaren, J. (1983). Behavior disturbances since childhood among a 5-year birth cohort of all mentally retarded young adults. *American Journal of Mental Deficiency, 87,* 386–395.

Kolvin, I., Garside, R.F., Humphrey, M., Kidd, J.S.H., McNay, A., Ounstead, C., Richardson, L.M., & Roth, M. (1971). Studies in the childhood psychoses I–VI. *British Journal of Psychiatry, 118,* 318–340.

Leck, I., Gordon, W.I., & McKeown, T. (1967). Medical and social needs of patients in hospitals for the mentally ill. *British Journal of Preventive and Social Medicine, 21,* 115–121.

Lund, J. (1985). The prevalence of psychiatric morbidity in mentally retarded adults. *Acta Psychiatrica Scandinavica, 72,* 563–570.

Lund, J. (1988). Psychiatric aspects of Down's syndrome. *Acta Psychiatrica Scandinavica, 78,* 369–374.

McLaughlin, M. (1987). Bipolar affective disorder in Down's syndrome. *British Journal of Psychiatry, 151,* 116–117.

Menolascino, F.J. (1965). Psychiatric aspects of mongolism. *American Journal on Mental Deficiency, 69,* 653–660.

Menolascino, F.J. (1970). Down's syndrome: Clinical and psychiatric findings in an institutionalized sample. In F.J. Menolascino (Ed.), *Psychiatric approaches to mental retardation* (pp. 191–204). New York: Basic Books.

Moore, B.C., Thuline, H.C., & Capes, L. (1968). Mongoloid and non-mongoloid retardates: A behavioral comparison. *American Journal on Mental Deficiency, 73,* 433–436.

Morgan, J.R. (1989). A case of Down's syndrome, insulinoma, and anorexia. *Journal of Mental Deficiency Research, 33,* 185–187.

Myers, B.A. (1990). Psychiatric problems in mental retardation. In A.J. Capute & P.J. Accardo (Eds.), *Developmental disabilities in infancy and childhood* (pp. 455–474). Baltimore: Paul H. Brookes Publishing Co.

Myers, B.A. (1991). Treatment of pedophilia in the developmentally disabled. *American Journal on Mental Retardation, 95,* 5–8.

Myers, B.A., & Pueschel, S.M. (1991a). *Obsessive-compulsive disorder in a population with Down syndrome*. Manuscript submitted for publication.

Myers, B.A., & Pueschel, S.M. (1991b). Psychiatric disorders in a population with Down syndrome. *Journal of Nervous and Mental Disease, 179,* 609–613.

Oliver, C., & Holland, A.J. (1986). Down's syndrome and Alzheimer's disease. *Psychological Medicine, 16,* 307–322.

Oliver, C., Murphy, G.H., & Corbett, J.A. (1987). Self-injurious behaviour in people with mental handicap: A total population study. *Journal of Mental Deficiency Research, 31,* 147–162.

Penrose, L.S. (1938). *A clinical and genetic study of 1280 cases of mental defect (Colchester survey)* [Medical Research Council Special Report, No. 229]. London: Her Majesty's Stationery Office.

Primrose, D.A. (1971). A survey of 502 consecutive admissions to a subnormality hospital from 1st January 1968 to 31st December 1970. *British Journal of Mental Subnormality, 17,* 25–28.

Rasmussen, S.A. (1990). Epidemiology of obsessive-compulsive disorder. *Journal of Clinical Psychiatry, 51,* 10–14.

Regier, D.A., & Burke, J.D. (1985). Epidemiology. In B.J. Sadock (Ed.), *Comprehensive textbook of psychiatry* (4th ed., pp. 295–312). Baltimore: Williams & Wilkins.

Reid, A.H. (1972). Psychoses in adult mental defectives: I. Manic depressive psychosis. *British Journal of Psychiatry, 120,* 205–212.

Reiss, S. (1982). Psychopathology and mental retardation: Survey of a developmental disabilities mental health program. *American Journal on Mental Deficiency, 20,* 128–132.

Reiss, S. (1990). Prevalence of dual diagnosis in community-based day programs in the Chicago metropolitan area. *American Journal on Mental Retardation, 94,* 578–585.

Roith, A.I. (1961). Psychotic depression in a mongol. *Journal of Mental Subnormality, 7,* 45–47.

Rutter, M., Graham, P., & Yule, W. (1970). A neuropsychiatric study in childhood. In *Clinics in developmental medicine*. London: SIMP with Heineman Medical.

Sachs, O.W. (1982). Acquired Tourettism in adult life. In A.J. Friedhoff & T.N. Chase (Eds.), *Advances in neurology* (Vol. 35). New York: Raven Press.

Sovner, R., & Hurley, A.D. (1983). Do the mentally retarded suffer from affective illness? *Archives of General Psychiatry, 40,* 61–67.

Sovner, R., Hurley, A.N., & Labrie, R. (1985). Is mania incompatible with Down's syndrome? *British Journal of Psychiatry, 146,* 319–320.

St. Clair, D. (1987). Chromosome 21, Down's syndrome, and Alzheimer's disease. *Journal of Mental Deficiency Research, 31,* 213–214.

Stein, G.F., & Susser, M. (1975). Public health and mental retardation: New power and new problems. In M.J. Begab & S.A. Richardson (Eds.), *The mentally retarded and society*. Baltimore: University Park Press.

Storm, W. (1990). Differential diagnosis and treatment of depressive features in Down's syndrome: A case illustration. *Research in Developmental Disabilities, 11,* 131–137.

Szymanski, L.S. (1984). Depression and anorexia nervosa of persons with Down syndrome. *American Journal on Mental Deficiency, 89,* 246–251.

Tredgold, A.F., & Soddy, K. (1956). *Textbook of mental deficiency*. Baltimore: Williams & Wilkins.

Vitiello, B., Spreat, S., & Behar, D. (1989). Obsessive-compulsive disorder in mentally retarded patients. *Journal of Nervous and Mental Disease, 177,* 232–236.

Volkmar, F.R. (1991). Autism and pervasive developmental disorders. In M. Lewis (Ed.), *Child and adolescent psychiatry: A comprehensive textbook* (pp. 499–508). Baltimore: Williams & Wilkins.

Wakabayashi, S. (1979). A case of infantile autism associated with Down's syndrome. *Journal of Autism and Developmental Disorders, 9,* 31–36.

Warren, A.C., Holroyd, S., & Folstein, M.P. (1990). Major depression in Down's syndrome. *British Journal of Psychiatry, 155,* 202–205.

Williams, C.E. (1971). A study of the patients in a group of mental subnormality hospitals. *British Journal of Mental Subnormality, 17,* 29–41.

Wright, E.C. (1982). The presentation of mental illness in mentally retarded adults. *British Journal of Psychiatry, 141,* 496–502.

Zigman, W.B., Schupf, N., Lubin, R.A., & Silverman, W.P. (1987). Premature regression of adults with Down syndrome. *American Journal of Mental Deficiency, 92,* 161–168.

Dermatologic Findings

Paul M. Benson and James M. Scherbenske

Dermatologic findings in individuals with Down syndrome are not specific for the syndrome but are seen with an increased frequency (see Table 19.1). Commonly seen conditions include dry skin (xerosis), atopic dermatitis, fungal infections of the feet (tinea pedis) and nails (onychomycosis), and various mucosal anomalies (scrotal tongue, cheilitis). Many other conditions are seen in a minority of persons with Down syndrome and include alopecia areata, syringomas, seborrheic dermatitis, and elastosis perforans, among others.

Some dermatologic conditions, such as atopic dermatitis or severe xerosis, may have a significant impact on the health and daily living of persons with Down syndrome. Other conditions such as scrotal tongue or palmar crease are interesting medical curiosities. Lastly, disorders such as Norwegian scabies or carotenemia are relics of the past when many persons with Down syndrome were institutionalized. The shift in emphasis to community living for most individuals

with Down syndrome has virtually eliminated this last group of dermatologic problems.

COMMON CONDITIONS

Dermatologic conditions often observed in persons with Down syndrome include xerosis, atopic dermatitis, cheilitis, and scrotal tongue. Bacterial folliculitis and other bacterial infections of the perigenital and perianal areas, thighs, and buttocks have been observed with an increased frequency in these persons (S.M. Pueschel, personal communication, 1991). Cutaneous fungal infections such as onychomycosis (nail infection), tinea pedis, and tinea corporis were previously common in postpubertal institutionalized patients with Down syndrome as a result of communal living (Moschella & Hurley, 1985). In persons living in the community, the prevalence is not known but these infections are probably no more common than in the general population. Ichthyosis-like changes in the skin and rupial psoriasis (thickened, hyperkeratotic crustaceous lesions) also have been reported in persons with Down syndrome (Kopec & Levine, 1979; Rotchford & Hyman, 1961).

Xerosis

In the infant with Down syndrome, the skin is soft, velvety, and appears otherwise normal. In later childhood, the skin becomes dry, pale, and lax. By the age of 15, over 70% of persons show mild to moderate generalized xerosis (Burton & Rook, 1986).

Xerosis is best managed by the limited use of nondrying or oilated soaps and adding oils to the bath water or applying to hydrated skin after

Table 19.1. Cutaneous manifestations of Down syndrome

Common (≥50% frequency)	Less common (<50% frequency)
Xerosis	Alopecia areata
Atopic dermatitis	Syringomas
Scrotal tongue	Acrocyanosis
Cheilitis	Cutis marmorata
Onychomycosis	Vitiligo
Tinea pedis	Seborrheic dermatitis
	Ichthyosis
	Norwegian scabies
	Elastosis perforans serpiginosa
	Psoriasis

Modified from Carter and Jegasothy (1976).

bathing. Numerous lubricating creams, moisturizers, and emollients are commercially available. Emollients that are particularly effective in the management of xerosis include those containing as ingredients 10% urea, 5% lactic acid, or 12% ammonium lactate (Arnold, Odom, & James, 1990).

Atopic Dermatitis

Atopic dermatitis usually presents during the 1st year of life as scaly, erythematous, and crusted symmetric patches on the cheeks and lower extremities, and occasionally other areas. The hair is often dry and the scalp scaly. During childhood, flexural areas including the antecubital and popliteal fossae, the neck, the wrists, and the ankles are commonly involved. The lesions are very pruritic, lichenified patches; plaques with excoriations and pigmentary changes are especially common in dark-skinned persons. In postpubertal individuals, the eruption becomes less exudative and more scaly with areas of lichenification (thickened skin with exaggerated skin folds) secondary to rubbing and scratching (Krafchik, 1988).

Management of atopic dermatitis is quite variable as a result of differing opinions regarding its pathogenesis. In general, measures that alleviate itching, dryness, and inflammation are most helpful. Mild, nonperfumed soaps should be used sparingly and bath oils may be added to lukewarm or room temperature bath water to improve hydration. Oilated oatmeal added to the water is particularly soothing (Krafchik, 1988). Cetaphil lotion, a lipid-free hydrophilic lotion, can be used without water for both cleansing and lubrication. Soft cotton clothing, avoidance of wool and other scratchy fabrics, and air conditioning during the summer months are other general measures of benefit (Hurwitz, 1981).

Oral antihistamines, such as hydroxyzine, are of value in the relief of pruritus. Atopic skin is frequently colonized by *Staphylococcus aureus* and scratching leads to secondary bacterial infections (impetigo, folliculitis). Localized areas of infection can be managed with topical therapy, such as 2% topical mupirocin ointment applied three times daily. More widespread involvement usually responds to long-term oral erythromycin (Arnold et al., 1990).

Topical corticosteroids are the mainstay of therapy to reduce the inflammation in atopic dermatitis. In children, only low-potency topical steroids should be used to minimize the possibility of cutaneous atrophy or percutaneous absorption. For health care providers unfamiliar with these agents or in cases of severe, chronic, or treatment-refractory atopic dermatitis, the advice of a dermatologist should be sought.

Cheilitis

Cheilitis occurs with greater frequency in persons with Down syndrome than in the general population (Figure 19.1). Infants with Down syndrome have smooth red lips that are similar in appearance to those of "normal" infants. During the first few years of life, one may observe whitening and thickening of the mucous membrane. Vertical fissures often occur, followed by gradual but persistent enlargement of the lips, associated with scaling and crusting. Cheilitis is more often seen in males, with the majority exhibiting mild to severe cheilitis. The etiology of the disorder is unknown. Sun exposure may play a role. However, the equal prevalence of lip changes among those persons who are primarily indoors and those who spend much time outdoors tends to minimize the role of sunlight as a factor (Butterworth, Leoni, Beerman, Wood, & Strean, 1960).

Scrotal Tongue

Scrotal tongue or lingua fissurata is a common developmental anomaly in which the dorsal surface of the tongue has numerous deep grooves and fissures (Figure 19.2). It is present in 3%–

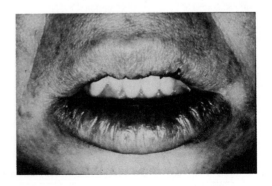

Figure 19.1.   Vertical fissures with mild scaling in a person with cheilitis and Down syndrome.

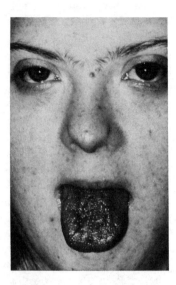

Figure 19.2. Scrotal tongue showing multiple fissures on the dorsal surface.

5% of the general population but occurs in almost all persons with Down syndrome (Zeligman & Scalia, 1954). The majority of cases of scrotal tongue are asymptomatic (Moschella & Hurley, 1985).

LESS COMMON CONDITIONS

Seborrheic Dermatitis

Seborrheic dermatitis is seen in about a third of persons with Down syndrome (Carter & Jegasothy, 1976). The condition is often present in infants as a scaly, erythematous dermatitis of the scalp known as "cradle cap." In adolescents and adults, seborrheic dermatitis is a chronic condition and is located on the scalp, eyebrows, nasal folds, ears, presternal area, and, occasionally, in skin folds. It presents as an erythematous, greasy, scaly, or crusting eruption (Hurwitz, 1981).

Treatment of seborrheic dermatitis in adolescents and adults consists of shampoos containing zinc pyrithione, selenium sulfide, or the recently introduced ketoconazole shampoo. Topical steroid solutions applied to the scalp and low-potency topical steroid creams applied to other areas provide relief of the dermatitis (Arnold et al., 1990). Recently, topically applied ketoconazole cream, an antifungal agent, has been shown to be very effective, presumably by suppressing skin con-

centrations of the lipophilic yeast Pityrosporum. Use of this agent avoids the potential long-term complications of skin atrophy and steroid rosacea seen with topical steroid use.

Multiple Syringomas

Syringomas are benign appendigeal tumors derived from eccrine sweat ducts and occur with a frequency of 20%–40% in persons with Down syndrome (Figure 19.3). Syringomas develop during puberty or adolescence and present as multiple 1 mm–3 mm skin-colored to yellowish firm papules located on the eyelids, neck, and upper anterior chest (Moschella & Hurley, 1985).

Syringomas were found in 18% of 200 institutionalized persons with Down syndrome (Butterworth, Strean, Beerman, & Wood, 1964). Another survey of cutaneous abnormalities in 214 individuals with Down syndrome found almost 60% of females and 27% of males to be affected with syringomas (Carter & Jegasothy, 1976). As in the general population, females are affected twice as often as males. The presence of syringomas does not appear to be related to the IQ of the individual or to any other manifestation of Down syndrome (Butterworth et al., 1964.)

In those persons desiring treatment, removal can be accomplished with light electrodessication, CO_2 laser ablation, or shave or scissor excision performed under local anesthesia.

Alopecia Areata

Alopecia areata is a condition in which there is rapid and complete loss of hair in one or more

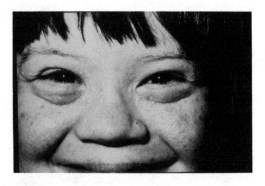

Figure 19.3. Skin-colored papules distributed symmetrically on the lower eyelids. Note the upper and outward slanting of the palpebral fissures and the epicanthal folds.

round or oval patches. These patches of alopecia areata may develop on the scalp, the beard area, eyebrows, eyelashes, and, only rarely on other hairy areas of the body. The patches vary in size from 1 cm–5 cm in diameter. "Exclamation point hairs" are found at the periphery of the bald patch and are tapered and attenuated at the point where they break off near the scalp.

The etiology is unknown but autoimmune and genetic factors are felt to play a role. It occurs with increased frequency in persons with autoimmune thyroiditis, pernicious anemia, vitiligo, and adrenal insufficiency as well as in persons with Down syndrome. In most individuals, especially those with minor involvement and in those whose onset was after puberty, there is a tendency for spontaneous recovery (Arnold et al., 1990).

The prevalence of alopecia areata in the general population has been estimated to be less than 1%, but it is found to be increased in Down syndrome (Carter & Jegasothy, 1976). Carter and Jegasothy reported 19 individuals with alopecia areata among 214 institutionalized persons with Down syndrome (8%). Three of these 19 persons with alopecia areata were also noted to have vitiligo. Another large survey of 1,000 persons with Down syndrome found a prevalence of alopecia areata of 6% (du Vivier & Munio, 1975).

When only one or a few patches are present, complete regrowth usually occurs within about 1 year in 95% of individuals (Hurwitz, 1981). In persons with earlier age of onset or in persons with more extensive or total hair loss, complete and permanent recovery occurs less than 30% of the time (Hurwitz, 1981).

Numerous therapies have been suggested for treatment of this condition including intralesional steroids (triamcinolone acetonide, 5–10 mg/cc); topical steroids with or without occlusion utilizing plastic wrap or bathing cap; and in severe, carefully selected cases, oral prednisone for 4–6 weeks followed by alternate-day therapy (Hurwitz, 1981). As discussion of therapy with other modalities is beyond the scope of this chapter, the reader is referred to Mitchell and Krull (1984) and Tosti, DePadova, Minghetti, and Veronesi (1986) for further recommendations.

Cutis Marmorata and Acrocyanosis

Cutis marmorata (a reticulated bluish mottling of the skin of the trunk and extremities) (Hurwitz, 1981) and acrocyanosis (Zeligman & Scalia, 1954) occur with greater frequency in persons with Down syndrome than in the general population. This may be due to poor peripheral circulation and the increased incidence of congenital heart disease (see Figure 19.4). Cutis marmorata is a physiologic response to chilling, with dilatation of the capillaries and venules. It usually disappears upon rewarming the skin. Cutis marmorata is seen in normal infants and the phenomenon usually ceases within weeks to months after birth. However, in persons with Down syndrome, trisomy 18, and Cornelia de Lange syndrome, the tendency to develop this vascular pattern often persists (Behrman, Vaughan, & Nelson, 1983; Hurwitz, 1981).

Elastosis Perforans Serpiginosa

Elastosis perforans serpiginosa is a rare disorder in which thickened elastic fibers from the papillary dermis are extruded through epidermal channels to produce keratotic papules on the skin. Clinically, these lesions are scaling 2 mm–5 mm papules that may be grouped or arranged in an annular pattern. Lesions are located most commonly on the nape of the neck, the face, or the arms (Figure 19.5). There is a male-to-female ratio of 4:1 (Lever & Schaumburg-Lever, 1990; Patterson, 1984).

In most individuals, elastosis perforans serpiginosa is not associated with any other med-

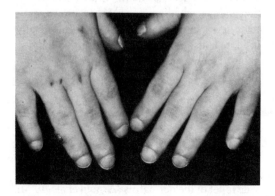

Figure 19.4. Clubbed, blue fingernails. Incidental angiokeratoma of the right fourth digit.

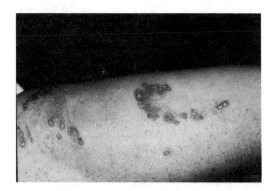

Figure 19.5. Multiple erythematous, keratotic papules in a serpiginous array on the upper arm.

ical conditions. However, 25% of individuals have an underlying condition that may include Down syndrome, Ehlers-Danlos syndrome, Marfan syndrome, osteogenesis imperfecta, acrogeria, Rothmund-Thompson syndrome, pseudoxanthoma elasticum, penicillamine therapy, or the nephrotic syndrome (Patterson, 1984; Schamroth, Kellen, & Grieve, 1986). It has been estimated that 1% of persons with Down syndrome have elastosis perforans serpiginosa (Arnold et al., 1990).

Idiopathic elastosis perforans serpiginosa and elastosis perforans serpiginosa associated with Down syndrome demonstrate some similarities and differences. In both instances, the lesions spontaneously resolve, leaving an atrophic scar; also, the lesions tend to develop in the 2nd decade of life. However, in persons with Down syndrome and elastosis perforans serpiginosa, the cutaneous lesions tend to be more extensive and the duration of the condition is longer (>10 years) than in the idiopathic cases (average 5 years) (Crotty, Bell, Estes, & Kitzmiller, 1983).

Most elastosis perforans serpiginosa lesions resolve without treatment. In those persons where treatment is desired, freezing with liquid nitrogen has been reported to be successful (Rosenblum, 1983).

RARE CONDITIONS

Norwegian (Crusted) Scabies

Norwegian (crusted) scabies is an uncommon form of scabies characterized by massive infesta-

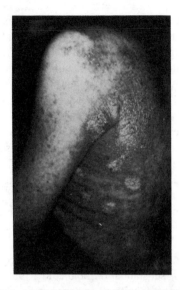

Figure 19.6. Multiple hyperkeratotic plaques of Norwegian (crusted) scabies in a person with Down syndrome. (Photograph courtesy of James Rotchford, M.D.)

tion of the skin surface by mites (Figures 19.6 and 19.7). It is highly contagious, and in contrast to the common form of scabies, many hundreds or thousands of Sarcoptes mites are present on the skin surface. The condition has been rarely reported to occur in the general population, but it is usually associated with immunosuppression or with mental or neurologic impairment (Glover, Young, & Goltz, 1987). Early reports of Norwegian scabies were in persons with Down syndrome, syphilitic tabes dorsalis, and syringomyelia (Glover et al., 1987). More recently, it has been reported to occur in immunocompromised

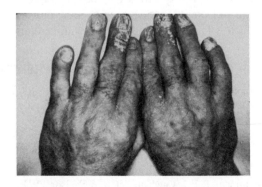

Figure 19.7. Hyperkeratotic crusting with pronounced nail dystrophy in a person with Down syndrome and Norwegian scabies. (Photograph courtesy of James Rotchford, M.D.)

individuals including those with leukemia or acquired immunodeficiency syndrome, and those receiving immunosuppressive therapy (Evans, 1973; Glover et al., 1987; Suzumiya, Sumiyoshi, Kuroki, & Inoue, 1985; Youshock & Glazer, 1981). The reason for the development of this form of scabies is unknown.

Clinically, individuals present with widespread crusted skin lesions resembling psoriasis or severe atopic dermatitis with thickened hyperkeratotic areas on the scalp, face, and pressure-bearing areas such as the elbows, knees, palms, soles, and buttocks. The tips of the fingers may be swollen and distorted, and the nails are dystrophic. The risk to medical attendants, family members, and other patients for acquiring scabies is substantial (Arnold et al., 1990).

Treatment is with permethrin cream, lindane lotion, or other effective scabicidal preparations. The addition of a mild keratolytic preparation such as urea cream may facilitate removal of excessive scale and reduce mite populations quickly (Arnold et al., 1990).

Carotenemia

In institutionalized persons with mental retardation, including those with Down syndrome, carotenemia occurs with increased frequency (Patel, Dunn, Tischler, McBurney, & Hach, 1973). The prevalence of carotenemia is thought to be due to two factors: 1) the high level of carotene products in the institutionalized diet (Barden, 1977), and 2) secondary to hypothyroidism. Persons with Down syndrome have been reported to have an increased incidence of hypothyroidism, which is known to be associated with caroten-

emia (Cohen, 1958; Cutler, Obeiter, & Brink, 1986).

CONCLUSION

Down syndrome presents a constellation of clinical findings of interest to specialists in many fields. Some of the dermatologic findings help to define the syndrome: epicanthal folds, single palmar crease, and characteristic facies. Other dermatologic manifestations such as alopecia areata, elastosis perforans serpiginosa, and syringomas may be found with increased frequency and merit special attention.

Awareness of the nature and prevalence of certain skin disorders in persons with Down syndrome ensures accurate and timely diagnosis and treatment. On the one hand, several frequently encountered conditions such as seborrheic dermatitis, ichthyosis, and tinea pedis are easily recognized and managed with available medications. On the other hand, atopic dermatitis may be severe enough to interfere with daily living and considerable skill is required to manage difficult cases. Lifestyle modifications are often necessary and include changes in bathing habits, clothing, and use of lubricants and topical corticosteroids.

Lastly, conditions such as vitiligo and alopecia areata may be cosmetically objectionable to persons with Down syndrome but pose no threat to health. This group of skin disorders can be therapeutically challenging to manage and results of treatment are often inconsistent or unsatisfactory. Considerable research efforts are being directed toward understanding the pathogenesis of these skin conditions and more effective treatments will undoubtedly follow.

REFERENCES

Arnold, H.L., Odom, R.B., & James, W.D. (Eds.). (1990). *Andrew's diseases of the skin* (8th ed.). Philadelphia: W. B. Saunders.

Barden, H.S. (1977). Vitamin A and carotene values of institutionalized mentally retarded subjects with and without Down's syndrome. *Journal of Mental Deficiency Research, 21,* 63–72.

Behrman, R.E., Vaughan, V.C., & Nelson, W.E. (Eds.). (1983). *Textbook of pediatrics* (12th ed.). Philadelphia: W.B. Saunders.

Burton, J.L., & Rook, A. (1986). Genetics in der-

matology. In A. Rook, F.J.G. Ebling, D.S. Wilkinson, R.H. Champion, & J.L. Burton (Eds.), *Textbook of dermatology* (p. 115). Oxford: Blackwell.

Butterworth, T., Leoni, E.P., Beerman, H., Wood, M.G., & Strean, L.P. (1960). Cheilitis of mongolism. *Journal of Investigative Dermatology, 35,* 347–352.

Butterworth, T., Strean, L.P., Beerman, H., & Wood, M.G. (1964). Syringoma and mongolism. *Archives of Dermatology, 90,* 483–487.

Carter, D.M., & Jegasothy, B.V. (1976). Alopecia

areata and Down's syndrome. *Archives of Dermatology*, *112*, 1397–1399.

Cohen, L. (1958). Observations on carotenemia. *Annals of Internal Medicine*, *48*, 218–227.

Crotty, G., Bell, M., Estes, S.A., & Kitzmiller, K.W. (1983). Cytologic features of elastosis perforans serpiginosa (EPS) associated with Down's syndrome [Letter to the editor]. *Journal of the American Academy of Dermatology*, *8*, 255–256.

Cutler, A., Obeiter, R., & Brink, S. (1986). Thyroid function in young children with Down's syndrome. *American Journal of Diseases of Children*, *140*, 479–483.

du Vivier, A., & Munio, D.D. (1975). Alopecia areata, autoimmunity and Down's syndrome. *British Medical Journal*, *1*, 191–192.

Evans, D.I. (1973). Norwegian scabies and monocytic leukemia. *British Medical Journal*, *4*, 613.

Glover, R., Young, L., & Goltz, R.W. (1987). Norwegian scabies in acquired immunodeficiency syndrome. *Journal of the American Academy of Dermatology*, *16*, 396–399.

Hurwitz, S. (1981). *Clinical pediatric dermatology*. Philadelphia: W.B. Saunders.

Kopec, A.V., & Levine N. (1979). Generalized connective tissue nevi and ichthyosis in Down's syndrome. *Archives of Dermatology*, *115*, 623–624.

Krafchik, B.R. (1988). Eczematous dermatitis. In L.A. Schachner & R.C. Hansen (Eds.), *Pediatric dermatology* (pp. 695–708). New York: Churchill Livingstone.

Lever, W.F., & Schaumburg-Lever, G. (Eds.). (1990). *Histopathology of the skin* (7th ed.). Philadelphia: J.B. Lippincott.

Mitchell, A.J., & Krull, E.A. (1984). Alopecia areata: Pathogenesis and treatment. *Journal of the American Academy of Dermatology*, *11*, 763–775.

Moschella, S.L., & Hurley, H.J. (Eds.). (1985). *Dermatology* (2nd ed.). Philadelphia: W.B. Saunders.

Patel, H., Dunn, H.G., Tischler, B., McBurney, A.K., & Hach, E. (1973). Carotenemia in mentally retarded children: I. Incidence and etiology. *Canadian Medical Association Journal*, *108*, 848–852.

Patterson, J.W. (1984). The perforating disorders. *Journal of the American Academy of Dermatology*, *10*, 561–584.

Rosenblum, G.A. (1983). Liquid nitrogen cryotherapy in a case of elastosis perforans serpiginosa. *Journal of the American Academy of Dermatology*, *8*, 718–721.

Rotchford, J.P., & Hyman, A.B. (1961). Extreme hyperkeratotic psoriasis in a mongoloid. *Archives of Dermatology*, *83*, 973–976.

Schamroth, J.M., Kellen, P., & Grieve, T.P. (1986). Elastosis perforans serpiginosa in a patient with renal disease. *Archives of Dermatology*, *122*, 82–84.

Suzumiya, J., Sumiyoshi, A., Kuroki, T., & Inoue, S. (1985). Crusted (Norwegian) scabies with adult T-cell leukemia. *Archives of Dermatology*, *121*, 903–904.

Tosti, A., DePadova, M.P., Minghetti, G., & Veronesi, S. (1986). Therapies versus placebo in the treatment of alopecia areata. *Journal of the American Academy of Dermatology*, *15*, 209–210.

Youshock, E., & Glazer, S.O. (1981). Norwegian scabies in a renal transplant patient. *Journal of the American Medical Association*, *246*, 2608–2609.

Zeligman, I., & Scalia, S.P. (1954). Dermatologic manifestations of mongolism. *Archives of Dermatology and Syphilology*, *69*, 342–344.

CHAPTER 20

Immunologic Features

Alberto G. Ugazio, Rita Maccario, and G. Roberto Burgio

Down syndrome is associated with a high incidence of viral and bacterial infections, autoimmune phenomena, malignancies, and hematologic disorders. The high incidence of serious infections, particularly of the respiratory tract, was first reported by Oster, Mikkelsen, and Nielsen (1964) and thereafter confirmed by several studies (Deaton, 1973; Mikkelsen, 1981; Oster, Mikkelsen, & Nielsen, 1975). The mortality and morbidity from infectious diseases are still high in persons with Down syndrome as compared to age- and sex-matched controls living in the same environmental conditions, in spite of the advances in chemotherapy and health care.

A high frequency of chronic carriers of the hepatitis B virus (HBV) (Figure 20.1), often associated with abnormalities of liver function and liver histology, has been reported in persons with Down syndrome (Hawkes, Boughton, Schroeter, Decker, & Overby, 1980; Sutnick, London, Gerstley, Cronolund, & Blumberg, 1968; Ugazio et al., 1977). This finding does not result from a higher rate of infection among persons with Down syndrome, with or without clinical disease.

Institutionalization is known to increase the risk of HBV infection; however, the frequency of chronic carriers among institutionalized persons at various ages is significantly higher in persons with trisomy 21 than in "normal" individuals (Ugazio et al., 1977). Taken together, these data suggest that the immune system of persons with Down syndrome is poorly efficient in eradicating HBV.

Hematologic abnormalities in persons with Down syndrome include the following:

- A high incidence of acute leukemia (Table 20.1) demonstrated by several epidemiologic investigations (Bernard, Mathè, Delorme, & Barnond, 1955; Fabia & Drolette, 1970; Fraumeni, Manning, & Mitus, 1971; Gunz, 1974; Hayashi et al., 1988; Kardos et al., 1983; Krivit & Good, 1957; R.W. Miller, 1970; Robinson & Neglia, 1987; Wong, Jones, Strivastava, & Gruppo, 1988). In the different studies, the frequency of acute leukemia was 7–50 times higher in persons with Down syndrome than in the general population. In contrast, the risk of chronic leukemia is not increased in persons with trisomy 21 (Rosner & Lee, 1972).

- A high incidence of transient myeloproliferative disorder during the neonatal period (Domenico et al., 1989; Hayashi et al., 1988; Wong et al., 1988) characterized by an abnormal proliferation (recovering spontaneously within a few weeks or months) of cells of the megakaryocytic lineage or of a myeloid progenitor committed to megakaryocytic differentiation. The same defect has been found in persons with Down syndrome with acute nonlymphoid leukemia, which, however, is characterized by monoclonality and clone chromosome abnormality (Hayashi et al., 1988).

- The number of granulocytic progenitor cells is reduced by more than 70% when compared to karyotypically "normal" controls. This decrease is not compensated by an increased proliferation (Standen, Philip, & Fletcher, 1979). (See also Lubin, Kahn, & Scott, chap. 21; this volume.)

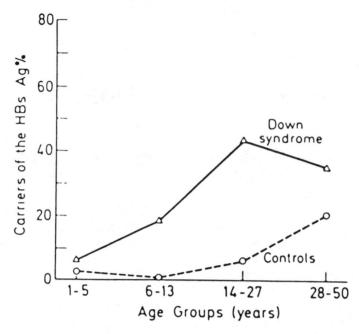

Figure 20.1. Frequency of carriers of the hepatitis B surface antigen (HBsAg) in persons with Down syndrome (△) and controls (O). Controls were carefully matched for age, sex, and socioenvironmental conditions. (Adapted from Ugazio et al., 1977.)

Many studies have reported a high frequency of autoantibodies, mainly antithyroid antibodies, in children with Down syndrome (Burgio, Severi, Rossoni, & Vaccaro, 1965; Fialkow, 1970; Ido & Green, 1977; Kanavin et al., 1988; Mellon, Pay, & Greene, 1963; Ugazio et al., 1977). These are associated with evidence of thyroid disturbances (Blumberg & AvRuskin, 1987; Culter, Benezra-Obeiter, & Brink, 1986), chronic active hepatitis, and alopecia areata (Du-Vivier & Munro, 1975; Ruch, Schurmann, Gordon, Burgin-Wolff, & Girard, 1985).

The high susceptibility to infections, high risk of malignancies, and increased frequency of autoantibodies have suggested that derangements of humoral and/or cell-mediated immunity may contribute to the clinical picture of Down syndrome (Burgio, Ugazio, Nespoli, & Maccario, 1983; Levin, 1987; Ugazio, 1981; Ugazio, Maccario, Notarangelo, & Burgio, 1990).

THYMUS

The thymus plays a crucial role in the maturation, differentiation, and selection of lymphoid precursors committed to the T-cell lineage. In

Table 20.1. Age distribution of acute lymphocytic leukemia (ALL) and acute nonlymphocytic leukemia (ANLL) in persons with or without Down syndrome

Age at diagnosis (years)	ALL (%)		ANLL (%)	
	Down syndrome ($n = 95$)	Non-Down syndrome ($n = 4,360$)	Down syndrome ($n = 20$)	Non-Down syndrome ($n = 931$)
<1	1	3	10	11
1–2	28	21	65	14
3–6	43	44	15	21
7–9	12	12	5	13
>10	16	20	5	41

Adapted from Robinson and Neglia (1987).

particular, under the influence of the thymic environment, T-cell precursors rearrange the T-cell receptor (TCR) genes and learn how to discriminate between self- and nonself-antigens (Benda & Strassmann, 1965; Fowlkes & Pardoll, 1989).

Morphologic derangements of the thymus were first reported by Benda and Strassmann (1965) and confirmed thereafter by several authors who showed that thymic abnormalities include small size; poor corticomedullary differentiation; severe reduction of the cortical area; increased number of large and degenerate Hassall corpuscles, most of which calcified; and a defective capacity of producing thymic hormonal factors (Duse et al., 1980; Fabris, Mocchegiani, & Amadio, 1984; Franceschi et al., 1978; Levin et al., 1979). It has been suggested that impairment of thymic function resulting from failure of epithelial cells to promote T-cell differentiation and selection may account for most of the immunologic anomalies of Down syndrome (Ugazio, 1981). This hypothesis has been strengthened by the recent observation that several T-cell differentiation antigens are poorly expressed by thymocytes of persons with Down syndrome. In particular, LaRocca et al. (1988) have reported that the population of thymocytes expressing CD1, CD3, CD4, and CD8 antigens—namely, "mature" thymocytes—is severely reduced, whereas Murphy and Epstein (1990) have demonstrated an impaired expression by thymocytes from persons with Down syndrome of the cell surface complex CD3/TCRα,β. The CD1, CD3, CD4, and CD8 antigens are crucial for the maturation and functional activity of T cells (Fowlkes & Pardoll, 1989) and the CD3/TCR receptor is essential for antigen recognition by T cells. Therefore, the findings by LaRocca et al. and Murphy and Epstein strongly suggest that intrathymic T-cell differentiation is severely impaired in persons with Down syndrome, possibly leading to the release of phenotypically and functionally immature T cells. Because Cossarizza et al. (1989) have found no phenotypic or functional alterations of thymocytes in fetuses with Down syndrome, it is conceivable that thymic impairment is the result of a progressive, age-dependent deterioration.

Murphy and Epstein (1990) have hypothesized that overexpression of genes located on chromosome 21—in particular, those coding for the β-chain (CD18) of the lymphocyte function-associated antigen-1 (LFA-1) and for the interferon receptor (Springer, Dustin, Kishimoto, & Marlin, 1987; Y.H. Tan, 1975)—may, in part, be responsible for the impairment of intrathymic maturation. Lymphocyte function-associated antigen-1, a receptor expressed on the surface of immature thymocytes (Bierer & Burakoff, 1988; Singer, Smith, Tuck, Denning, & Haynes, 1989; Springer et al., 1987), is crucial for the binding of human-activated thymocytes to thymic epithelial cells (Singer et al., 1989), and is known to play an important role in the interaction between T lymphocytes and several antigen-presenting cells (Bierer & Burakoff, 1988; Springer et al., 1987). Interferon-gamma can be produced by immature thymocytes (Ransom et al., 1987) and is known to increase the expression of class I and class II human leukocyte antigen (HLA) molecules as well as of the intercellular adhesion molecule-1 (ICAM-1), which is a ligand for LFA-1 (Bierer & Burakoff, 1988; Dustin, Rothlein, Bhan, Dinarello, & Springer, 1986; Singer et al., 1989; Springer et al., 1987). Overexpression of the interferon receptor and of LFA-1 increases the sensitivity to interferon-gamma and enhances the LFA-1–mediated adhesion capacity of lymphoid cells from persons with Down syndrome (Cupples & Tan, 1977; Epstein & Epstein, 1980; Funa, Anneren, Alm, & Björksten, 1984; Morgenesen, Vignaux, & Gresser, 1982; Nair & Schwartz, 1984; Revel, Bash, & Ruddle, 1976; Tan, 1976; Taylor, 1987; Taylor, Haigh, Williams, D'Souza, & Harris, 1988; Taylor, Williams, & D'Souza, 1986; Taylor et al., 1988; Weil, Epstein, & Epstein, 1980). Overexpression of ICAM-1 and HLA class I and II molecules induced on thymic cells by interferon together with overexpression of the LFA-1 receptor may ultimately result in an abnormal interaction between thymocytes and thymic epithelial cells, thus resulting in aberrant T-cell maturation and selection.

T-CELL–MEDIATED IMMUNITY

The number of circulating T lymphocytes, identified by means of monoclonal antibodies specific for the CD3 antigen, a molecule associated

Table 20.2.   Membrane phenotype of circulating T lymphocytes in persons with Down syndrome

Subset	Percentage	References
Total T cells (CD3+, CD2+)	Normal	Burgio, Ugazio, Nespoli, and Maccario (1983) Franceschi et al. (1978) Gupta, Fikrig, Mariano, and Quazi (1983)
Helper T cells (CD4+)	Normal	Burgio, Ugazio, Nespoli, and Maccario (1983) Kabelits (1990)
Helper/inducer T cells (CD4/CDW29+)	Low	Raziuddin and Elawad (1990)
Suppressor/inducer T cells (CD4/CD45R+)	High	Raziuddin and Elawad (1990)
Suppressor T cells (CD8+)	High/normal	Burgio, Ugazio, Nespoli, and Maccario (1983) Maccario et al. (1984)

with the TCR, is either normal or slightly depressed in persons with Down syndrome (Table 20.2). A normal percentage of total T cells has also been reported using monoclonal antibodies specific for the CD2 antigen (sheep erythrocytes receptor), expressed on the surface of T cells since the earliest stages of maturation and involved in a pathway of T-cell activation that is alternative/accessory to the "classical pathway" triggered via the CD3/TCR complex (Kabelits, 1990). However, early reports on the distribution of T-cell subsets in persons with Down syndrome had shown that, in spite of a normal percentage of CD3- and CD2-positive lymphocytes, a high proportion of cells express low-avidity receptors for sheep erythrocytes (Burgio et al., 1978; Burgio et al., 1983).

Although the proportion of T lymphocytes expressing the CD4 antigen, associated with helper function, is normal in persons with Down syndrome (Burgio et al., 1983; Maccario et al., 1984), Raziuddin and Elawad (1990) have recently reported that, within the CD4 subset, the proportion of helper/inducer (CD4+, CDW29+) lymphocytes is significantly decreased and the proportion of suppressor/inducer (CD4+, CD45R+) cells is markedly increased. This imbalance may contribute to the alteration of immunoregulatory mechanisms in persons with Down syndrome.

The percentage of lymphocytes expressing the CD8 antigen, known to be associated with

cytotoxic/suppressive activity, is markedly increased in most individuals with Down syndrome (Burgio et al., 1983; Maccario et al., 1984). This finding is likely to result, at least in part, from the presence in the peripheral blood of a high percentage of natural killer (NK) cells (discussed later in this chapter), partly expressing the CD8 antigen (Maccario et al., 1984; Montagna et al., 1988).

Defective proliferative capacity in vitro of T lymphocytes from persons with Down syndrome has been reported in several studies, using different experimental designs (Table 20.3). Early reports on mitogen-induced proliferation showed that the response to phytohemagglutinin and concanavalin A are within the normal range in the 1st decade of life and decline thereafter progressively (Burgio et al., 1975; Epstein & Epstein, 1980; Gershwin, Crinella, Castles, & Trent, 1977; Melman, Younkin, & Baker, 1970; Philip et al., 1986; Schechter, Handzel, Altmain, Nir, & Levin, 1977; Whittingham, Pitt, Sharma, & Mackay, 1977).

Recent reports by Bertotto et al. (1987), Bertotto, Crupi, Arcangeli, Gerli, Marinelli et al. (1989), and Bertotto, Crupi, Arcangeli, Gerli, Scalise, et al. (1989) have extended these observations by demonstrating a defective response of T lymphocytes to other T-cell mitogens such as monoclonal antibodies specific for the CD3 and CD2 antigens. These results are in keeping with the finding by the same authors of an abnormal

Table 20.3.   Evaluation of in vivo and in vitro T-cell functions in persons with Down syndrome

Function	Activity	References
Mitogen-induced proliferation:		
Phytohemagglutinin, concanavalin A	Low/normal	Epstein and Epstein (1980); Melman, Younkin, and Baker (1970); Philip et al. (1986); Whittingham, Pitt, Sharma, and Mackay (1977)
α-CD3, α-CD2	Low	Bertotto et al. (1987); Bertotto, Crupi, Arcangeli, Gerli, Marinelli, et al. (1979); Bertotto, Crupi, Arcangeli, Gerli, Scalise, et al. (1989)
Phorbol ester +A23187	Normal	Bertotto, Crupi, Arcangeli, Gerli, Scalise, et al. (1989)
Allogenic mixed lymphocyte culture:		
Proliferation	Low/high	Franceschi et al. (1980); Gupta, Fikrig, Mariano, and Quazi (1983); Raziuddin and Elawad (1990); Sasaki and Yoshitaka (1969); Walford et al. (1981)
Cytotoxic activity	Low	Ugazio, Maccario, Notarangelo, and Burgio (1990)
Antigen-induced proliferation:		
Staphilococcus, streptococcus, Sendai virus	Normal	Funa, Annerén, Alm, and Björksten (1984)
Tetanus toxoid, influenza virus	Low	Boxer and Yokoyama (1972); Philip et al. (1986)
Interleukin 2 production:		
Mitogen induced	Low/normal	Bertotto, Crupi, Arcangeli, Gerli, Marinelli, et al. (1989); Gupta, Fikrig, Mariano, and Quazi (1983); Karttunen, Nurmi, Ilonen, and Surcel (1984); Ugazio, Maccario, Notarangelo, and Burgio (1990)
Allo–mixed lymphocyte culture induced	Low/normal	Grupta, Fikrig, Mariano, and Quazi (1983); Ugazio, Maccario, Notarangelo, and Burgio (1990)
Antigen induced	Low	Philip et al. (1986)
	Low/normal	Funa, Annerén, Alm, and Björksten (1984); Levin et al. (1979); Nair and Schwartz (1984)

expression of the CD2 and CD3 antigens on the surface of T lymphocytes of persons with Down syndrome (LaRocca et al., 1988; Murphy & Epstein, 1990) as well as with the earlier findings of CD2-positive T cells with an abnormally low avidity for sheep erythrocytes (Burgio et al., 1978; Burgio et al., 1983). These data suggest that impairment of CD2- and CD3-mediated pathways of T-cell activation may contribute to the immunodeficiency of persons with Down syndrome. The same authors (Bertotto, Crupi, Arcangeli, Gerli, Marinelli, et al., 1989) have reported that the proliferative response to some polyclonal activators such as phorbol ester and calcium ionophore A23187 is normal in persons with Down syndrome. Because stimulation with phorbol ester and A23187 activates T cells by bypassing the early steps of the activation process required by other polyclonal activators, these data suggest that T-cell responses are impaired in

persons with Down syndrome due to a defective transmembrane signal transduction.

Conflicting results have been reported concerning T-cell proliferation induced in allogenic mixed lymphocyte culture (MLC). Some groups have found an abnormally high proliferation (Franceschi et al., 1980; Gupta, Fikrig, Mariano, & Quazi, 1983; Sasaki & Yoshitaka, 1969), whereas others have shown depressed response (Raziuddin & Elawad, 1990; Walford et al., 1981). In a recent study, Ugazio et al. (1990) reported defective proliferative response in MLC with decreased expression of the membrane receptor (CD25) for interleukin 2, the lymphokine necessary to promote antigen- and mitogen-induced T-cell growth. Low secretion of interleukin 2 in the supernatant (Table 20.4) and depressed allo-specific cytotoxic activity (Figure 20.2) have also been recorded in this study.

Analysis of the proliferative response in vitro

Table 20.4.   Lymphocyte proliferation, interleukin 2 production, and interleukin 2 receptor (TAC-Antigen) expression induced in the mixed lymphocyte reaction (MLR) in 15 persons with Down syndrome (4–15 years) compared to 15 age-matched karyotypically "normal" controls

Subjects	Proliferation[a] (cpm/culture)	Interleukin 2 production (units/ml)	Expression of CD25 (% positive cells)
Down syndrome	9150 ± 2412	4.3 ± 2.9	8 ± 3
Control	37069 ± 8486	29.4 ± 12.2	39 ± 8
p	<0.001	<0.001	<0.001

Adapted from Ugazio, Maccario, Notarangelo, and Burgio (1990).

[a]Results are expressed as mean ± 1 standard deviation; the mean of the three assays are obtained by subtracting the background values (without stimulator cells) from the values obtained from allo–mixed lymphocyte reaction (MLR)–induced cultures. Tac expression and lymphocyte proliferation were evaluated after 3 days of culture, as was interleukin 2 production in the supernatants after 5 days of activation.

of lymphocytes from persons with Down syndrome to antigenic stimuli has given different results, depending on the antigen used (Table 20.3). In particular, normal responses have been reported to staphylococcal and streptococcal antigens as well as to Sendai virus (Funa et al., 1984), whereas stimulation with tetanus toxoid and influenza virus has given low proliferative responses (Boxer & Yokoyama, 1972; Philip et al., 1986). The impaired T-lymphocyte response to certain antigens only may suggest that the "repertoire" of T cells is more limited in persons

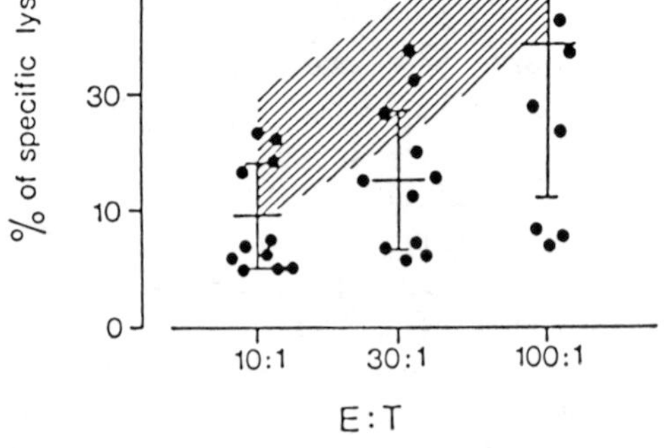

Figure 20.2. Cytotoxic T-lymphocyte activity of peripheral blood mononuclear cells of 11 persons with Down syndrome, at various effector to target ratios (E:T). Shaded area represents mean value ± SD of cytotoxic T-lymphocyte activity in "normal" controls. (Adapted from Montagna et al., 1988.)

with Down syndrome than in karyotypically "normal" individuals, possibly due to deranged intrathymic differentiation and selection of T-cell clones.

Production and secretion of lymphokines by T lymphocytes in persons with Down syndrome has been investigated by several authors with contradictory results (Table 20.3). In particular, some groups have reported defective production of interleukin 2 in response to phytohemagglutinin (Ugazio et al., 1990), anti-CD3 or anti-CD2 monoclonal antibodies (Bertotto, Crupi, Arcangeli, Gerli, Marinelli, et al., 1989), and allogeneic stimuli (Ugazio et al., 1990); in other studies, interleukin 2 production induced by phytohemagglutinin or in the MLC has been normal (Gupta et al., 1983; Karttunen, Nurmi, Ilonen, & Surcel, 1984). In one study (Philip et al., 1986), antigen-induced production of interleukin 2 by T lymphocytes of persons with Down syndrome was markedly reduced in response to influenza virus and bacterial antigens such as tetanus toxoid. Recently, a severe impairment of interleukin 2 gene expression has been reported in persons with Down syndrome (Gerez et al., 1991).

Defective production of interferon in persons with Down syndrome was first described in vivo at the onset of viral infections (Boyer & Fontes, 1975), and then confirmed in vitro in different experiments involving measurement of both interferon-alfa and interferon-gamma (Levin et al., 1979; Nair & Schwartz, 1984). However, in some studies, normal levels of interferon-alfa and interferon-gamma were observed using concanavalin A or Sendai virus as activators (Funa et al., 1984).

A number of studies have shown that cells belonging to different lineages such as fibroblasts, monocytes, and T and NK cells have an enhanced sensitivity to the effect of interferon in Down syndrome (Cupples & Tan, 1977; Epstein & Epstein, 1980; Funa et al., 1984; Morgenesen et al., 1982; Nair & Schwartz, 1984; Revel et al., 1976; Tan, 1976; Weil et al., 1980), probably due to overexpression of the interferon receptor coded for by the IfRec gene located on chromosome 21 (Tan, 1975). These data suggest that abnormal interaction of interferon with its own receptor may be one of the factors that impair the immune response in persons with Down syndrome.

Low serum zinc levels have been reported in most persons with Down syndrome (Björksten et al., 1980). Because zinc is an important cofactor in T-cell–mediated responses, it is also conceivable that zinc deficiency may contribute to the impairment of T-cell function. However Lockitch et al. (1989) have recently reported no effect of long-term, low-dose oral zinc supplementation on several immunologic functions, including number and proportion of T-lymphocyte subset and in vitro response to polyclonal activators. Other groups have reported an improvement of phytohemagglutinin-induced lymphocyte proliferation in persons with Down syndrome after 2 months of zinc therapy (Stabile et al., 1991). Further studies are needed to clarify the reasons for these discrepancies.

NATURAL KILLER CELLS: PHENOTYPE AND FUNCTION

The absolute number and proportion of NK cells expressing the CD57 and/or CD16 surface antigens are elevated in the peripheral blood of persons with Down syndrome (Burgio et al., 1983; Maccario et al., 1984; Raziuddin & Elawad, 1990; Stabile et al., 1991). Most of these cells coexpress the CD57 and CD3 or CD8 antigens: This phenotypic feature is characteristically associated with immature stages of differentiation and low cytotoxic capacity of NK cells (Abo, Cooper, & Balch, 1982). These data are in keep-

ing with the observation that NK activity of lymphocytes is depressed in persons with Down syndrome (Figure 20.3), in spite of the elevated number of cells with the NK phenotype (Raziuddin & Elawad, 1990).

Natural killer lymphocytes are likely to be involved in vivo in the defense against viral infections and neoplastic cells (Ortaldo & Herbermann, 1984). Because it has been shown that NK cells also play an important role in the regulation of the immune response and of hematopoiesis, probably through the secretion of various lymphokines, alterations in the number and function of NK cells may contribute to the immunologic and hematologic derangements in persons with Down syndrome.

The low spontaneous activity of trisomic NK cells can be improved in vitro by the addition of interferon (Nurmi, Huttunen, et al., 1982). The enhancing capacity of interferon is more pronounced in children than in adults: Indeed, NK cells from adults with Down syndrome respond poorly to the boosting effect of interferon (Funa et al., 1984). Much in the same way as T-cell function, NK activity also may be affected in vivo and in vitro by overexpression of the inter-

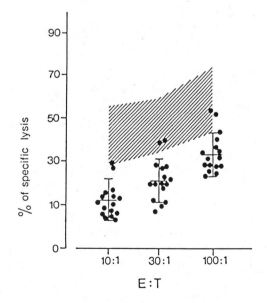

Figure 20.3. Natural killer activity of peripheral blood mononuclear cells from 16 persons with Down syndrome at various effector to target ratios (E:T). Vertical bars represent mean values ± 1 SD. Shaded area represents mean value ± 1 SD in karyotypically "normal" controls. (Adapted from Montagna et al., 1988.)

feron receptor on the membrane and by defective capacity to produce interferon.

Another factor that may potentially affect NK activity in persons with Down syndrome, is overexpression of the β-chain (CD18) of the LFA-1 molecule, encoded on chromosome 21 (Suomalainen, Gahmberg, Patarroyo, Beatty, & Schoder, 1986). The already-mentioned LFA-1 is a member of the integrin family, a group of cell-adhesion molecules promoting aggregation of leukocytes (homotypic adhesion) and their adhesion to accessory, target, and endothelial cells (Pardi, Bender, Dettori, Giannazza, & Engleman, 1989; Springer et al., 1987). In particular, LFA-1 can increase the strength of the binding between cytotoxic cells (either cytotoxic T lymphocytes or NK) and their targets. Its overexpression on lymphocytes of persons with Down syndrome may result in an abnormal pattern of adhesion between cytotoxic cells and their targets, thus contributing to hamper cytotoxic function. The impairment of cytotoxic activity also involves antibody-mediated cell cytotoxicity (ADCC), which is reduced in persons with Down syndrome as compared to karyotypically "normal" controls (Nair & Schwartz, 1984; Warren et al., 1987).

The evaluation of the "activated" NK cytotoxicity has given different results depending on the stimulus used for induction: Lectin-induced cellular cytotoxicity was found to be low (Nair & Schwartz, 1984) and the NK-like activity measured in MLC was in the normal range (Montagna et al., 1988). Contradictory results have been reported for lymphokine-activated killing (LAK) activity, with some studies showing low levels of cytotoxicity (Nair & Schwartz, 1984) and others a normal response (Montagna et al., 1988). These discrepancies may result from differences in the concentrations of interleukin 2 used in the assay and/or incubation time.

Natural killer cells represent a heterogeneous population, initially defined on the basis of their functional activity: the capacity of killing spontaneously neoplastic or virus-infected target cells (Ortaldo & Herbermann, 1984). The differentiation pathway followed by NK cells during their ontogeny has not been fully clarified so far. Also, the membrane receptor employed by NK

lymphocytes to recognize target cells is presently unknown. There is evidence that part of the cells displaying NK activity may share a common progenitor with the T-cell lineage and that a small proportion of circulating lymphocytes coexpress T-cell and NK-cell markers (Ortaldo & Herbermann, 1984; Yonagi et al., 1985). This is also in keeping with the findings in persons with Down syndrome and suggests that the thymic derangement observed not only may result in impaired maturation of T cells but also may affect the differentiation of NK cells.

ANTIBODY-MEDIATED IMMUNITY

Impairment of the immune system in persons with Down syndrome also involves antibody-mediated responses, including some abnormalities in the distribution of serum immunoglobulins (Ig) and defective capacity to produce antibodies in response to certain antigens (Table 20.5).

Immunoglobulin serum levels are usually low in infants with Down syndrome, turn to normal within the first 5 years, and increase thereafter in adults to reach mean values that are higher than in "normal" adults (Burgio et al., 1975; Miller, Mellman, Cohen, Kohn, & Dietz, 1969; Ugazio et al., 1978). In a recent study, Avanzini et al. (1988) observed an anomalous distribution of IgG subclasses, with some subjects showing high levels of IgG1 and IgG3 and low or undetectable levels of IgG2 and IgG4 (Table 20.6). Immunoglobulin G2 are known to be primarily involved in the response to bacterial polysaccharide antigens: Defective production of IgG2 may be responsible for the low antibody response to pneumococcal vaccine in persons with Down syndrome, as reported by Nurmi, Huttunen, et al. (1982). In spite of high values of IgG1 and IgG3, defective antibody response to some viral antigens such as OX174 and influenza virus has been reported, both in vitro and in vivo (Epstein & Philip, 1987; Gordon, Sinha, & Carlson, 1971; Lopez, Ochs, Thuline, Davis, & Wedgwood, 1975; Philip et al., 1986), whereas stimulation with other antigens has resulted in normal antibody responses (Table 20.5). Conflicting results have been also obtained after vac-

Table 20.5. B-cell phenotype and function in Down syndrome

Phenotype/function	Activity	References
Total B cell number	Normal	Burgio, Ugazio, Nespoli, and Maccario (1983); Franceschi et al. (1978)
Serum immunoglobulins:		
IgG	Abnormal	Burgio, Ugazio, Nespoli, and Maccario (1983); Miller et al. (1969); Ugazio et al. (1978)
IgM	Low/normal	Burgio, Ugazio, Nespoli, and Maccario (1983)
IgA	Abnormal	Burgio, Ugazio, Nespoli, and Maccario (1983); Miller et al. (1969); Ugazio et al. (1978); Whittingham, Pitt, Sharmay, and Mackay (1977)
IgD	High	Rundle, Clothier, and Sudell (1971)
IgE	Low/normal	Jacobs, Burdash, Manos, and Duncan (1978); Whittingham, Pitt, Sharmay, and Mackay (1977)
IgG subclasses:		
IgG1 and IgG3	High	Avanzini et al. (1988)
IgG2 and IgG4	Low	Avanzini et al. (1988)
Serum antibodies:		
Bacterial antigens	Low/normal	Hawkes, Boughton, Schroeter, Decker, and Overby (1980); Nurmi, Huttunen, et al. (1982)
Viral antigens	Low/normal	Gordon et al. (1971); Hawkes, Boughton, Schroeter, Decker, and Overby (1980)
Production of Ig in vitro	Low	Philip et al. (1986)

cination with hepatitis B surface antigen (HBsAg). In one study, the antibody response was six-fold lower than in controls (Hawkes et al., 1980), whereas other studies showed normal rates of seroconversion and antibody titers (Heitjtink, de Jong, Schalm, & Masurel, 1984; Troisi, Heiberg, & Hollingerr, 1985). An abnormal response to the hepatitis B vaccine reported by Avanzini et al. (1988) and Avanzini, Monafo, De Amici, Maccario, and Burgio (1990) showed low IgG subclass responses in adults with Down syndrome (Table 20.7). In spite of normal or even high levels of IgG1, the overall response was impaired due to low titers of hepatitis B virus–specific IgG1 antibodies. Because vaccination

with HBsAg induces a predominant response in the IgG1 subclass in karyotypically "normal" individuals, the low titers of IgG1 antibodies observed in this study may in part account for the high frequency of chronic carriers of the virus among persons with Down syndrome. The abnormal pattern of IgG also includes low levels of "natural antibodies" to E. coli antigens in children less than 5 years old and in adults (Ugazio et al., 1978).

Serum IgA levels are within the normal range until the age of 5 years and increase thereafter (Burgio et al., 1975; Miller et al., 1969; Ugazio et al., 1978; Whittingham et al., 1977) while IgM levels decrease during adolescence and are

Table 20.6. Deranged IgG subclass levels of children and adults with Down syndrome

Subjects	Number with elevated levels		Number with decreased levels	
	IgG1	IgG3	IgG2	IgG4
Children (n = 21)	2 (9.5%)	5 (24%)	2 (9.5%)	4 (19%)
Adults (n = 36)	15 (41.6%)	28 (77.8%)	11 (30%)	11 (30%)
p	0.02	0.002	0.13	0.52

Adapted from Avanzini, Monafo, De Amici, Maccario, and Burgio (1990).

Table 20.7.   Responders to hepatitis B vaccine among adults with Down syndrome and controls

Subjects	Number of responders			
	IgG1	IgG2	IgG3	IgG4
Controls (16)	12 (75)	4 (25%)	2 (37.5%)	9 (56.2%)
Down syndrome	2 (16.7%)	2 (16.7%)	2 (16.7%)	0
p	0.007	0.94	0.43	0.006

Adapted from Avanzini, Monafo, De Amici, Maccario, and Burgio (1990).

lower than normal in the majority of adults with Down syndrome (Burgio et al., 1975). Serum IgE levels were low in one study (Whittingham et al., 1977) and higher than normal in another report (Jacobs, Burdash, Manos, & Duncan, 1978). High levels of IgD have been reported (Rundle, Clothier, & Sudell, 1971).

In spite of the abnormalities of serum immunoglobulin levels and of various antibody responses, the proportion of circulating B lymphocytes expressing the different surface Ig is substantially normal in persons with Down syndrome (Table 20.5). In children with Down syndrome, Gupta et al. (1984) have observed a B-cell subset that is highly represented only in aging, karyotypically "normal" individuals.

It is well known that B-cell differentiation to antibody-secreting cells is controlled by a network of cytokines and cellular interactions and that T lymphocytes play a crucial regulatory role. Therefore, it is conceivable that the impairment of humoral immunity observed in persons with Down syndrome may result from abnormalities in the T–B-cell cooperation mechanisms due to the deranged differentiation and function of T cells.

NEUTROPHIL AND MONOCYTE FUNCTION

Because polymorphonuclear and mononuclear phagocytes play an important role in the defense against microorganisms, several authors have investigated their distribution and function in persons with Down syndrome, in order to correlate possible defects of phagocyte activity with the high incidence of infections. With the exception of one study (Spina, Smith, Korn, Fahey, & Grossman, 1981), a normal proportion of neutro-

phils has been reported, whereas functional activity in vitro has been found to be defective (Levin, 1987).

Crucial events of phagocyte-mediated defense that can be evaluated in vitro include the capacity of migration in response to adequate stimuli (chemotaxis), phagocytosis of microorganisms, and activation of the oxidative metabolism with production of oxygen radicals (e.g., superoxide) that cause killing of the ingested microorganisms. Both neutrophil and monocyte chemotaxis are depressed in persons with Down syndrome (Barking, Weston, Humbert, & Maire, 1980; Barroeta et al., 1983) and this can also affect the phagocytosis and killing capacity of these cells. As it is well known that zinc is necessary to promote chemotactic responsiveness, low levels of serum zinc may be one of the factors affecting chemotactic activity in persons with Down syndrome. Furthermore, chemotaxis may be impaired because of overexpression of LFA-1 or of a defective production of cytokines involved in the chemotactic process.

Phagocytosis and killing of microorganisms susceptible to superoxide, such as *Candida albicans* and *Staphylococcus aureus*, are defective in persons with Down syndrome (Costello & Wabber, 1976; Gregory, Williams, & Thompson, 1972). Superoxide is converted to hydrogen peroxide by superoxide dismutase-1 (SOD-1) (McCord & Fridovich, 1969), which is coded for by a gene located on chromosome 21 (V.H. Tan, Tischfield, & Ruddle, 1973). Superoxide dismutase-1 activity in persons with Down syndrome is, on the average, 150% of that found in karyotypically "normal" individuals (Baetman, Mattei, Baret, & Mattei, 1984), resulting in a high rate of conversion of superoxide into peroxide. The intracellular levels of superoxide are consequently low (Annerén & Björksten, 1984) and do not allow efficient killing. This anomaly may contribute to increase the susceptibility of persons with Down syndrome to bacterial infections, particularly those caused by microorganisms (such as staphylococci) that strictly require superoxide in order to be killed efficiently. With the exception of chemotactic activity, few data are available on the functional activity of mononuclear phagocytes in the defense against protozoa and fungi (Cline, 1970).

Monocytes/macrophages also play a central role as antigen-presenting cells in the activation of T lymphocytes. Moreoever, they secrete a number of cytokines (e.g., interleukin 1 and interleukin 6) involved in the modulation of the immune response and of inflammatory processes. Epstein and Philip (1987) have reported that monocytes from persons with Down syndrome have a normal capacity of producing interleukin 1 in vitro in response to various stimuli such as lipopolysaccharide and interferon.

CONCLUSION

Many factors have been shown to contribute to the immune deficiency that results in the high susceptibility to infections and high rate of malignancies and autoimmune phenomena in persons with Down syndrome.

Gene coding for molecules that plays an important role in various immune mechanisms, such as the β-chain of LAF-1 and interferon receptor are located on chromosome 21. Their overexpression is likely to affect the function of both T and NK lymphocytes as well as of polymorphonuclear cells and monocytes. Overexpression of the two molecules also may contribute to the thymic derangement that ultimately results in an anomalous maturation and selection of T-cell clones leading to a limited "repertoire" of functionally impaired T cells.

T lymphocytes play a central role, not only in the effector phase of cell-mediated immune response, but also in controlling the differentiation and activity of other cellular subpopulations such as B and NK lymphocytes, monocytes, and hematopoietic precursors. It is conceivable that

defective differentiation of the T-cell lineage during intrathymic maturation may account for the majority of the immunologic abnormalities of persons with Down syndrome. In fact, anomalies in the cooperation between T and B lymphocytes, resulting from the low number and activity of helper/inducer T-cell subsets, may result in the defective production of antibodies directed against certain antigens. Furthermore, the high number of NK cells with low cytotoxic activity may also be related to the thymic derangement resulting from abnormal intrathymic maturation of a precursor common to both T and NK cells. Overexpression of LFA-1 and interferon receptor, depressed capacity to produce lymphokines, and persistence of viral infections also may be involved in the impairment of NK activity. Overexpression of the gene coding for superoxide dismutase-1, also located on chromosome 21, may ultimately lead to impairment of neutrophil killing activity, thus contributing to the high susceptibility to bacterial infections. Finally, low serum zinc levels may also contribute to the impairment of the immune response.

In spite of major advances in the understanding of the cellular and molecular defects underlying the immunodeficiency of persons with Down syndrome, therapeutic options are still limited and controversial. Because the immune defect is relatively mild, an aggressive use of appropriate antibiotics is usually sufficient to control most bacterial infections. Furthermore, although the specific antibody response to HBV antigens is partly impaired and deranged, vaccination with HBsAg usually results in protective immunity and is therefore highly advisable in persons with Down syndrome.

The mildness of the immune defect, which is certainly not among the major handicaps of persons with Down syndrome, also raises ethical questions on the usefulness and advisability of clinical trials with potentially harmful modifiers of the immune response. Trials with thymic hormones have been suggested but are of doubtful significance, also in view of the multiplicity of the factors contributing to the immune deficiency in persons with Down syndrome. Therapeutic trials with zinc have given contradictory results both in vitro and in vivo.

REFERENCES

Abo, T., Cooper, M.D., & Balch, C.M. (1982). Characterization of HNK-1 + (Leu-7) human lymphocytes I. Two distinct phenotypes of human NK cells with different cytotoxic capability. *Journal of Immunology*, *129*, 1752–1757.

Annerén, G., & Björksten, B. (1984). Low superoxide levels in blood phagocytic cells in Down's syndrome. *Acta Paediatrica Scandinavica*, *73*, 345–348.

Avanzini, M.A., Monafo, V., De Amici, M., Maccario, R., & Burgio, G.R. (1990). Humural immunodeficiencies in Down syndrome: Serum IgG subclass and antibody response to hepatitis B vaccine. *American Journal of Medical Genetics Supplement*, *7*, 231–233.

Avanzini, M.A., Soderstrom, T., Wahl, M., Plebani, A., Burgio, G.R., & Hanson, L.A. (1988). IgG subclass deficiency in patients with Down's syndrome and aberrant hepatitis B vaccine response. *Scandinavian Journal of Immunology*, *28*, 465–470.

Baetman, M.A., Mattei, M.G., Baret, A., & Mattei, J.F. (1984). Immunoreactive copper-zinc superoxide-dismutase (SOD-1) in mosaic trisomy 21 and normal subjects. *Acta Paediatrica Scandinavica*, *73*, 341–344.

Barking, R.M., Weston, W.L., Humbert, J.R., & Maire, F. (1980). Phagocytic function in Down's syndrome: I. Chemotaxis; II. Bactericidal activity and phagocytosis. *Journal of Mental Deficiency Research*, *24*, 243–256.

Barroeta, O., Nungaray, M., Luyez-Osana, M., Armendares, S., Salamanca, F., & Kretsahmer, R.R. (1983). Defective monocyte chemotaxis in children with Down syndrome. *Pediatric Research*, *17*, 292–295.

Benda, C.E., & Strassmann, G.S. (1965). The thymus in mongolism. *Journal of Mental Deficiency Research*, *9*, 109–177.

Bernard, J., Mathè, G., Delorme, J.C., & Barnond, O. (1955). Les leucoses des très jeunes enfants [Leukemias in infancy]. *Archives Francaises de Pédiatrie*, *12*, 470–477.

Bertotto, A., Arcangeli, C., Crupi, S., Marinelli, I., Gerli, L., & Vaccaro, R. (1987). T cell response to anti-CD3 antibody in Down's syndrome. *Archives of Disease in Childhood*, *62*, 1148–1151.

Bertotto, A., Crupi, S., Arcangeli, C., Gerli, R., Marinelli, I., Verlardi, A., & Vaccaro, R. (1989). T-cell response to anti-CD2 monoclonal antibodies in Down's syndrome. *Scandanavian Journal of Immunology*, *30*, 39–43.

Bertotto, A., Crupi, S., Arcangeli, C., Gerli, R., Scalise, F., Fabietti, G., Agea, E., & Vaccaro, R. (1989). T-cell response to phorbol ester PMA and calcium inophore A23187 in Down's syndrome.

Scandinavian Journal of Immunology, *30*, 583–586.

Bierer, B.E., & Burakoff, S.J. (1988). T cell adhesion molecules. *Federation of European Biochemical Societies Journal*, *192*, 2584–2590.

Björksten, B., Back, O., Gustavson, H., Hallmans, G., Hogglof, B., & Tarnvick, A. (1980). Zinc and immune function in Down's syndrome. *Acta Paediatrica Scandinavica*, *69*, 183–187.

Blumberg, D., & AvRuskin, T. (1987). Down's syndrome, autoimmune hypothyroidism, and hypoparathyroidism: A unique triad. *American Journal of Diseases of Children*, *141*, 11–49.

Boxer, L.A., & Yokoyama, M. (1972). Lymphocyte antigens in patients with Down's syndrome. *Vox Sanguinis*, *22*, 539–543.

Boyer, J.M., & Fontes, A.K. (1975). Interferon levels in Down's syndrome. *Journal of the American Osteopathic Association*, *75*, 437–441.

Burgio, G.R., Lanzavecchia, A., Maccario, R., Vitiello, A., Plebani, A., & Ugazio, A.G. (1978). Immunodeficiency in Down's syndrome: T lymphocyte subset imbalance in trisomic children. *Clinical and Experimental Immunology*, *33*, 298–301.

Burgio, G.R., Severi, F., Rossoni, R., & Vaccaro, R. (1965). Mongolism and thyroid autoimmunity. *Lancet*, *i*, 166–167.

Burgio, G.R., Ugazio, A.G., Nespoli, L., & Maccario, R. (1983). Down syndrome: A model of immunodeficiency. *Birth Defects: Original Article Series*, *19*, 325–327.

Burgio, G.R., Ugazio, A.G., Nespoli, L., Marcioni, A.F., Bottelli, A.M., & Pasquali, F. (1975). Derangements of immunoglobulin levels, phytohemagglutinin responsiveness, and T and B cell markers in Down's syndrome at different ages. *European Journal of Immunology*, *5*, 600–603.

Cline, M.J. (1970). Monocytes and macrophages. Differentiation and functions. In T.J. Greenwalt & G.A. Jameson (Eds.), *Formation and destruction of blood cells* (pp. 222–239). Philadelphia: J.B. Lippincott.

Cossarizza, A., Mundi, D., Montagnani, G., Furabusco, A., Dagna-Bricarelli, F., & Franceschi, C. (1989). Fetal thymic differentiation in Down's syndrome. *Thymus*, *14*, 163–170.

Costello, C., & Wabber, A. (1976). White cell function in Down's syndrome. *Clinical Genetics*, *9*, 603–605.

Culter, A.T., Benezra-Obeiter, R., & Brink, S.J. (1986). Thyroid function in young children with Down syndrome. *American Journal of Diseases of Children*, *140*, 479–483.

Cupples, C.G., & Tan, Y.H. (1977). Effect of human interferon preparations on lymphoblastogenesis in Down's syndrome. *Nature*, *267*, 165–167.

Deaton, J.G. (1973). The mortality rate and causes of death among institutionalized mongols in Texas. *Journal of Mental Deficiency Research, 17*, 117–122.

Domenico, D.R., Dizikes, G.J., Melnyk, A.R., Bird, M.L., Suarez, C.R., & Schumacher, H.R. (1989). Pseudoleukemia in Down's syndrome. Analysis of immunophenotype and gene rearrangement. *American Journal of Clinical Pathology, 9*, 709–714.

Duse, M., Brugo, M.A., Martini, A., Tassi, C., Ferrario, C., & Ugazio, A.G. (1980). Immunodeficiency in Down's syndrome: Low levels of serum thymic factor in trisomic children. *Thymus, 2*, 127–131.

Dustin, M.L., Rothlein, R., Bhan, A.K., Dinarello, C.A., & Springer, T.A. (1986). Induction by IL 1 and interferon-gamma: Tissue distribution, biochemistry, and function of a natural adherence molecule (ICAM-I). *Journal of Immunology, 137*, 247–254.

DuVivier, A., & Munro, D. (1975). Alopecia areata, autoimmunity and Down's syndrome. *British Medical Journal, 1*, 191–192.

Epstein, L.B., & Epstein, C.J. (1980). T-lymphocyte function and sensitivity to IFN in trisomy 21. *Cellular Immunology, 51*, 303–318.

Epstein, L.B., & Philip, R. (1987). Abnormalities of the immune response to influenza antigen in Down syndrome (trisomy 21). In E. McCoy & C. Epstein (Eds.), *Oncology and immunology of Down syndrome* (pp. 163–182). New York: Alan R. Liss.

Fabia, J., & Drolette, M. (1970). Malformations and leukemia in children with Down syndrome. *Pediatrics, 45*, 60–70.

Fabris, N., Mocchegiani, E., & Amadio, L. (1984). Thymic hormone deficiency in normal aging and Down's syndrome: Is there a primary failure of the thymus? *Lancet, i*, 983–986.

Fialkow, P.J. (1970). Thyroid autoimmunity and Down's syndrome. *Annals of the New York Academy of Sciences, 171*, 500–511.

Fowlkes, B.J., & Pardoll, D.M. (1989). Molecular and cellular events of T cell development. *Advances in Immunology, 44*, 207–264.

Franceschi, C., Licastro, F., Chisicolo, M., Bonetti, F., Zanotti, M., Fabbris, N., Macchegiani, E., Fantini, M.P., Paolucci, P., & Masi, M. (1980). Deficiency of autologous mixed lymphocyte reaction and serum thymic factor levels in Down's syndrome. *Journal of Immunology, 126*, 2162–2167.

Franceschi, C., Licastro, F., Paolucci, P., Masi, M., Cavicchi, S., & Zanotti, M. (1978). T and B lymphocyte subpopulations in Down's syndrome. A study on non-institutionalized subjects. *Journal of Mental Deficiency Research, 22*, 179–191.

Fraumeni, J.F., Manning, M.D., & Mitus, W.J. (1971). Acute childhood leukemia: Epidemiological study by cell type in 1263 cases at the Children's Cancer Research Foundation in Boston, 1947–1965. *Journal of the National Cancer Institute, 46*, 461–470.

Funa, K., Annerén, G., Alm, G.V., & Björksten, B. (1984). Abnormal interferon production and NK cell responses to interferon in children with Down's syndrome. *Clinical and Experimental Immunology, 56*, 493–500.

Gerez, L., Madar, L., Arad, G., Sharav, T., Reshef, A., Ketzinel, M., Sayer, D., Silberger, C., & Kaempfer, R. (1991). Aberrant regulation of interleukin-2 but not of interferon-gamma gene expression in Down syndrome (trisomy 21). *Clinical Immunology and Immunopathology, 58*, 251–266.

Gershwin, M.E., Crinella, F.M., Castles, J.J., & Trent, J.K. (1977). Immunologic characteristics of Down's syndrome. *Journal of Mental Deficiency Research, 21*, 237–249.

Gordon, M.C., Sinha, S.K., & Carlson, S.D. (1971). Antibody responses to influenza vaccine in patients with Down's syndrome. *American Journal of Mental Deficiency, 75*, 391–399.

Gregory, L., Williams, R., & Thompson, E. (1972). Leukocyte function in Down's syndrome and acute leukemia. *Lancet, i*, 1359–1361.

Gunz, F.W. (1974). Genetics of human leukemia. *Seminars in Haematology, 7*, 164–191.

Gupta, S., Fikrig, S.M., Mariano, E., & Quazi, Q. (1983). Monoclonal antibody defined T-cell subsets and autologous mixed lymphocyte reaction in Down's syndrome. *Clinical and Experimental Immunology, 53*, 25–30.

Gupta, S., Zola, H., Brooks, D.A., Bradley, J., Fikrig, S.M., Mariano, E., & Quazi, Q. (1984). Monoclonal antibody defined B cell subset in aging humans and Down's syndrome. *Gerontology, 30*, 388–392.

Hawkes, R.A., Boughton, C.R., Schroeter, D.R., Decker, R.H., & Overby, L.R. (1980). Hepatitis B infection in institutionalized Down's syndrome inmates: A longitudinal study with five hepatitis B virus markers. *Clinical and Experimental Immunology, 40*, 478–486.

Hawkes, R.A., Boughton, C.R., & Schroeter, D.R. (1978). The antibody response of institutionalized Down's syndrome patients to seven microbial antigens. *Clinical and Experimental Immunology 31*, 298–304.

Hayashi, Y., Eguchi, M., Sugita, K., Nakazawa, S., Sato, T., Kojima, S., Bessho, F., Konishi, S., Inaba, T., Hanada, R., & Yamamoto, K. (1988). Cytogenetic findings and clinical features of acute leukemia and transient myeloproliferative disorder in Down's syndrome. *Blood, 72*, 15–23.

Heitjtink, R.A., de Jong, P., Schalm, S.W., & Masurel, L. (1984). Hepatitis B vaccination in Down's syndrome and other mentally retarded patients. *Hepatology, 4*, 611–614.

Ido, Y., & Green, P. (1977). Down's syndrome and autoimmunity. *American Journal of Medical Sciences*, *273* (1), 95–99.

Jacobs, P.F., Burdash, N.M., Manos, J.P., & Duncan, R.C. (1978). Immunological parameters in Down's syndrome. *Annals of Clinical and Laboratory Science*, *8*, 17–22.

Kabelits, J. (1990). Do CD2 and CD3-TCR T-cell activation pathways function independently? *Immunology Today*, *11*, 44–47.

Kanavin, O., Scott, H., Fausa, O., Ek, J., Gaarder, P.I., & Brandtzaeg, P. (1988). Immunological studies of patients with Down's syndrome. *Acta Medica Scandinavica*, *244*, 473–477.

Kardos, G., Révèsz, T., Bulin, A., Fekete, G., Vargha, M., Schuler, D., & Hungarian Working Party on Childhood Leukemia. (1983). Leukemia in children with Down's syndrome. *Oncology*, *40*, 280–283.

Karttunen, R., Nurmi, T., Ilonen, J., & Surcel, H.M. (1984). Cell-mediated immunodeficiency in Down's syndrome: Normal IL-2 production but inverted ratio of T-cell subsets. *Clinical and Experimental Immunology*, *55*, 257–263.

Krivit, W., & Good, R.A. (1957). Simultaneous occurrence of monogolism and leukemia. *American Journal of Diseases of Children*, *94*, 289–293.

LaRocca, L.M., Piantelli, M., Valitutti, S., Castellino, F., Maggiomo, N., & Musiani, P. (1988). Alterations on thymocyte subpopulations in Down's syndrome (trisomy 21). *Clinical Immunology and Immunopathology*, *49*, 175–186.

Levin, S. (1987). The immune system and susceptibility to infections in Down syndrome. In E. McCoy & C. Epstein (Eds.), *Oncology and immunology of Down syndrome* (pp. 143–162). New York: Alan R. Liss.

Levin, S., Schlesinger, M., Handzel, Z.T., Hahn, T., Altman, Y., Czernobilsky, B., & Boss, J. (1979). Thymic deficiency in Down's syndrome. *Pediatrics*, *63*, 80–83.

Lockitch, G., Puterman, M., Godolphin, W., Sheps, S., Tingle, A.J., & Quigley, G. (1989). Infection and immunity in Down syndrome: A trial of long-term low oral doses of zinc. *Journal of Pediatrics*, *114*, 781–787.

Lopez, V., Ochs, H.D., Thuline, H.C., Davis, S.D., & Wedgwood, R.J. (1975). Defective antibody response to bacteriophase ΦX 174 in Down syndrome. *Journal of Pediatrics*, *86*, 207–211.

Maccario, R., Ugazio, A.G., Nespoli, L., Albertini, C., Montagna, D., Porta, F., Bonetti, F., & Burgio, G.R. (1984). Lymphocyte subpopulations in Down's syndrome: High percentage of circulating HNK-1 + Leu2a + cells. *Clinical and Experimental Immunology*, *57*, 222–226.

McCord, R., & Fridovich, I. (1969). The utility of superoxide dismutase in studying free radical reactions. *Journal of Chemistry*, *244*, 6056–6063.

Mellon, J.P., Pay, B.Y., & Greene, D.M. (1963). Mongolism and thyroid antibodies. *Journal of Mental Deficiency Research*, *7*, 31–47.

Mellman, W.J., Younkin, L.H., & Baker, D. (1970). Abnormal lymphocyte function in trisomy 21. *Annals of the New York Academy of Sciences*, *117*, 537–542.

Mikkelsen, M. (1981). Epidemiology of trisomy 21. Population peri and antenatal data. In G.R. Burgio, M. Fraccaro, L. Tiepolo, & U. Wolf (Eds.), *Trisomy 21* (pp. 211–226). Berlin-Heidelberg: Springer-Verlag.

Miller, M.E., Mellman, W.J., Cohen, M.M., Kohn, G., & Dietz, W.H., Jr. (1969). Depressed immunoglobulin G in newborn infants with Down's syndrome. *Journal of Pediatrics*, *75*, 996–1000.

Miller, R.W. (1970). Neoplasia and Down's syndrome. *Annals of the New York Academy of Sciences*, *171*, 637–644.

Montagna, D., Maccario, R., Ugazio, A.G., Nespoli, L., Pedroni, E., Faggiano, P., & Burgio, G.R. (1988). Cell-mediated cytotoxicity in Down syndrome: Impairment of allogeneic mixed lymphocyte reaction, NK and NK-like activities. *European Journal of Pediatrics*, *148*, 53–57.

Morgenesen, K.E., Vignaux, F., & Gresser, I. (1982). Enhanced expression of cellular receptors for human interferon alpha on peripheral lymphocytes from patients with Down's syndrome. *Federation of the European Biochemical Societies*, *104*, 285–287.

Murphy, M., & Epstein, L.B. (1990). Down syndrome (trisomy 21) thymuses have a decreased proportion of cells expressing high levels of TCR alfa, beta and CD3. *Clinical Immunology and Immunopathology*, *55*, 453–467.

Nair, M.P.N., & Schwartz, S.A. (1984). Association of decreased T cell mediated natural cytotoxicity and interferon production in Down's syndrome. *Clinical Immunology and Immunopathology*, *33*, 412–424.

Nurmi, T., Huttunen, K., Lassila, O., Hen Honen, M., Sakkinen, A., Linna, S.L., & Tijlikainen, A. (1982). Natural killer cell function in trisomy 21 (Down's syndrome). *Clinical and Experimental Immunology*, *47*, 735–741.

Nurmi, T., Leinonen, M., Haiva, M., Tijlikainen, A., & Kouvalainen, K. (1982). Antibody response to polysaccharide vaccine in patients with trisomy 21 (Down's syndrome). *Clinical and Experimental Immunology*, *48*, 485–490.

Ortaldo, J.R., & Herbermann, R.B. (1984). Heterogeneity of natural killer cells. *Annual Review of Immunology*, *2*, 359–394.

Öster, J., Mikkelsen, M., & Nielsen, A. (1964). The mortality and causes of death in patients with Down's syndrome (mongolism). *Proceedings of the International Copenhagen Congress on Scientific Studies of Mental Retardation*, *1*, 410–414.

Öster, J., Mikkelsen, M., & Nielsen, A. (1975). Mortality and lifetable in Down's syndrome. *Acta Pediatrica Scandinavica*, *64*, 322–326.

Pardi, R., Bender, J.R., Dettori, C., Giannazza, E., & Engleman, E.G. (1989). Heterogenus distribution and transmembrane rigualing properties of lymphocyte functives associated antigen (LFA-1) in human lymphocytes subsets. *Journal of Immunology*, *143*, 3157–3166.

Philip, R., Berger, A.C., McManus, N.H., Warner, N.H., Peacock, M.A., & Epstein, L.B. (1986). Abnormalities of the in vitro cellular and humoral responses to tetanus and influenza antigens with concomitant numerical alterations in lymphocyte subsets in Down syndrome (trisomy 21). *Journal of Immunology*, *136*, 1661–1667.

Ransom, J., Fischer, M., Mosman, T., Yokota, T., DeLuca, D., Schumacher, J., & Zlotnick, A. (1987): Interferon-gamma is produced by activated immature mouse thymocytes and inhibits the interleukin 4-induced proliferation of immature thymocytes. *Journal of Immunology*, *139*, 4102–4108.

Raziuddin, S., & Elawad, M.E. (1990). Immunoregulatory CD4 + CD45R + suppressor/inducer T lymphocyte subsets and impaired cell-mediated immunity in patients with Down's syndrome. *Clinical and Experimental Immunology*, *79*, 67–71.

Revel, M., Bash, D., & Ruddle, F.H. (1976). Antibodies to cell surface component coded by human chromosome 21 inhibit action of interferon. *Nature*, *260*, 139–141.

Robinson, L., & Neglia, J.P. (1987). Epidemiology of Down syndrome and childhood acute leukemia. In E. McCoy & C. Epstein (Eds.), *Oncology and immunology of Down syndrome* (pp. 19–32). New York: Alan R. Liss.

Rosner, F., & Lee, S.L. (1972). Down's syndrome and acute leukemia: Myeloblastic or lymphoblastic? Report of 43 cases and review of the literature. *American Journal of Medicine*, *53*, 203–218.

Ruch, W., Schurmann, K., Gordon, P., Burgin-Wolff, A., & Girard, J. (1985). Coexistent coeliac disease, Graves disease and diabetes mellitus type 1 in a patient with Down syndrome. *European Journal of Pediatrics*, *144*, 89–90.

Rundle, A.T., Clothier, B.O., & Sudell, B. (1971). Serum IgD levels and infections in Down's syndrome. *Clinica Chimica Acta*, *35*, 489–493.

Sasaki, M., & Yoshitaka, O. (1969). Hypersensitivity of leukocyte in Down's syndrome by mixed leukocyte culture experiments. *Nature*, *222*, 596–598.

Schechter, B., Handzel, Z.T., Altmain, Y., Nir, E., & Levin, S. (1977). Cellular immunity in newborn infants and children: Stimulation of lymphocyte protein synthesis as a measure of immune competence. *Clinical and Experimental Immunology*, *27*, 478–484.

Singer, K.H., Smith, J.L., Tuck, D.T., Denning, S.M., & Haynes, B.F. (1989). The role of LFA-1

and ICAM-1 in the binding of Con-A activated human thymocytes to thymic epithelial cells (TE). *Federation of the American Societies for Experimental Biology Journal*, *3*, 784.

Spina, C.A., Smith, D., Korn, E., Fahey, J.L., & Grossman, H.J. (1981). Altered cellular immune functions in patients with Down's syndrome. *American Journal of Diseases of Children*, *135*, 251–255.

Springer, T.A., Dustin, M.L., Kishimoto, T.K., & Marlin, S.D. (1987). The lymphocyte function-associated LFA-1, CD2 and LFA-3 molecules: Cell adhesion receptors of the immune system. *Annual Review of Immunology*, *5*, 223–252.

Stabile, A., Pesaresi, M.A., Stabile, A.M., Pastore, M., Sopo, S.M., Ricci, R., Celestini, E., & Segni, G.P. (1991). Immunodeficiency and plasma zinc levels in children with Down's syndrome: A long-term follow-up of oral zinc supplementation. *Clinical Immunology and Immunopathology*, *58*, 207–216.

Standen, G., Philip, M.A., & Fletcher, J. (1979). Reduced number of peripheral blood granulocytic progenitor cells in patients with Down's syndrome. *British Journal of Haematology*, *42*, 417–423.

Stutman, O. (1978). Intrathymic and extrathymic T cell maturation. *Immunological Review*, *42*, 138–184.

Suomalainen, H.H., Gahmberg, C.G., Patarroyo, M., Beatty, P.G., & Schoder, J. (1986). Genetic assignment of Gp90, leucocyte adhesion glycoprotein to human chromosome 21. *Somatic Cell Molecular Genetics*, *12*, 297–302.

Sutnick, A.I., London, W.T., Gertsley, B.J.S., Cronolund, M.N., & Blumberg, B.S. (1968). Anicteric hepatitis associated with Australia antigen. *Journal of the American Medical Association*, *205*, 670–674.

Tan, V.H. (1976). Chromosome 21 and cell growth inhibitory effect of human interferon preparations. *Nature*, *260*, 141–143.

Tan, V.H., Tischfield, J., & Ruddle, F.H. (1973). The linkage of genes for the human interferon induced antiviral protein and indophenol oxidase-B traits to chromosome G-21. *Journal of Experimental Medicine*, *137*, 317–330.

Tan, V.H. (1975). Chromosome 21 dosage effect on inducibility of anti-viral gene(s). *Nature*, *253*, 280–282.

Taylor, G.M. (1987). Altered expression of lymphocyte functional antigen in Down syndrome. *Immunology Today*, *8*, 366–369.

Taylor, G.M., Haigh, H., Williams, A., D'Souza, S.W., & Harris, R. (1988). Down's syndrome lymphoid cell lines exhibit increased adhesion due to the over-expression of lymphocyte function-associated antigen (LFA-1). *Journal of Immunology*, *64*, 451–456.

Taylor, G.M., Williams, A., & D'Souza, S.W.

(1986). Increased expression of lymphocyte functional antigen in Down syndrome. *Lancet, ii,* 740.

Taylor, G.M., Williams, A., D'Souza, S.W., Fergusson, W.F., Douai, D., Fennel, J., & Harris, R. (1988). The expression of CD18 is increased in trisomy 21 (Down syndrome) lymphoblastoid cells. *Clinical and Experimental Immunology, 71,* 324–328.

Troisi, C.L., Heiberg, D.A., & Hollingerr, F.B. (1985). Normal immune response to hepatitis B vaccine in patients with Down's syndrome. *Journal of the American Medical Association, 254,* 3196–3199.

Ugazio, A.G. (1981). Down's syndrome: Problems of immunodeficiency. In G.R. Burgio, M. Fraccaro, L. Tiepolo, & U. Wolf (Eds.), *Trisomy 21* (pp. 33–39). Berlin-Heidelberg: Springer-Verlag.

Ugazio, A.G., Jayakar, S., Marcioni, A.F., Duse, M., Monafo, V., Pasquali, F., & Burgio, G.R. (1977). Immunodeficiency in Down's syndrome. Relationship between presence of human thyroglobulin anti-bodies and HBsAG carrier status. *European Journal of Pediatrics, 126,* 139–146.

Ugazio, A.G., Lanzavecchia, A., Jayakar, S., Plebani, A., Duse, M., & Burgio, G.R. (1978). Immunodeficiency in Down syndrome. *Acta Pediatrica Scandinavica, 67,* 705–708.

Ugazio, A.G., Maccario, R., Notarangelo, L.D., & Burgio, G.R. (1990). Immunology of Down syndrome. A review. *American Journal of Medical Genetics Supplement, 7,* 204–212.

Walford, R.L., Gessett, T.C., Naeim, F., Tam, C.F., Van Laucher, J.L., Barnett, E.V., Chia, D., Sparkers, R.S., Fahey, J.L., Spina, C., Gatti, R.A., Media, M.A., Grossman, H., Hibraur, H., & Motola, M. (1981). Immunological and biological and biochemical studies of Down's syndrome as a model of accelerated aging. In D. Segre & L. Smith (Eds.), *Immunological aspects of aging* (pp. 479–488). New York: Dekker.

Warren, R.P., Healey, M.C., Johnston, A.V., Sidwell, R.W., Radov, L.A., Murray, R.J., & Kinsolving, C.R. (1987). PR 879-317A enhances in vitro immune activity of peripheral blood mononuclear cells from patients with Down syndrome. *International Journal of Immunopharmacology, 9,* 919–926.

Weil, J., Epstein, L.B., & Epstein, C.J. (1980). Synthesis of interferon induced polypeptides in normal and chromosome 21-aneuploid human fibroblasts: Relationship to relative sensitivities in antiviral assays. *Journal of Interferon Research, 1,* 111–119.

Whittingham, S., Pitt, D.B., Sharma, D.L.B., & MacKay, I.R. (1977). Stress deficiency of the T-C lymphocyte system exemplified by Down's syndrome. *Lancet, i,* 163–166.

Wong, K.Y., Jones, M.M., Strivastava, A.K., & Gruppo, R.A. (1988). Transient myeloproliferative disorder and acute non lymphoblastic leukemia in Down syndrome. *Journal of Pediatrics, 112,* 18–22.

Yonagi, Y., Caccia, N., Kroanenberg, M., Chin, B., Roder, J., Rohel, D., Kiyohara, T., Lanzon, R., Toyonaga, B., Rosenthal, K., Dennert, G., Acha-Orbea, H., Hangartzer, H., Hood, L., & Mark, T.W. (1985). Gene rearrangement in cells with natural killer activity and expression of beta-chain of T-cell antigen receptor. *Nature, 314,* 631–633.

CHAPTER
21

Hematologic Manifestations

Bertram H. Lubin, Sarah Cahn, and Mark Scott

Abnormalities in almost every cellular component of the hematopoietic system have been reported in persons with Down syndrome (Dewald et al., 1990; Ganick, 1986; Ibarra et al., 1990). Although it is likely that the genetic imbalance created by the trisomic chromosome is responsible for many of these aberrations, little information is known in regard to specific mechanisms (Scroggin & Patterson, 1982; Shapiro, 1983). Table 21.1 illustrates a list of the genes that have been mapped to chromosome 21. It is estimated that 900 genes are located on this chromosome. At present, 39 of these have been identified and 4 have been shown to be disease related. None has been clearly associated with a specific hematologic abnormality. Future molecular studies, including analysis of persons who have partial trisomy 21 and identification of new genes located on chromosone 21, eventually may make it possible to define relationships between gene dose and hematopathology.

In general, persons with Down syndrome can have the same types of hematologic complications as those without Down syndrome. However, it should be noted that several hematologic abnormalities are unique. These include transient myelodysplasia in infancy (Weinberg, Schiller, & Windmiller; 1982; Weinstein, 1978); red cell macrocytosis (Akin, 1988; Easthman & Jancar, 1983; Roizen & Amarose, 1991; Wachtel & Pueschel, 1991); and increased susceptibility to leukemia (Kalwinsky et al., 1990; Mitelman, Heim, & Mandahl, 1990; Robinson et al., 1984), particularly the acute megakaryocytic type (J. Suda et al., 1988; Zipursky, Peeters, & Poon,

Table 21.1. Genes and expressed sequences on chromosome 21

Genes	Expressed sequences
RNA4	Ribosomal 4
AD1	Alzheimer disease 1 (by linkage)
APP	Amyloid beta (A4) precursor protein
SOD1	Cu-Zn superoxide dismutase 1, soluble
IFNAR	Interferon, alpha; receptor
IFNBR	Interferon, beta; receptor
IFNTI	Interferon, gamma; transducer 1
IFNGR2	Interferon, gamma; receptor 2 (confers antiviral resistance)
ALS	Amyotrophic lateral sclerosis (by linkage)
PAIS	Phosphoribosylaminoimidazole synthetase
PGFT	Phosphoribosylglycinamide formyl transferase
PRGS	Phosphoribosylglycinamide synthetase
ERG	Avian erythroblastosis virus E26 oncogene-related
ETS 2	Avian erythroblastosis virus E26 oncogene homolog2
HMG 14	High mobility group protein 14
MX1.2	Myxovirus influenza resistance homolog of murine
BCEI	Breast cancer, estrogen-inducible sequence
CBS	Cystathionine beta synthetase
EPM1	Progressive myoclonus epilepsy (by linkage)
CRYA1	Crystallin, alpha polypeptide
PFKL	Phosphofructakinase, liver type
CD18	Antigen CD18 (p95) lymphocyte function associated antigen 1
COL6A1	Collagen, type VI, alpha 1
COL6A2	Collagen, type VI, alpha 2
S100B	S100 protein, beta polypeptide (neural)

The authors wish to acknowledge the outstanding secretarial and graphic support provided by Klara Kleman, Shirley Thomas, and Carolyn Znoj in the preparation of this chapter.

1987). Unfortunately, limited information is available in regard to the mechanisms for any of these abnormalities.

This chapter reviews the hematologic abnormalities that have been reported in persons with Down syndrome and discusses their potential mechanisms. These are categorically listed in Table 21.2. The laboratory and clinical findings associated with each are discussed and speculations regarding the etiology of several of the disorders are presented. The authors wish to emphasize that few studies have been conducted to explore potential relationships between gene dosage and specific hematopoietic defects. As new genes are identified on chromosome 21, investigations of their role in hematopathology should be encouraged, not only to understand better the cause and treatment of hematopoietic dysplasia in persons with Down syndrome, but

Table 21.2. Hematologic abnormalities in persons with Down syndrome

Red blood cells
  Erythrocytosis in the newborn
  Erythrocytosis secondary to cyanotic heart disease
  Increased mean cell volume
  Alteration in intracellular enzymes
  Membrane protein abnormalities
  Cation transport defects
Platelets
  Neonatal thrombocytopenia
  Neonatal thrombocytosis
  Decreased serotonin levels
  Decreased calcium levels
  Abnormal calcium transport
  Acute megakaryocytic leukemia
White blood cells
  Increased turnover of peripheral granulocyte pool
  Decreased number of circulating granulocytic
    progenitors
  Functional defects
  Abnormal enzyme content
  Abnormal morphology
  Abnormal cellular immunity
  Transient myelodysplasia in infancy
  Increased incidence of congenital leukemia
  Increased incidence of acute leukemia
Bone marrow
  Myelofibrosis
  Aplastic anemia

also, perhaps, to provide new insights into molecular factors that regulate and/or disturb ordered hematopoiesis.

RED CELL ABNORMALITIES

Abnormalities of production, volume regulation, enzyme content, membrane cation transport, and membrane protein structure have been reported in persons with Down syndrome. Indeed, given that almost every aspect of red cell biology is affected, it is surprising that persons with Down syndrome are rarely anemic. Each of these abnormalities is briefly discussed, with emphasis placed on the most common ones.

Erythrocytosis

Erythrocytosis appears to be a common event in newborns with Down syndrome. Although often referred to as polycythemia, the authors refer to this complication as erythrocytosis rather than polycythemia, as the red cell series is primarily involved. The incidence of erythrocytosis has not been documented in large clinical surveys as blood counts are not routinely determined in newborns who are diagnosed with Down syndrome. In at least two studies, erythrocytosis, as defined by hematocrit levels over 65%, was detected in 16%–20% of otherwise healthy newborns (Lappalainen & Kouvalainen, 1972; Weinberger & Oleinick, 1971). There was no evidence for hypoxia in these infants and the mechanism for erythrocytosis was not established. When compared to infants who had perinatal complications frequently associated with erythrocytosis, such as maternal diabetes or respiratory distress, the hematocrits in newborns with Down syndrome were consistently higher. Hematocrit values returned to normal by 3 weeks of age and there was no suggestion that these infants had more medical complications than expected (Miller & Cosgriff, 1983).

The factor or factors responsible for erythrocytosis in newborns with Down syndrome have not been established. In contrast to most newborns, where the etiology of erythrocytosis is due to passive transfusion (Oski & Naiman,

1982), a direct effect on erythropoiesis appears to be involved in Down syndrome. One explanation could be a transient alteration in sensitivity of erythroid progenitors to erythropoietin. If this were the case, the in vitro response of erythroid progenitors to erythropoietin should be increased. This possibility has not been explored.

Another mechanism could be an abnormality in placental function. When oxygen transport from mother to fetus is compromised by placental dysplasia or dysmaturity, the resulting fetal hypoxia stimulates erythropoietin production and results in secondary erythrocytosis (Naveh, Schwart, & Pang, 1971). Although placental weights appear to be normal, histologic findings consistent with placental dysplasia have been noted (Kouvalainen & Osterlund, 1967; Labbe, Copin, Choiset, Girard, & Barbet, 1989). The abnormal levels of estriol and human gonadotropin (Brock et al., 1990; Chard, 1991) in pregnancies associated with Down syndrome could be due, at least in part, to a defect in placental function.

The most likely mechanism, however, to explain neonatal erythrocytosis is a transient dysregulated state of erythropoiesis. This hypothesis is based upon the observation that several defects in hematopoietic regulation are noted in persons with Down syndrome and that most of these are prominent in the neonatal period. One could also speculate that the avian erythroblastosis virus oncogene, which is located on chromosome 21, could be involved. The reports of erythroleukemia in children with Down syndrome suggest a potential relationship to this oncogene (Juberg & Jones, 1970).

The evaluation of newborns who have erythrocytosis should include exclusion of cyanotic heart disease. This is particularly important in infants with Down syndrome due to the high incidence of congenital heart disease. Cardiopulmonary status should be carefully evaluated and the arterial blood gas and oxygen saturation determined. Additional laboratory tests such as a reticulocyte count and erythropoietin level help to distinguish infants who have been passively transfused from those who have active erythrocytosis. In the passively transfused infant, the reticulocyte count and erythropoietin level are normal or low whereas in the hypoxic infant with secondary erythrocytosis both are generally elevated.

A wide variety of complications, called the hyperviscosity syndrome, occur in newborns when the hematocrit exceeds 65% (Phibbs, 1991). The pathophysiology of this syndrome is related to the effect that hematocrit has on whole blood viscosity; as the hematocrit increases, whole blood viscosity increases. When blood viscosity reaches a critical level, blood flow is impaired. Depending upon the extent of circulatory compromise, organ damage and death can occur. Current recommendations are to treat symptomatic infants with a partial exchange transfusion using plasma or an equivalent fluid. In older children with cyanotic heart disease, the hematocrit level correlates well with the arterial oxygen saturation (Gidding, Bessel, & Liao, 1990). As with the newborn, hyperviscosity in older children can result in major complications, in particular, stroke, and interventions to maintain the hematocrit below 55% (rather than 65%, as recommended for infants) are recommended.

Children with cyanotic heart disease often develop iron deficiency as a consequence of stress erythropoiesis. This complication is not unique to children with Down syndrome. Progressive depletion of iron stores results in abnormalities of red cell size and shape as well as systemic signs of iron deficiency. Although microcytic, hypochromic red blood cells would be expected, macrocytic red cells have been reported in many phenotypically "normal" children with cyanotic heart disease (Gidding et al., 1990).

Since an adequate supply of iron is required to sustain erythropoiesis, it was once felt that iron deficiency was an effective means to inhibit erythropoiesis in persons with cyanotic heart disease. However, iron-deficient red cells are less deformable than normal red cells and the combination of increased blood viscosity and decreased red cell deformability, created by an iron-deficient state, was found to increase the risk of stroke in persons with cyanotic heart disease (Linderkamp et al., 1979). At present, most physicians recommend treatment of iron deficiency and use of phlebotomy when the hematocrit exceeds 60%, or at lower levels if the individual has signs of hyperviscosity. Persons with Down syndrome usually have no difficulty with this procedure and feel much better post-phlebotomy.

Fetal hemoglobin levels may be abnormal in persons with Down syndrome. Low fetal hemoglobin levels have been reported in newborns. This finding could result from a developmental abnormality in erythropoiesis (Wilson, Schroeder, & Graves, 1968). One hypothesis is that low fetal hemoglobin levels are a sign of postmaturity or premature aging. An alternate hypothesis is that the switch from fetal to adult hemoglobin occurs earlier in gestation than expected due to a molecular regulatory defect. Further studies should be performed to document the frequency and biologic significance of this observation as well as a potential relationship to the previously described erythrocytosis. In older children with Down syndrome, initial studies demonstrating increased levels of fetal hemoglobin have not been confirmed (Ibarra et al., 1990).

Macrocytosis

By far the most common abnormality of red blood cells in both children and adults with Down syndrome is an increase in the mean red cell volume (Akin, 1988; Easthman & Jancar, 1983; Roizen & Amarose, 1991; Wachtel & Pueschel, 1991). The authors refer to the increase in red cell volume as macrocytosis. It is estimated that as many as 65% of persons with Down syndrome have macrocytic red cells. It is not known if this finding is manifested in the newborn or if it develops later in life. The differential diagnosis of macrocytosis in children and adults is shown in Table 21.3.

There have been several hypotheses that have attempted to explain the macrocytosis in persons with Down syndrome. One is that the red cells are large as a result of a mild hemolytic anemia due to an acquired intracellular red cell defect (Wachtel & Pueschel, 1991). In this case, the elevated mean cell volume would be a reflection of a young red cell population. In support of this hypothesis is the shortened red cell survival noted in persons with Down syndrome (22.6 days) compared to persons without Down syndrome (26–30 days). The increased activity of several age-dependent red cell enzymes, particularly the erythrocyte glutamic oxalacetic transaminase, is

Table 21.3.   Differential diagnosis of macrocytosis

Down syndrome
Chronic liver disease
Hypothyroidism
Folic acid deficiency
Vitamin B_{12} deficiency
Hemolytic anemia
Bone marrow dysplasia–preleukemia
Drug toxicity (anticonvulsants)
Neonatal red cells
Overhydrated cells

consistent with a young red cell population (Bartosz & Kedziora, 1983; C.J. Epstein, 1989; Mattei, Baetman, & Baret, 1982; Naiman, Oski, & Mellman, 1965; Stocchi, Magnani, Cuchiarini, Novelli, & Dallapiccola, 1985). Reports of subtle red cell membrane protein abnormalities characteristic of premature cell aging are also consistent with an intraerythrocytic defect (Bartosz, Seszynski, & Kedziora, 1982; Kedziora et al., 1981). Since accelerated aging, accompanied by lipid peroxidation, is a histopathologic characteristic of the brain in persons with Down syndrome (Brooksbank & Balázs, 1984; Lott, 1982), it is quite possible that the red cell could be used as a model to study these molecular events.

However, these results do not necessarily dictate the conclusion that a hemolytic process is the only explanation for the increase in the red cell volume in persons with Down syndrome. Indeed, reticulocyte counts are not elevated; haptoglobin levels, which are low in persons with hemolytic anemia, are normal; and several explanations could account for the increased activity of certain red cell enzymes.

Hypothyroidism is often considered in the differential diagnosis of macrocytosis. Because the frequency of hypothyroidism in persons with Down syndrome is increased compared to controls (Baxter et al., 1975; Pueschel & Pezzullo, 1985), thyroid function tests have been performed in the evaluation of many people who have macrocytosis. In several large series, however, thyroid function studies were normal. This is not surprising since the anemia associated with hypothyroidism is usually hypochromic and microcytic and not macrocytic. Only in rare cases where thyroid deficiency is secondary to a generalized immune disorder is a macrocytic anemia noted (Tudhope & Wilson, 1960). Under these circumstances, measurements of antibody against thyroid as well as intrinsic factor should be performed as macrocytosis is often secondary to acquired vitamin B_{12} deficiency. Thus, unless clinical signs of hypothyroidism exist, persons with Down syndrome who have macrocytic red cells do not require analysis of thyroid function.

Given the high frequency of both leukemia and preleukemia in persons with Down syndrome, a preleukemic condition should be considered in the differential diagnosis of macrocytosis. The abnormalities in hematopoiesis that accompany the preleukemic state include nucleated red cells, megaloblastic red cells, and alterations in red cell size and shape (Linman & Bagby, 1976). Since most persons with Down syndrome who have macrocytosis are otherwise healthy, unless additional hematologic signs such as abnormalities in granulocytes and/or platelets are noted, this diagnosis need not be extensively pursued.

Several red cell cation transport defects have been reported in persons with Down syndrome. It is remotely possible that macrocytosis results from a defect in cell water and cation regulation (Baar & Gordon, 1963). The mechanism for this abnormality is not known although oxidation of cation transport proteins in the red cell membrane could be a plausible explanation (Gerli et al., 1990; Sinet, 1982). Studies of red cell oxidation, membrane proteins, cation transport, and cell water content in persons with Down syndrome who have increased red cell volume, compared to those with normal values, could address this hypothesis.

Except for the rare circumstance noted with immune thyroid disease, there is no evidence that macrocytosis in persons with Down syndrome is due to either vitamin B_{12} or folic acid deficiency. Several studies reported that red cell and serum folate levels were normal in persons with Down syndrome who had macrocytic red cells (Roizen & Amarose, 1991; Wachtel & Pueschel, 1991). Earlier studies, however, suggested that children with Down syndrome could have abnormal red blood cell folate metabolism in the presence of normal serum folate levels

(Gericke, Hesseling, Brink, & Tiedt, 1977). Three genes involved in purine synthesis have been located on chromosome 21 (Hards et al., 1986; Patterson, Graw, & Jones, 1981). These genes may alter folic acid requirements and produce subtle abnormalities in its metabolism. The increase in purine nucleoside phosphorylase activity (Bartosz & Kedziora, 1983; Stocchi et al., 1985) is consistent with this hypothesis. It is possible that differences between individuals in regard to expression of these three genes may explain the variations in red cell volume observed in persons with Down syndrome.

Superoxide Dismutase

Since the gene for superoxide dismutase (SOD) is located on chromosome 21, the intracellular concentration of superoxide dismutase is increased by 50% in all erythroid as well as non-erythroid cells (Crosti, Serra, Rigo, & Viglino, 1976). This enzyme converts superoxide anion into hydrogen peroxide and water. Cells with elevated superoxide dismutase have lower quantities of superoxide anion and higher hydrogen peroxide levels. Intracellular hydrogen peroxide can damage the red cell by causing lipid peroxidation and protein oxidation. The increase in activity of both glucose-6-phosphate dehydrogenase and glutathione peroxidase may represent a compensatory response to the elevated intracellular levels of hydrogen peroxide (C.J. Epstein, 1989; Frischer, Chu, Ahmad, Justice, & Smith, 1981; Gerli et al., 1990; Gustavson, 1989; Ibarra et al., 1990; Mattei et al., 1982; Michelson, Puget, Durosay, & Bonneau, 1977; Sinet, Lejeune, & Jerome, 1979).

Figure 21.1 schematically illustrates the potential consequences of elevated SOD in persons with Down syndrome and the relationships between intracellular enzymes involved in oxidant–antioxidant pathways. Hydrogen peroxide can react with cellular iron stores and generate a highly toxic free radical called the hydroxyl radical or ·OH. Theoretically, widespread toxicity could result from the excess generation of hydrogen peroxide within the cell, including damage to DNA, to critical intracellular and membrane enzymes involved in metabolism, and to processes involved in cell renewal. The latter could

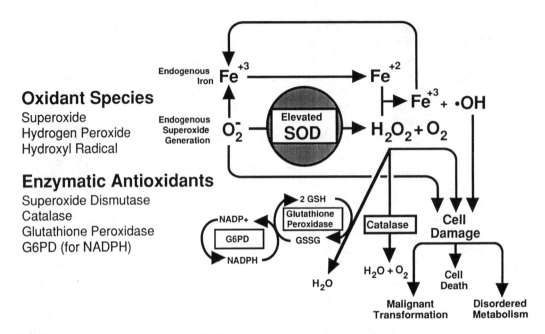

Oxidant Species
Superoxide
Hydrogen Peroxide
Hydroxyl Radical

Enzymatic Antioxidants
Superoxide Dismutase
Catalase
Glutathione Peroxidase
G6PD (for NADPH)

Figure 21.1.   Potential consequences of elevated SOD in trisomy 21.

result in premature aging and cell death. Given the enzymes involved in protecting cells against oxidative damage shown on the bottom of Figure 21.1, it would be of interest to determine the consequences of glucose-6-phosphate dehydrogenase deficiency in persons with Down syndrome. One might expect these individuals to demonstrate more evidence of oxidant toxicity. Since the role of oxidative injury in the pathobiology of human disease, including mental retardation and "Alzheimer-like" brain pathology, has recently received considerable attention, these findings may have broad biologic significance (Brooksbank & Balázs, 1984; Cutler, Heston, Davies, Haxby, & Schapiro, 1985; Sinet et al., 1979).

Additional red cell enzymes such as glutamic oxalacetic transaminase (SGOT), phosphokinase, 6-phosphogluconate dehydrogenase, adenosine deaminase, and catechol-O-methyltransferase are increased 15%–60% (Brahe, Serra, & Morton, 1985; C.J. Epstein, 1989; Hsia, Smith, Dowben, & Justice, 1971; Layzer & Epstein, 1972; Puukka, Puukka, Leppilampi, Linna, & Kouvalainen, 1982). As previously discussed, the elevated SGOT may be a marker of young red cell age associated with hemolysis. The conse-

quences of most of these enzyme abnormalities are unknown and further studies to determine their role are to be encouraged.

GRANULOCYTE ABNORMALITIES

Persons with Down syndrome have been reported to have a greater susceptibility to bacterial and viral infections than age-matched controls. The incidence of infectious complications appears to decrease with age, with the highest frequency noted during the first 5 years of life. It is important to recognize that many of the infectious disease studies performed on institutionalized individuals may have little relevance to the types of clinically significant infections seen in persons who are living in the community. Furthermore, since there are no recent studies to document the frequency and clinical course of bacterial or viral infections, use of modern antibiotics and immunization procedures may have made a significant impact on this problem.

Functional Defects in Granulocytes

There are a number of defects in immunity that could classify the person with Down syndrome as an "immuno-compromised host." These include abnormalities in granulocyte kinetics and function and defects in cellular and circulating immunity. Although defects in granulocyte functions such as phagocytosis and bactericidal activity have been reported (Barkin, Weston, Humbert, & Maire, 1980; Barkin, Weston, Humbert, & Sunada, 1980; Mellman, Oski, Tedesco, Maciera-Coelho, & Harris, 1964; Mellman, Raab, & Oski, 1967; Pearson, 1967; Rosner, Ong, Mahanand, Paine, & Jacobsen, 1964; Standen, Philip, & Fletcher, 1979), many of these studies were done prior to current knowledge of biochemical and molecular pathways essential for host defense. Re-evaluation of granulocyte function in persons with Down syndrome using modern technology is warranted. It is possible that careful studies to identify specific granulocyte defects could provide new strategies to treat persons who have recurrent infections.

Excess activity of superoxide dismutase has been implicated as one of the factors contributing to the bactericidal defect reported in granulocytes from persons with Down syndrome (Anneren & Björksten, 1984; Mills & Quie, 1980). Superoxide dismutase is an enzyme that plays an important role in the granulocytes' response to ingested bacteria. In normal granulocytes, superoxide anion, which participates in bacterial killing, is generated after granulocytes ingest bacteria. One might think that "bigger would be better" and that excess production of superoxide dismutase would be beneficial. However, excess superoxide dismutase activity decreases the intracellular concentration of superoxide anion and this imbalance could interfere with intracellular killing of certain pathogens (Scott, Meshnick, & Eaton, 1987). Studies of granulocyte function in persons with Down syndrome have revealed a number of similarities to studies of granulocyte function in persons who have chronic granulomatous disease (Curnutte, 1988). These include low superoxide anion levels following ingestion of bacteria (Anneren & Björksten, 1984) and abnormal nitroblue tetrazolium dye reduction (Mellman et al., 1964). Furthermore, *Staphylococcal aureus* and *Candida albucans* infections, all characteristic of chronic granulomatous disease, have been reported in persons with Down syndrome.

The severity of infectious complications in persons with chronic granulomatous disease is much greater than that seen in persons with Down syndrome. However, a mild bactericidal killing defect might occur in some individuals and, if this were detected, appropriate therapeutic intervention could be considered. For example, use of prophylactic antibiotics such as trimethoprim/sulfamethoxazole (5 mg/kg/day of trimethoprim) could be evaluated in persons who have recurrent staphylococcal infections. Recent reports on the efficacy of recombinant interferon gamma in persons with chronic granulomatous disease raise the possibility that this therapy could also be of value under certain circumstances (Newburger & Ezekowitz, 1988). However, the potential side effects of administering interferon to persons who have increased copies of a transducer for the interferon gamma receptor on target cells, as well as the reported stimulation of superoxide dismutase activity by interferon gamma, appear to exclude this potential therapy (L.B. Epstein, Lee, & Epstein, 1980; Jung et al., 1987; Pottathil & Lang, 1983).

Enzymes and Morphology

A number of additional defects in granulocyte function have been reported. Several enzymes' activities are increased such as acid phosphatase, galactose-1-phosphate uridyltransferase, and glucose-6-phosphate dehyrogenase (C.J. Epstein, 1989). Abnormalities in phagocytosis and chemotaxis have been reported, although their significance has not been determined (Khan, Evans, Glass, Skin, & Almonte, 1975). Leukocyte alkaline phosphatase levels are elevated in the absence of infection (O'Sullivan & Pryles, 1963). It is of interest that leukocyte alkaline phosphatase levels are also affected, although in the reverse direction, in persons with paroxysmal nocturnal hemoglobinuria, a condition characterized by a predisposition to leukemia, myelofibrosis, and aplastic anemia (Burroughs, Devine, Browne, & Kaplan, 1988). Perhaps there are molecular similarities between persons with Down syndrome who develop myelodysplastic complications and persons with paroxysmal nocturnal hemoglobinuria.

Morphologic abnormalities in the neutrophils

of persons with Down syndrome include hyposegmented polymorphonuclear cells and a decreased number of nuclear appendages in females (Mittwoch, 1964). These morphologic changes have no known clinical significance. Studies of granulocyte kinetics have revealed increased turnover of circulating granulocytes (Mellman et al. 1967). Although leukopenia has been reported, the absolute neutrophil counts are most often in the normal range.

Granulocytopoiesis

Besides abnormalities in granulocyte structure, function, and kinetics, defects in granulocytopoiesis also occur in persons with Down syndrome. In general, granulocytopoiesis is studied by placing either peripheral blood or bone marrow samples, which contain primitive granulocyte precursors, into specific culture media and observing the number and morphology of granulocyte colonies after stimulation by a variety of growth factors. Although strong correlations between in vitro results and in vivo granulocytopoiesis do not always exist, studies of granulocytopoiesis may provide insights into the mechanisms underlying defects in neutrophil production. As such, they have been used to evaluate persons who have neutropenia and persons with transient myelodysplasia on preleukemic states.

Studies of granulocytopoiesis in persons with Down syndrome have demonstrated several abnormalities. Measurements of colony-forming units obtained from peripheral blood samples revealed a decreased number of circulating granulocyte progenitors when compared to age-matched, "normal" controls (Standen et al., 1979). The in vitro response of bone marrow–derived granulocyte precursors to growth factors, as well as the morphology of granulocyte colonies, have also been reported to be abnormal. Nevertheless, persons with Down syndrome appear to have normal neutrophil response to bacterial infections with an appropriate elevation in the granulocyte count and shift to the left in the granulocyte series.

Attempts have been made to differentiate the transient myelodysplasia, seen in infants with Down syndrome, from leukemia based upon the morphology and number of granulocyte precursor colonies observed when bone marrow is grown in vitro (de Alarcon, Patil, Goldberg, Allen, & Shaw, 1987; Denegri, Rogers, Chan, Sadoway, & Thomas, 1981). In some cases, bone marrow culture techniques have been used to attempt to identify persons with preleukemia (Hoelzer, Ganser, & Heimpel, 1984). The results of these studies indicate that in vitro characteristics of granulocyte colony formation can provide supportive but not diagnostic information and that additional laboratory and clinical evaluation are always needed to confirm a diagnosis.

Cellular Immunity

Abnormalities in both cellular and humoral immunity have been reported in persons with Down syndrome (Miale, Nasrallah, Lobel, Demian, & Bowman, 1986; Philip et al., 1986). Defects in thymic development and abnormal interactions between immature thymic-based lymphocytes may be responsible for these findings (Burgio, Ugazio, Nespoli, & Maccario, 1983; C.J. Epstein, Weiol, & Epstein, 1987; Levin et al., 1979; Spina et al., 1981). Studies of the thymus obtained from persons with Down syndrome who have undergone cardiac surgery have shown a decreased proportion of cells expressing particular membrane receptors. The decreased acquisition of molecules that are critical for antigenspecific recognition by T cells suggests a possible mechanism for the abnormal T-cell function found in individuals with Down syndrome (Murphy & Epstein, 1990; Murphy, Lempert, & Epstein, 1990). (For a more detailed description of the immune abnormalities in persons with Down syndrome, see Ugazio, Maccario, & Burgio, chap. 20, this volume.)

PLATELET ABNORMALITIES

Alterations in both number and function of platelets as well as susceptibility of platelet progenitors to malignant transformation have been reported in persons with Down syndrome. It is quite possible that these abnormalities reflect a disturbance in hematopoiesis involving megakaryocytic progenitors. For example, the thrombocytopenia and thrombocytosis reported in newborns could represent a progenitor cell defect similar to that responsible for erythrocytosis or transient myelodysplasia.

Thrombocytopenia

Thrombocytopenia, as an isolated hematologic finding, has been reported in newborns with Down syndrome (Thuring & Tonz, 1979). In most cases, it is mild and has no clinical significance. The differential diagnosis of neonatal thrombocytopenia includes immune and infectious causes. Persons with cyanotic heart disease can also become thrombocytopenic, often as a result of mild disseminated intravascular coagulation (Pochedly & Ente, 1968). Thrombocytopenia can also be the initial sign of transient myelodysplasia or congenital leukemia. A prospective study in which platelet counts are determined on all newborns should be undertaken if the prevalence of thrombocytopenia in newborns with Down syndrome is to be established.

In older children, a low platelet count is usually due to idiopathic thrombocytopenic purpura —just as it is in "normal" children. Although the frequency of certain autoimmune disorders, such as immune thyroiditis, is increased in people with Down syndrome, the incidence of idiopathic thrombocytopenia does not appear to be increased.

There have been several case reports of leukemia in children with Down syndrome following prolonged periods of thrombocytopenia (Sumi et al., 1990). Interpretation of the initial bone marrow aspirate in these individuals was consistent with idiopathic thrombocytopenic purpura. After months of persistent thrombocytopenia and failure to respond to treatment, these persons demonstrated evidence of leukemia in the peripheral blood and bone marrow. In most cases, the diagnosis was acute nonlymphoblastic leukemia. Appropriate studies often were not performed to determine if the leukemia could be classified as acute megakaryocytic.

Thrombocytosis

Thrombocytosis has also been reported in infants with Down syndrome. In some infants, it is associated with a transient myeloproliferative disorder (Miller, Sherrill, & Hathaway, 1967) whereas in others it occurs as an isolated event. The authors of this chapter analyzed the platelet counts in 30 infants with Down syndrome admitted to the Children's Hospital of Oakland, California, for evaluation of cardiac disease. They found a marked increase in thrombocytosis in children with Down syndrome compared to controls (Figure 21.2). Twenty percent had platelet counts above $400,000/mm^3$. This was most evident in children below 6 months of age. The etiology of the thrombocytosis was not determined and there was no correlation between the type of heart defect and thrombocytosis. The platelet counts were never greater than 1 million, there were no thrombotic complications, and the platelet counts returned to normal over a 1-month period. Considering the frequency of megakaryocytic leukemia in persons with Down syndrome, it is possible that thrombocytosis represents a form of transient hematodysplasia localized to the megakaryocyte series. Although this study was performed on children with Down syndrome who had congenital heart disease, thrombocytosis is not a common finding in children who do not have Down syndrome but have similar heart defects. It would be important to determine if thrombocytosis occurs in infants with Down syndrome who do not have congenital heart disease.

Functional platelet defects are quite rare in children with Down syndrome and only a few examples have been reported in the literature. These are often associated with disseminated intravascular coagulation and appear to represent the result of in vivo platelet activation and not a primary platelet defect.

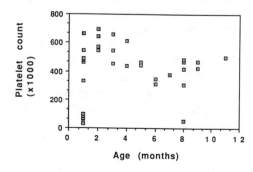

Figure 21.2.   Platelet counts in children with Down syndrome.

Biochemistry

Several laboratories have reported biochemical alterations in platelets in persons with Down syndrome, including decreased calcium and decreased serotonin content (Lott, Chase, & Murphy, 1972; McCoy & Sneddon, 1984). Platelet cation levels are also abnormal, with an increase in sodium and a decrease in potassium (McCoy & Enns, 1978). The low levels of serotonin within platelets appears to be due to the inability of platelets to incorporate serotonin from the plasma. This defect has been localized to the dense granule transport system of the platelet (Schickler, Knobler, Avraham, Elroy-Stein, & Groner, 1989).

The development of a transgenic mouse, in which superoxide dismutase levels are increased due to insertion of the human gene for copper/zinc superoxide dismutase into a fertilized mouse egg, has facilitated studies on the effects of excess gene dosage for superoxide dismutase (C.J. Epstein et al., 1987; Groner, Avraham, Schickler, Yaroml, & Knobler, 1990; Groner, Elroy-Stein, et al., 1990). Since a similar gene-dosage effect exists in persons with Down syndrome, this model has great potential to study the pathobiology of Down syndrome.

Surprisingly, investigation of the platelets from these transgenic mice revealed decreased uptake of serotonin secondary to an abnormal pH gradient across the membranes of intracellular storage granules (Groner, Elroy-Stein, et al., 1990). Similar abnormalities in pH gradient and serotonin uptake are seen in platelets from persons with Down syndrome. This suggests that, in some manner, excess superoxide dismutase affects amine transport across intracellular membranes of the platelet. Since the transport mechanisms for serotonin within the nervous system are similar, the defect in platelet serotonin transport may reflect a generalized defect in amine transport. This defect could contribute to the developmental and neurologic abnormalities observed in persons with Down syndrome. Although these findings probably have minimal significance in regard to platelet function, they illustrate that the transgenic mouse and the platelet are useful models to investigate the effects of overexpression of genes located on chromosome 21.

LEUKEMIA

Leukemia and Chromosome 21

The most clinically significant of the hematologic abnormalities associated with Down syndrome is leukemia. It is estimated that the frequency of acute leukemia in children with Down syndrome is increased approximately 10- to 30-fold over that in "normal" children. Children with Down syndrome account for 2% of all cases of acute childhood leukemia (Fong & Brodeur, 1987; Rosner & Lee, 1972). Furthermore, there is a 200-fold increase in the incidence of acute megakaryocytic leukemia in persons with Down syndrome compared to controls (Lewis, 1983; Lewis, Thompson, Hudson, Liberman, & Samson, 1983; Mitelman et al., 1990; Pui et al., 1982; Zipursky et al., 1987). This striking susceptibility to leukemia is primarily noted during the 1st decade of life. In contrast to leukemia, the incidence of solid tumors and lymphomas in persons with Down syndrome is similar to that noted in the general population.

A strong relationship between trisomy 21 and leukemia is not only suggested by the frequency of acute leukemia in persons with Down syndrome but by the identification of trisomy 21 in phenotypically "normal" individuals who develop acute leukemia (Rowley, 1981). Although in the former case a causal relationship between chromosome 21 and leukemia has been proposed, in the latter case it is difficult to know if the trisomy 21 represents a primary mutagenic event or if it represents an epiphenomenon that has no relationship to leukemogenesis.

Chromosome analysis is currently performed on all persons with leukemia, as an abnormal karyotype can serve as a marker of the leukemic cell line and have prognostic significance. The trisomy 21 karyotype is often noted in phenotypically "normal" children who develop acute lymphocytic leukemia. In several studies, 14%–19% of persons who had an aneuploid or hyperdiploid karyotype associated with acute lymphocytic anemia had trisomy 21 as part of the karyotypic abnormality (Golomb & Rowley, 1981; Mitelman et al., 1990; Rowley, 1981). The trisomy was only found in the leukemic clone and disappeared following remission (Ferster, Verhest,

Vamos, DeMaertelaere, & Otten, 1986; Sikand, Taysi, Strandjord, Griffith, & Vietti, 1980). The incidence of an acquired trisomy 21 karyotype in persons with acute nonlymphocytic leukemia was much lower, being found in 4.1%–6.7% of the aneuploid children. Numeric and/or structural chromosome changes in addition to trisomy 21 were frequently noted in both types of leukemia. Additional evidence for the involvement of chromosome 21 in acute leukemia is the identification of chromosome translocations involving chromosome 21 in a number of individuals (Rowley, 1981).

Studies on children with mosaic forms of trisomy 21 have provided important information in regard to the relationship between chromosome 21 and hematopoietic dysplasia. In such children, trisomy 21 can be detected in skin fibroblasts but not bone marrow cells. The number of trisomic cells in the peripheral blood may be very low, making the diagnosis difficult at times. This is especially true in the child who has minimal physical findings and is mildly retarded. If these children develop leukemia, trisomy 21 can be found within the leukemic cells of the bone marrow. Following remission, the karyotype of bone marrow cells returns to normal (Ferster et al., 1986).

A similar situation exists when acute megakaryocytic leukemia occurs in persons who are mosaic for trisomy 21. The megakaryoblast is the only hematopoietic cell line that contains the supernumerary chromosome (Koike et al., 1990). There have been several case reports in which persons were not considered to have Down syndrome but were diagnosed with acute megakaryocytic leukemia. Subsequently, a mosaic form of Down syndrome was diagnosed. Since acute megakaryocytic leukemia is rare in children (Cairney, McKenna, Arthur, Nesbit, & Woods, 1986; Chan et al., 1983), a karyotype analysis should be considered on skin fibroblasts, peripheral blood lymphocytes, and bone marrow on all children with this diagnosis.

Leukemogenesis

Several hypotheses have been proposed to explain the increased susceptibility to leukemia in persons with Down syndrome (Fong & Brodeur,

1987; Sutnick, London, Blumberg, & Gerstley, 1971). Most of these suggest that primary or secondary effects related to the extra complement of genes located on chromosome 21 (Table 21.4) are involved. In considering these hypotheses, a number of important questions must be answered, including:

Why does the extra dose of genes on chromosome 21 cause leukemia in some but not others?
Is the susceptibility to oxidative damage a factor?
Is the parental origin of the trisomic chromosome important?
What role does immune deficiency play?

As more of the genes located on chromosome 21 are identified, it may become possible to answer these and perhaps other broader biologic questions regarding leukemogenesis.

Excess expression of oncogenes and abnormalities in the regulation of tumor-suppressor genes are theories that have been proposed to explain the susceptibility to acute leukemia in persons with Down syndrome. Molecular investigations lend support to this hypothesis. In a child with Down syndrome who developed acute megakaryocytic leukemia, the expression of the c-*sis* oncogene was amplified (Sunami et al., 1987). This gene encodes for the β chain of platelet-derived growth factor and is the cellular counterpart of the transforming gene v-*sis* of simean sarcoma virus. The fibrosis seen in bone marrow of persons with acute megakaryocytic leukemia may be due, in part, to platelet-derived growth factor released from megakaryoblasts (Bain et al., 1981; Bennett et al., 1985; Doolittle et al., 1983; Nordan & Humbert, 1979). It seems likely

Table 21.4. Susceptibility to leukemia in persons with Down syndrome

Oncogenes or tumor suppressor genes on chromosome 21
DNA damage secondary to oxidant injury
Genetic imprinting
Abnormal susceptibility to viral transformation
Defects in DNA repair
Abnormal cell cycle kinetics
Defects in immune surveillance

that the c-*sis* messenger RNA detected in blasts from this child has biologic relevance to the pathophysiology of acute megakaryocytic leukemia and perhaps to myelofibrosis, which has also been reported in persons with Down syndrome (D.I.K. Evans, 1975; Nordan & Humbert, 1979). As the c-*sis* gene is located on chromosome 22 and not 21, transacting factors regulated by genes on chromosome 21 could explain its activation.

There are many examples of in vitro DNA alterations, which could relate to the increased susceptibility to leukemia in persons with Down syndrome. Several reports have suggested that there is a decreased rate of DNA synthesis or cell doubling in cultured fibroblasts obtained from persons with Down syndrome (Kaback & Bernstein, 1970; Segal & McCoy, 1973). In addition, there is increased sensitivity of fibroblast DNA to radiation and chemical damage in persons with Down syndrome (C.J. Epstein, 1989). The cell transformation induced by transforming virus, simian virus 40, is increased two- to threefold in fibroblasts prepared from persons with Down syndrome compared to controls (Aaronson, 1970; Lubiniecki et al., 1979; Todaro & Martin, 1967). Viral infections, such as measles, have been reported to increase the number of chromosome breaks in fibroblasts from persons with Down syndrome 4.8 times compared to 1.2 times in "normal" persons (Higurashi, Tamura, & Nakatake, 1973). These findings suggest that abnormalities in DNA stability exist in persons with Down syndrome. It remains to be established how or if these abnormalities contribute to the susceptibility to leukemia.

The parental origin of the trisomic chromosome may have biologic significance in regard to the predisposition to leukemia in persons with Down syndrome. Although the extra chromosome in 95% of persons with Down syndrome is maternal in origin (Antonarakis & Down Syndrome Collaborative Group, 1991), studies to determine parental origin of the trisomic chromosome in persons who have leukemia have not been reported. Since genetic imprinting may contribute to the susceptibility to malignant transformation, this information could be quite important (Hall, 1990; Little, Van Heyningen, & Hastie, 1991; Reik, Collick, Norris, Barton, & Surani, 1987). If studies demonstrate that persons with leukemia have a paternally duplicated chromosome 21, knowledge of the origin of the trisomic chromosome in young children who develop the transient myelodysplasia syndrome might have clinical significance.

Although oxidation has been considered primarily in relationship to premature aging in persons with Down syndrome, it has also been recognized for its potential to cause DNA damage and predispose to leukemia (Ames, 1989). There is considerable experimental evidence that hydrogen peroxide can cause DNA damage and alter DNA structure (Cerutti, 1985). Normally, such alterations would be repaired. However, persons with Down syndrome have a defect in DNA repair (Athanasiou, Sideris, & Bartsocas, 1980). Abnormalities in folate metabolism may also contribute to chromosome fragility and susceptibility to leukemia (Gericke et al., 1977). A recent report suggesting that there is increased expression of chromosomal fragile sites in persons with Down syndrome is consistent with this hypothesis (Roizen & Amarose, 1991). Since it is now possible to detect products of DNA oxidation by analysis of urine samples, this oxidation-based theory could be investigated in persons with leukemia (Fraga, Shigenaga, Park, Degan, & Ames, 1990).

The defect responsible for the susceptibility to leukemia in persons with Down syndrome may reside in the immune regulatory system (Noble & Warren, 1987). It is possible that the immune response to abnormal glycoproteins on the surface of leukemic cells may not be intact. Theoretically, such a defect would permit the leukemic clone to proliferate, eventually resulting in leukemia. Transient abnormalities in immune surveillance could also explain the myeloproliferative response seen in young children (Miale et al., 1986). A similar mechanism has been proposed to explain the clinical course of infants who have stage IVS neuroblastoma (C.E. Evans, 1980). Although this type of neuroblastoma is metastatic, patients often have a complete remission without chemotherapy.

There is considerable evidence that a basic defect in immunity exists in children with Down syndrome (Noble & Warren, 1987). As previously discussed, histologic examinations of thymic tissue from children with Down syndrome demonstrate a number of significant changes. Some of these resemble the changes observed in children with severe combined immunodeficiency. Although children with Down syndrome do not have immune defects as severe as those associated with severe combined immune deficiency, these findings suggest that a defect in thymic-regulated immune function could alter immune surveillance and natural resistance to leukemia. Abnormalities in the interactions between immune regulatory cells and hematopoietic stem cells could also contribute to defects in hematopoiesis.

Classification, Clinical Manifestations, and Laboratory Diagnosis

The classification and age distribution of children with Down syndrome who develop acute leukemia is similar to that found in "normal" children (Robinson et al., 1984). During the first 3 years of life, acute nonlymphocytic leukemia predominates. After age 3, approximately 80% have acute lymphocytic leukemia and 20% have acute nonlymphocytic leukemia. As previously noted, within the acute nonlymphocytic category, there is a high frequency of acute megakaryocytic leukemia in all age groups.

Comparison of the clinical and hematologic findings in children with Down syndrome who had acute lymphocytic leukemia to a group of children who also had acute lymphocytic leukemia but did not have Down syndrome revealed no statistically significant differences (Robinson et al., 1984). This analysis included laboratory parameters at presentation, immunologic markers, and cytochemical findings.

For the most part, the clinical and laboratory manifestations reported in persons with Down syndrome who had acute nonlymphocytic leukemia are also similar to those noted in children who did not have Down syndrome (Rosner, Kozinn, & Jervis, 1973). However, within this category of leukemia, biphenotypic patterns demonstrating erythroid and megakaryocytic characteristics were noted, children with erythroleukemia were reported, and the incidence of acute megakaryocytic leukemia was dramatically increased (Juberg & Jones, 1970; Suarez, LeBan, Silberman, Fresco, & Rowley, 1985). It is difficult to document precisely the incidence of acute megakaryocytic leukemia from these retrospective studies, as appropriate immunologic and cytochemical analyses to demonstrate megakaryoblasts were often not used (Bennett et al., 1985).

Acute megakaryocytic leukemia should be suspected if the bone marrow aspirate is difficult to obtain and a "dry tap" occurs. Histologic examination of bone marrow biopsy specimens may reveal fibrosis. Since acute megakaryocytic leukemia is so unique in persons with Down syndrome, some diagnostic guidelines are listed in Table 21.5 (Bennett et al., 1985; Cairney et al., 1986; Chan et al., 1983; Saribam et al., 1984). Using flow cytometry, several immunologic markers can identify megakaryocytic precursors in peripheral blood or bone marrow samples. Cytochemical stains show that blasts are positive for platelet peroxidase and α-napthyl acetate esterase but negative for α-napthyl butyrate esterase. Platelet peroxidase stains on electron micrograph preparations of blasts reveal a pattern consistent with megakaryoblasts. Bone marrow fibrosis can be detected using a reticulin stain on bone marrow biopsy specimens. As with other leukemias, cytogenetic analysis should be performed to determine if chromosome markers in addition to trisomy 21 are present. Studies to identify amplification of c-sis oncogene are recommended.

Therapy

Although earlier reports suggested that children with Down syndrome respond poorly to chemotherapy and that chemotherapy is excessively toxic, more recent studies have suggested that, except for the induction phase, the response to chemotherapy is quite similar to that observed in children who do not have Down syndrome (Lampkin et al., 1983; Ragab et al., 1991). In cases where acute megakaryocytic leukemia is diagnosed, the response of children with Down

Table 21.5.   Laboratory diagnosis of acute megakaryocytic leukemia: M7

Morphology
  Highly polymorphic
  20%–30% of the blasts are two to three times larger
    than the rest of the cells
  Small rim of deeply basophilic cytoplasm with
    distinctive blebs
  Megakaryocytic fragments may be noted in the
    peripheral blood
  Nucleus contains several nucleoli and chromatin is in
    a fine reticular pattern
Cytochemistry
  Peroxidase negative
  Sudan black negative
  Alpha-napthol-butyrate esterase negative
  Nonspecific esterase-positive
  Acid phosphatase positive
  Periodic acid schiff-negative to granular
Immunologic
  Positive reaction against anti-platelet glycoprotein
    antibodies
    glycoprotein Ib
    glycoprotein IIb/IIIa
    Factor VIII antigen
    additional monoclonal antibodies
Bone marrow
  Difficult aspiration due to fibrosis
  Reticulin stain positive
  Myelofibrosis
Electron microscopy
  Positive platelet peroxidase reaction
  Reactivity exclusively on nuclear membrane and
    endoplasmic reticulum
Cytogenetics
  Association with trisomy 21 (constitutional or
    acquired)
  Other chromosomal abnormalities

Adapted from Bennett et al. (1985).

syndrome to chemotherapy appears to be similar
to that for children with acute nonlymphocytic
leukemia. This is in contrast to adults who have
acute megarkaryocytic leukemia, where the response to therapy is often poor.

The two most frequent complications in children with Down syndrome undergoing chemotherapy for acute leukemia are methotrexate
toxicity involving the skin, gastrointestinal mucosa, and bone marrow; and infections, particularly during induction. A decrease in methotrexate dose may be required to prevent severe

gastrointestinal and myelosuppressive toxicity.
However, such alterations should be made on an
individual basis as many persons tolerate full
doses of methotrexate without difficulty. Infectious complications may be due to the combination of drug toxicity and immune deficiency, as
previously described.

The abnormal sensitivity to methotrexate in
some persons with Down syndrome appears to
be secondary to a defect in methotrexate metabolism (Blatt, Albo, Prin, Orlando, & Wollman,
1986; Frankel, Pullen, & Boyett, 1986; Lejeune
et al., 1986; Peeters & Poon, 1987). Studies of
methotrexate clearance rates reveal prolonged
values in children with Down syndrome compared to controls. Abnormal methotrexate clearance correlates well with clinical toxicity (Garre
et al., 1987). Alterations in dose or duration of
leucovorin, which is given to prevent methotrexate toxicity, have not been very successful.

Three genes involved in purine metabolism
have been mapped to chromosome 21: phospho-
ribosylglycinamide synthetase, phosphoribosyl-
glycinamide formyl transferase, and phospho-
ribosylglycinamide synthetase (Hards et al.,
1986; Patterson et al., 1981). These genes may
alter purine metabolism and explain the elevated
purine and serum uric acid levels reported in persons with Down syndrome. As a consequence
of gene dosage, there is a greater demand for
tetrahydrofolic acid and greater sensitivity to an-
tifolate agents such as methotrexate. If a gene-
dosage effect were to be directly calculated,
methylation demands would have to be 1.5 times
normal and the maximum tolerated dose of
methotrexate reduced by 1.5 times (Peeters &
Poon, 1987). Variability in expression of these
three genes may explain why not all patients
have severe methotrexate toxicity.

It has been suggested that children with Down
syndrome who have acute nonlymphocytic leukemia may have a better prognosis than children
without Down syndrome (Lampkin et al., 1983).
One possible explanation for an improved outcome in these children is that the biologic characteristics of acute nonlymphocytic leukemia in
children with Down syndrome are unique. The
prevalence of acute megakaryocytic leukemia is
consistent with this hypothesis. Factors re-

sponsible for spontaneous remission in the transient myeloproliferative syndrome could also be involved.

Bone marrow transplantation is a well-accepted means to treat persons with certain types or stages of leukemia. It is usually reserved for clinical situations in which chemotherapy is inadequate. There are a number of life-threatening complications associated with bone marrow transplantation. Some of these can be minimized by selection of an immunologic compatible donor, which decreases the risk of graft versus host disease. Initial reports suggested that bone marrow transplantation should not be considered for children with Down syndrome primarily because children with Down syndrome did not tolerate the conditioning regimen required for transplantation (Robinson et al., 1984; Rubin, O'Leary, Koch, & Nesbit, 1986). However, more recent experience has indicated that the ability to tolerate the conditioning regimen in children with Down syndrome is similar to that in children without Down syndrome. An analysis of the number of patients with Down syndrome who underwent bone marrow transplantation compared to a calculated number of patients who would be expected to have this procedure revealed that only 20%–25% of eligible patients have been transplanted (Arenson & Forde, 1989). This study concluded that there is no justification for denial of bone marrow transplantation to otherwise appropriate candidates with Down syndrome and leukemia.

TRANSIENT MYELODYSPLASIA IN NEWBORNS

An unusual, severe transient myelodysplastic syndrome has been reported in infants with Down syndrome (de Castro et al., 1990; Weinberg et al., 1982; Weinstein, 1978). Within the first few months of life, these infants develop a marked elevation in the peripheral blood leukocyte count with a predominance of blasts. Immunologic studies may demonstrate that the blasts have megakaryocytic and/or basophil-like characteristics (Coulombel et al., 1987; J. Suda et al., 1988). A leukemoid reaction secondary to bacterial sepsis must be considered in the differential diagnosis. However, in most cases, bacteriologic studies are negative. The clinical presentation is often indistinguishable from congenital leukemia (de Castro et al., 1990).

The usual management of these infants, once an infection has been excluded, is to observe the patient and not give chemotherapy. In the majority of children, spontaneous remission occurs by 2–3 months of age, with the granulocyte count returning to normal and blasts disappearing from the peripheral blood. In some infants, the leukocyte count can exceed $100,000/mm^3$. If this occurs, an exchange transfusion should be considered as this degree of leukocytosis can increase whole blood viscosity and cause vascular obstruction (Jones, Waver, & Laug, 1987; Nakagawa et al., 1988). For the infant who does not have a spontaneous remission and appears to progress to leukemia, chemotherapy must be considered.

Distinguishing transient myelodysplasia from acute leukemia is difficult since morphologic markers, immunologic markers, and in vitro bone marrow culture characteristics are often inconclusive (de Alarcon et al., 1987; Denegri et al., 1981). Karyotypic analysis is extremely important as clonal chromosome abnormalities in addition to trisomy 21 are consistent with leukemia. Because of the many similarities to leukemia, the term "transient leukemia" is sometimes used to describe this myeloproliferative disorder (Fong & Brodeur, 1987; Lazarus, Heerema, Palmer, & Baehner, 1981; Mendelow, Krawitz, Cohn, & Bernstein, 1984; Wong, Jones, Srivastava, & Gruppo, 1988; Zipursky et al., 1987). In many cases, ultrastructural morphology and in vitro growth characteristics of blasts support this conclusion (Bessho, Hayashi, Hayashi, & Ohga, 1988; Coulombel et al., 1987). Approximately 20% of the infants who initially have spontaneous remission have a relapse several years later with a diagnosis of acute nonlymphocytic leukemia (Barnett, Clark, & Garson, 1990; Morgan, Hecht, Cleary, Sklar, & Link, 1985). These leukemias have frequently been classified as megakaryocytic. Unfortunately, there are no satisfactory techniques to identify the infant likely to have a relapse.

There have been several case reports of children with the mosaic form of trisomy 21 who develop this transient myeloproliferative disorder (Brodeur, Dahl, Williams, Tipton, & Kalwinsky, 1980; Heaton, Fitzgerald, Fraser, & Abbott, 1981; Seibel, Sommer, & Miser, 1984; Weinberg et al., 1982). In some of these children, the diagnosis of Down syndrome had not been made prior to the onset of the myelodysplastic syndrome. The blast cells in the peripheral blood and bone marrow contained the trisomy 21 karyotype whereas the normal hematopoietic progenitor cells did not. Following spontaneous remission, peripheral blood lymphocytes and hematopoietic progenitor cells within the bone marrow had a diploid karyotype. A typical pattern for such a child is shown in Table 21.6. Because of the unique association between transient myelodysplasia and trisomy 21, any phenotypically "normal" infant demonstrating transient myelodysplasia should be considered to have a mosaic form of trisomy 21 and have a karyotype analysis performed on peripheral blood, skin fibroblasts, and bone marrow (Jones, Waver, & Laug, 1987).

A study by Hayashi et al. (1988) compared the laboratory and clinical parameters in persons with transient myelodysplasia to those in persons with acute leukemia. The analysis of 28 persons with Down syndrome who had blasts in the peripheral blood showed that 13 had acute leukemia and 15 had a transient myeloproliferative disorder. The results of this study are shown in Table 21.7. The age range for the children with acute leukemia was 6–30 months and 0–34 days for the infants with transient myelodysplasia. Many of the children in the acute leukemia group had pancytopenia. This finding was not characteristic in the transient myelodysplasia group. In addition to being younger, the transient myelodysplasia group had higher hemoglobin levels as well as higher platelet and leukocyte counts. The detection of a clonal chromosome abnormality was strong evidence for leukemia rather than transient myelodysplasia. Similar conclusions in regard to detection of clonal chromosome abnormalities have been drawn by others (Hecht, Hecht, Morgan, Sandberg, & Link, 1986).

The immature leukocytic cells in both groups had immunologic and cytochemical characteristics similar to those of megakaryocytes, suggesting that the megakaryocyte line can be involved in both transient myelodysplasia and acute leukemia (J. Suda et al., 1988). Since immunologic studies may demonstrate basophil, erythrocyte, and megarkaryocyte markers on the blasts in these children, the progenitor cell proximal to the differentiation step for each cell type may be the point where the hematopoietic transformation occurs (T. Suda et al., 1985).

PRELEUKEMIA, APLASTIC ANEMIA, AND MYELOFIBROSIS

To complete the spectrum of hematopoietic dysplasia, a discussion regarding preleukemia, aplastic anemia, and myelofibrosis in persons with Down syndrome is necessary. A list of myeloproliferative abnormalities in Down syndrome is illustrated in Table 21.8. Their association with trisomy 21 provides additional support for disordered hematopoiesis in persons with Down syndrome.

Preleukemia is a disorder that affects primi-

Table 21.6. Cytogenetic data in a child with a mosaic form of trisomy 21 and transient myelodysplasia

Age (days)	Tissue sampled	Cells counted	Percentage of cells counted		
			Blasts	46,XY	47,XY, + 21
3	Blood	50	70	0	100
3	Marrow	22	50	0	100
8	Blood	50	80	0	100
8	Skin	100	NA	96	4
100	Blood	75	0	76	24
100	Marrow	34	9	100	0

NA = not applicable.

From Brodeur, G.M., Dahl, G.V., Williams, D.L., Tipton, R.E., & Kalwinsky, D.K. (1980). Transient leukemoid reaction and trisomy 21 mosaicism in a phenotypically normal newborn. *Blood, 55,* 692; reprinted with permission.

Table 21.7.   Acute leukemia (AL) versus transient myelodysplasia (TMD) in persons with Down syndrome

Condition	Age (mo)	Hb (g/dL)	Platelets ($\times$ 10⁹/L)	WBC ($\times$ 10⁹/L)	Blasts (%)
AL	19.2	9.6	3.1	14.4	30.5
(n = 13)	(6–30)	(7.6–14.9)	(1.0–5.6)	(1.8–40.6)	(0–68)
TMD	7.4	17.0	23.1	106.5	57.7
(n = 15)	(0–34)	(14.6–20)	(2.9–85.3)	(28–248.6)	(20–89)

Adapted from Hayashi et al. (1988).

tive cellular elements of the marrow with characteristics suggestive, but not diagnostic, of leukemia (Hoelzer et al., 1984; Linman & Bagby, 1976). The clinical course of persons with preleukemia varies, with some remaining in a relatively stable state for months to even years, whereas others rapidly progress to the full-blown leukemic picture in a short time period. As with acute leukemia, there are suggestions in the literature that this complication occurs more frequently in children with Down syndrome than in children without Down syndrome.

The laboratory parameters in preleukemia are rather characteristic. Either pancytopenia or abnormalities in one of the cellular elements of the marrow can be seen. In some individuals, for example, thrombocytopenia occurs weeks, months, or even years before the onset of leukemia. Macrocytosis and abnormalities in red cell shape are noted, nucleated red blood cells are seen, and alterations in granulocyte morphology and number can be observed. Analysis of bone marrow aspirates or biopsy specimens often show abnormalities in maturation of granulocytes, erythroid or megakaryocytic precursors. These are often suggestive, but not diagnostic, of leukemia. In vitro

Table 21.8.   Myeloproliferative disorders in persons with Down syndrome

Neonatal period
  Thrombocytosis
  Erythrocytosis
  Transient myelodysplasia
  Congenital leukemia
Childhood and adulthood
  Acute lymphocytic leukemia
  Acute nonlymphocytic leukemia
  Myelofibrosis
  Aplastic anemia

culture of bone marrow may reveal alterations in size and morphology of granulocyte colonies. In addition, chromosome changes similar to those associated with leukemia may be noted (Smith & Willoughby, 1981).

The treatment of persons who develop a preleukemic syndrome depends upon the clinical manifestations. If the individual is symptomatic as a result of anemia or thrombocytopenia, red cell or platelet transfusions can be given. Aggressive treatment for those suspected of having bacterial infections is warranted. In some cases, the decision to initiate chemotherapy is made based upon the "leukemia-like" clinical picture, even though the person does not have leukemia. In most situations, however, chemotherapy is not given until leukemia develops.

There have been several case reports of aplastic anemia in persons with Down syndrome (Erdogan, Akosy, & Dincol, 1967; Hanukoglu, Meytes, Fried, Rosen, & Shacked, 1987; McWilliams & Dunn, 1982; Weinblatt, Higgins, & Ortega, 1981). The relative infrequency of these reports suggests that persons with Down syndrome do not have an increased incidence of idiopathic aplastic anemia. It is possible that many of the reports of aplastic anemia in persons with Down syndrome represent part of the spectrum of myelodysplasia–myelofibrosis.

There are data to suggest that the frequency of acute myelofibrosis in persons with Down syndrome is increased compared to controls (D.I.K. Evans, 1975; Nordan & Humbert, 1979; Ueda et al., 1981). This complication most likely represents part of the spectrum of megakaryocytic leukemia (Bain et al., 1981). Analysis of bone marrow aspirates in these individuals demonstrates fibrosis, reticulum cells, and megakaryocytes, and no evidence of leukemia. Chromosome changes in bone marrow cells may be noted. These individuals often become pancytopenic and have clinical manifestations similar to aplastic anemia. The production of platelet-derived growth factor as a consequence of amplification of the c-*sis* gene in acute megakaryocytic leukemia results in marrow fibrosis. It is possible that a similar amplification can result in myelofibrosis and studies to measure the c-*sis* gene under these circumstances are to be encouraged. In general, the prognosis is poor for these patients and there are no recommendations in regard to specific treatment. If one considers myelofibrosis to be a consequence of acute megakaryocytic leukemia, chemotherapy is a possible option.

CONCLUSION

Insufficient evidence is available to describe the frequency of most of the hematologic abnormalities found in persons with Down syndrome. Furthermore, few studies to determine the relationship between gene dosage and clinical manifestation have been conducted. With the present advances in molecular biology—mapping the genes located on chromosome 21, and the development of appropriate transgenic mouse models—it is likely that new information will soon be generated to answer important questions related to leukemogenesis and the other hematologic manifestations in persons with Down syndrome.

The dysregulated hematopoiesis seen in many newborns with Down syndrome should be further explored. It is possible that new information in regard to relationships between cellular immunity and hematopoiesis may be uncovered in such investigations. This is particularly true in relationship to the unique transient myelodysplasia seen in persons with Down syndrome. Possible common pathophysiologic pathways involving erythroid or megakaryocytic precursors need to be explored and their relationships, if any, to transient myelodysplasia examined.

The unique susceptibility to leukemia, in particular to acute megakaryocytic leukemia, may involve alterations in oncogene expression as discussed in this chapter. However, many additional factors, particularly those involving susceptibility to oxidation, require further investigation. As newer approaches to prevent oxidation become available, attempts to evaluate these in persons with Down syndrome should be considered. It is apparent that aggressive treatment should be offered to persons with Down syndrome who have acute leukemia as the response to therapy is similar to that in "normal" individuals.

The significance of the most common hematologic abnormality in persons with Down syndrome, macrocytosis, remains to be determined. If hemolysis is the underlying cause, it is unclear why some persons are affected and others not. If oxidation and premature aging are underlying factors, perhaps evaluation of neurodevelopment in relationship to macrocytosis should be considered. Alternatively, subtle defects in intracellular metabolism of folic acid remain to be evaluated. Perhaps, inheritance of genes involved in purine metabolism on the trisomic chromosome is variable and this accounts for the range of red cell volume measurements noted in persons with Down syndrome.

The mechanism for susceptibility to infection in some individuals with Down syndrome also requires further investigation. Perhaps therapeutic interventions such as prophylactic antibiotics or antiviral therapies might be indicated. Immunologic studies in persons with Down syndrome may provide new insights into the role of thymic maturations and the cellular changes involved during thymic development.

It is apparent that hematologic studies of persons with Down syndrome have just begun to yield insights into the unique characteristics of hematopoiesis in persons with an extra chromosome 21 and that further studies of the effects of this genetic imbalance are warranted.

REFERENCES

Aaronson, S.A. (1970). Susceptibility of human cell strains to transformation by simian virus 40 and simian virus 40 deoxyribonucleic acid. *Journal of Virology*, 6(4), 470–475.

Akin, K. (1988). Macrocystosis and leukopenia in Down's syndrome. *Journal of the American Medical Association, 259*(6), 842.

Ames, B.N. (1989). Endogenous DNA damage as related to cancer and aging. *Mutation Research, 214,* 41–46.

Annerén, G., & Björksten, B. (1984). Low superoxide levels in blood phagocytic cells in Down's syndrome. *Acta Paediatrica Scandinavica, 73,* 373–348.

Antonarakis, S., & Down Syndrome Collaborative Group. (1991). Parental origin of the extra chromosome in trisomy 21 as indicated by analysis of DNA polymorphisms. *New England Journal of Medicine, 324,* 872–876.

Arenson, E., & Forde, M. (1989). Bone marrow transplantation for acute leukemia and Down syndrome: Report of a successful case and results of a national survey. *Journal of Pediatrics, 114,* 69–72.

Athanasiou, K., Sideris, E.G., & Bartsocas, C. (1980). Decreased repair of X-ray induced DNA single-strand breaks in lymphocytes in Down's syndrome. *Pediatric Research, 14,* 336–338.

Baar, H.S., & Gordon, M. (1963). Cation fluxes in erythrocytes of mongoloids. *Proceedings of the Second International Congress on Mental Retardation Research, 1,* 373–378.

Bain, B.J., Catovsky, D., O'Brien, M., Prentice, H.G., Lawlor, E., Kumaran, T.O., McCann, S.R., Matutes, E., & Galton, D.A.G. (1981). Megakaryoblastic leukemia presenting as acute myelofibrosis. *Blood, 58,* 206–213.

Barkin, R.M., Weston, W.L., Humbert, J.R., & Maire, R. (1980). Phagocytic function in Down syndrome: I. Chemotaxis. *Journal of Mental Deficiency Research, 24*(4), 243–249.

Barkin, R.M., Weston, W.L., Humbert, J.R., & Sunada, K. (1980). Phagocytic function in Down syndrome: II. Bactericidal activity and phagocytosis. *Journal of Mental Deficiency Research, 24*(4), 251–256.

Barnett, P., Clark, A., & Garson, O. (1990). Acute nonlymphocytic leukemia after transient myeloproliferative disorder in a patient with Down syndrome. *Medical and Pediatric Oncology, 18,* 347–353.

Bartosz, G., & Kedziora, J. (1983). Erythrocyte anomalies in Down's syndrome. *Medical Hypothesis, 11*(4), 471–477.

Bartosz, G., Seszynski, M., & Kedziora, J. (1982). Aging of the erythrocyte: VI. Accelerated red cell membrane aging in the Down's syndrome. *Cell Biology International, 6,* 73–77.

Baxter, R.G., Larkins, R.G., Martin, F.I., Heyma, P., Myles, K., & Ryan, L. (1975). Down syndrome and thyroid function in adults. *Lancet, ii,*(7939), 794–796.

Bennett, J.M., Catovsky, D., Daniel, M.T., Flandrin, G., Galton, D.A.G., Grainick, H., & Sultan, C.

(1985). Criteria for the diagnosis of acute leukemia of megakaryocyte lineage (M7). *Annals of Internal Medicine, 103,* 460–462.

Bessho, F., Hayashi, Y., Hayashi, Y., & Ohga, K. (1988). Ultrastructural studies of peripheral blood of neonates with Down's syndrome and transient abnormal myelopoiesis. *American Journal of Clinical Pathology, 89,* 627–633.

Blatt, J., Albo, V., Prin, W., Orlando, S., & Wollman, M. (1986). Excessive chemotherapy-related myelotoxicity in children with Down's syndrome and acute lymphoblastic leukemia [Letter]. *Lancet, ii,* (8514), 914.

Brahe, C., Serra, A., & Morton, N.E. (1985). Erythrocyte catechol-O-methyltransferase activity: Genetic analysis in nuclear families with one child affected by Down syndrome. *American Journal of Medical Genetics, 21*(2), 373–384.

Brock, D.J., Barron, L., Holloway, S., Liston, W.A., Hillier, S.G., & Seppala, M. (1990). Human Genetics Unit, University of Edinburg, U.K. *Prenatal Diagnosis, 10*(4), 245–251.

Brodeur, G.M., Dahl, G.V., Williams, D.L., Tipton, R.E., & Kalwinsky, D.K. (1980). Transient leukemoid reaction and trisomy 21 mosaicism in a phenotypically normal newborn. *Blood, 55,* 691–693.

Brooksbank, B.W.L., & Balázs, R. (1984). Superoxide dismutase, glutathione peroxidase and lipoperoxidation in Down's syndrome fetal brain. *Developmental Brain Research, 16,* 37–44.

Burgio, G.R., Ugazio, A., Nespoli, L., & Maccario, R. (1983). Down syndrome: A model of immunodeficiency. *Birth Defects, 19*(3), 325–327.

Burroughs, S.F., Devine, D.V., Browne, G., & Kaplan, M.E. (1988). The population of paroxysmal nocturnal hemoglobinuria netrophils deficient in decay accelerating factor is also deficient in alkaline phosphatase. *Blood, 71*(4), 1086–1089.

Cairney, A.E., McKenna, R., Arthur, D.C., Nesbit, M.E., & Woods, W.G. (1986). Acute megakaryoblastic leukaemia in children. *British Journal of Hematology, 63,* 541–554.

Cerutti, P.A. (1985). Prooxidant states and tumor promotion. *Science, 227,* 375–381.

Chan, W.C., Brynes, R.K., Kim, T.H., Verras, A., Schick, C., Green, R.J., & Ragab, A.H. (1983). Acute megakaryoblastic leukemia in early childhood. *Blood, 62*(1), 92–98.

Chard, T. (1991). Biochemistry and endocrinology of the Down's syndrome pregnancy. *Annals of the New York Academy of Sciences, 626,* 580–596.

Coulombel, L., Derycke, M., Villeval, J.L., Leonard, C., Breton-Gorius, J., Vial, M., Bourgeois, P., & Tchernia, G. (1987). Characterization of the blast cell population in two neonates with Down's syndrome and transient myeloproliferative disorder. *British Journal of Hematology, 66,* 69–76.

Crosti, N., Serra, A., Rigo, A., & Viglino, P. (1976).

Dosage effect of SOD-A gene in 21-trisomic cells. *Human Genetics, 31,* 197–202.

Curnutte, J.T. (1988). Classification of chronic granulomatous disease. *Hematology Oncology Clinics of North America, 2*(2), 241–252.

Cutler, N.R., Heston, L.L., Davies, P., Haxby, J.V., & Schapiro, M.B. (1985). NIH Conference. Alzheimer's disease and Down's syndrome: New insights. *Annals of Internal Medicine, 103,* 566–578.

de Alarcon, P.A., Patil, S., Goldberg, J., Allen, J.B., & Shaw, S. (1987). Infants with Down's syndrome. Use of cytogenic studies and in vitro colony assay for granulocyte progenitor to distinguish acute nonlymphocytic leukemia from a transient myeloproliferative disorder. *Cancer, 60,* 987–993.

de Castro, M., Salas, S., Martinez, A., Larrocha, C., Viloria, A., & Jimenez, M. (1990). Transitory T-lymphoblastic leukemoid reaction in a neonate with Down syndrome. *American Journal of Pediatric Hematology/Oncology, 12*(1), 71–73.

Denegri, J.F., Rogers, P.C., Chan, K.W., Sadoway, J., & Thomas, J.W. (1981). In vitro cell growth in neonates with Down's syndrome and transient myeloproliferative disorder. *Blood, 58*(4), 675–677.

Dewald, G., Diez-Martin, J., Steffen, S., Jenkins, R., Stupca, P., & Burgert, E. (1990). Hematologic disorders in 13 patients with acquired trisomy 21 and 13 individuals with Down syndrome. *American Journal of Medical Genetics Supplement, 7,* 247–250.

Doolittle, R.F., Hunkapiller, M.W., Hood, L.E., Devare, S.G., Robbins, K.C., Aaronson, S.A., & Antoniades, H.N. (1983). Simian sarcoma virus onc gene, v-sis, is derived from the gene (or genes) encoding a platelet-derived growth factor. *Science, 227,* 275–277.

Easthman, R.D., & Jancar, J. (1983). Macrocytosis and Down's syndrome. *British Journal of Psychology, 143,* 203–204.

Epstein, C.J. (1989). Down syndrome. In C.R. Scriver, A.L. Beaudet, W.S. Sly, & D. Valle (Eds.), *The metabolic basis of inherited disease* (6th ed., Vol. I, pp. 298–300). New York: McGraw-Hill.

Epstein, C., Avraham, K., Lovett, M., Smith, S., Elroy-Stein, O., Rotman, G., Bry, C., & Groner, Y. (1987). Transgenic mice with increased Cu/Zn-superoxide dismutase activity: Animal model of dosage effects in Down syndrome. *Proceedings of the National Academy of Sciences of the United States of America, 84,* 8044–8048.

Epstein, C.J., Weiol, J., & Epstein, L. (1987). Abnormalities in the interferon response and immune systems in Down syndrome: Studies in human trisomy 21 and mouse trisomy 16. In E.E. McCoy & C.J. Epstein (Eds.), *Oncology and immunology of Down syndrome* (pp. 191–209). New York: Alan R. Liss.

Epstein, L.B., Lee, S.H., & Epstein, C.J. (1980). Enhanced sensitivity of trisomy 21 monocytes to the maturation-inhibiting effect of interferon. *Cellular Immunology, 50*(1), 191–194.

Erdogan, G., Akosy, M., & Dincol, K. (1967). A case of idiopathic aplastic anemia associated with trisomy 21 and partial endoreduplication. *Acta Haematologica, 37,* 137–142.

Evans, C.E. (1980). Natural history of neuroblastoma. In E.A. Evans (Ed.), *Advances in neuroblastoma research* (pp. 3–11). New York: Raven Press.

Evans, D.I.K. (1975). Acute myelofibrosis in children with Down's syndrome. *Archives of Disease in Childhood, 50,* 458–462.

Ferster, A., Verhest, A., Vamos, E., DeMaertelaere, E., & Otten, J. (1986). Leukemia in a trisomy 21 mosaic: Specific involvement of the trisomic cells. *Cancer Genetics Cytogenetics, 20*(1–2), 109–113.

Fong, C.T., & Brodeur, G.M. (1987). Down's syndrome and leukemia: Epidemiology, genetics, cytogenetics and mechanisms of leukemogenesis. *Cancer Genetics Cytogenetics, 28*(1), 55–76.

Fraga, C.G., Shigenaga, M.K., Park, J.W., Degan, P., & Ames, B.N. (1990). Oxidative damage to DNA during aging: 8-hydroxy-2-deoxyguanosine in rat organ DNA and urine. *Proceedings of the National Academy of Sciences of the United States of America, 87,* 4533–4537.

Frankel, L.S., Pullen, J., & Boyett, J. (1986). Excessive drug toxicity in children with Down's syndrome treated for acute lymphocytic leukemia despite similarity of clinical and biological features to other patients. *Proceedings of American Society of Clinical Oncology, 5,* 631a.

Frischer, H., Chu, L.K., Ahmad, T., Justice, P., & Smith, G.F. (1981). Superoxide dismutase and glutathione peroxidase abnormalities in erythrocytes and lymphoid cells in Down syndrome. In G.J. Brewer (Ed.), *The red cell: Fifth Ann Arbor Conference* (pp. 269–283). New York: Alan R. Liss.

Ganick, D.J. (1986). Hematological changes in Down's syndrome. *CRC Critical Reviews in Oncology/Hematology, 6*(1), 55–69.

Garre, M., Relling, M., Kalwinsky, D., Dodge, R., Crom, W., Abromowitch, M., Pui, C.H., & Evans, W. (1987). Pharmacokinetics and toxicity of methotrexate in children with Down syndrome and acute lymphocytic leukemia. *Journal of Pediatrics, 111,* 606–612.

Gericke, G.S., Hesseling, P.B., Brink, S., & Tiedt, F.C. (1977). Leukocyte ultrastructure and folate metabolism in Down's syndrome. *South African Medical Journal, 51*(12), 369–373.

Gerli, G., Zenoni, L., Locatelli, G., Mongiat, R., Piattoni, F., Orsini, G., Montagnani, A., Gueli, M., & Gualandri, V. (1990). Erythrocyte antioxidant system in Down syndrome. *American Journal of Medical Genetics Supplement, 7,* 272–273.

Gidding, S.S., Bessel, M., & Liao, Y. (1990). Determinants of hemoglobin concentration in cyanotic heart disease. *Pediatric Cardiology, 11,* 121–125.

Golomb, H.M., & Rowley, J.D. (1981). Significance of cytogenetic abnormalities in acute leukemia. *Human Pathology, 12,* 515–522.

Groner, Y., Avraham, K., Schickler, M., Yarom, R., & Knobler, H. (1990). Clinical symptoms of Down syndrome are manifested in transgenic mice over-expressing the human Cu/Zn-superoxide dismutase gene. *Progress in Clinical and Biological Research, 360,* 233–262.

Groner, Y., Elroy-Stein, O., Avraham, K.B., Yarom, R., Schickler, M., Knobler, H., & Rotman, G. (1990). Down syndrome clinical symptoms are manifested in transfected cells and transgenic mice overexpressing the human Cu/Zn-superoxide dismutase gene. *Journal de Physiologie, 84*(1), 53–77.

Gustavson, K.H. (1989). Increased plasma and erythrocyte glutathione peroxidase. *Acta Paediatrica Scandinavica, 78,* 879–884.

Hall, J.G. (1990). Genomic imprinting: Review and relevance to human diseases. *American Journal of Human Genetics, 46,* 857.

Hanukoglu, A., Meytes, D., Fried, A., Rosen, N., & Shacked, N. (1987). Fatal aplastic anemia in a child with Down's syndrome. *Acta Paediatrica Scandinavica, 76,* 539–543.

Hards, R.G., Benkovic, S.J., Van Keuren, M.L., Graw, S.L., Drabkin, H.A., & Patterson, D. (1986). Assignment of a third purine biosynthetic gene (glycineamide ribonucleotide transformylase) to human chromosome 21. *American Journal of Human Genetics 39,* 179–195.

Hayashi, Y., Eguchi, M., Sugita, K., Nakazawa, S., Sato, T., Kojima, S., Bessho, F., Konishi, S., Inaba, T., Hanada, R., & Yamamoto, K. (1988). Cytogenetic findings and clinical features in acute leukemia and transient myeloproliferative disorder in Down's syndrome. *Blood, 72*(1), 15–23.

Heaton, D.C., Fitzgerald, P.H., Fraser, J., & Abbott, G.D. (1981). Transient leukemoid proliferation of the cytogenetically unbalanced +21 line of a constitutional mosaic boy. *Blood, 57,* 883–887.

Hecht, F., Hecht, B.K., Morgan, R., Sandberg, A.A., & Link, M.P. (1986). Chromosome clues to acute leukemia in Down's syndrome. *Cancer Genetics and Cytogenetics, 3,* 109–124.

Higurashi, M., Tamura, T., & Nakatake, T. (1973). Cytogenetic observations in cultured lymphocytes from patients with Down's syndrome and measles. *Pediatric Research, 7*(6), 582–587.

Hoelzer, D., Ganser, A., & Heimpel, H. (1984). "Atypical" leukemias: Preleukemia, smoldering leukemia and hypoplastic leukemia. *Recent Results of Cancer Research, 93,* 69–101.

Hsia, D.Y-Y., Smith, G.F., Dowben, R.M., & Justice, P. (1971). Down syndrome. A critical review of the biochemical and immunological data. *American Journal of Diseases of Children, 121,* 153–161.

Ibarra, B., Rivas, F., Medina, C., Franco, E.,

Romero-Garcia, F., Enriquez, C., Galarza, M., Hernandez-Cordova, A., & Hernandez, T. (1990). Hematological and biochemical studies in children with Down syndrome. *Annales de Genetique, 33*(2), 84–87.

Jones, G.R., Waver, M., & Laug, W.E. (1987). Transient blastemia in phenotypically normal newborns. *American Journal of Pediatric Hematology and Oncology, 9*(2), 153–157.

Juberg, R.C., & Jones, B. (1970). The Christchurch chromosome (Gp-): Mongolism, erythroleukemia and an inherited Gp- chromosome (Christchurch). *New England Journal of Medicine, 282*(6), 292–297.

Jung, V., Rashidbaigi, A., Jones, C., Tischfield, J.A., Shows, T.B., & Pesztka, S. (1987). Human chromosomes 6 and 21 are required for sensitivity to human interferon gamma. *Proceedings of the National Academy of Sciences of the United States of America, 84*(12), 4151–4155.

Kaback, M.M., & Bernstein, L.H. (1970). Biologic studies of trisomic cells growing in vitro. *Annals of the New York Academy of Sciences, 171,* 526.

Kalwinsky, D., Raimondi, S., Bunin, N., Fairclough, D., Pui, C.H., Relling, M., Ribeiro, R., & Rivera, G. (1990). Clinical and biological characteristics of acute lymphocytic leukemia in children with Down syndrome. *American Journal of Medical Genetics Supplement, 7,* 267–271.

Kedziora, J., Koter, M., Bartel, H., Bartosz, G., Leyko, W., & Jeske, J. (1981). Ultrastructural modifications of the erythrocyte membrane in Down syndrome. *Acta Biologica Hungarica, 40,* 423–428.

Khan, A.J., Evans, H.E., Glass, L., Skin, Y.H., & Almonte, D. (1975). Defective neutrophil chemotaxis in patients with Down syndrome. *Journal of Pediatrics, 87*(1), 87–89.

Koike, T., Urushiyama, M., Narita, M., Saitoh, H., Ishida, F., Imashuku, S., Morioka, Y., Utsumi, J., Ishizuka, T., Tsuruta, T., Takeuchi, Y., Kashimura, M., & Shibata, A. (1990). Target cell of leukemic transformation in acute megakaryoblastic leukemia. *American Journal of Hematology, 34,* 252–258.

Kouvalainen, K., & Osterlund, K. (1967). Placental weights in Down's syndrome. *Annales Medicinae Experimentalis et Biologiae Fenniae, 45*(3), 320–322.

Labbe, S., Copin, H., Choiset, A., Girard, S., & Barbet, J.P. (1989). Placenta and trisomies 3, 18, 21. *Journal de Gynecologie, Obstetrique et Biologie de la Reproduction, 18*(8), 989–996.

Lampkin, B.C., Woods, W., Strauss, R., Feig, S., Higgins, G., Bernstein, I., D'Angio, G., Chard, R., Bleyer, A., & Hammond, D. (1983). Current status of the biology and treatment of acute non-lymphocytic leukemia in children. *Blood, 61,* 215–228.

Lappalainen, J., & Kouvalainen, K. (1972). High hematocrits in newborns with Down's syndrome. *Clinical Pediatrics, 11*, 472–474.

Layzer, R.B., & Epstein, C.J. (1972). Phosphofructokinase and chromosome 21. *American Journal of Human Genetics 24*(5), 533–543.

Lazarus, K.H., Heerema, N.A., Palmer, C.G., & Baehner, R.L. (1981). The myeloproliferative reaction in a child with Down syndrome: Cytological and chromosomal evidence for a transient leukemia. *American Journal of Hematology, 11*, 417–423.

Lejeune, J., Rethore, M.O., de Blois, M.C., Maunoury-Burolla, C., Mir, M., Nicolle, L., Borowy, F., Borghi, E., & Recan, D. (1986). Metabolism of monocarbons and trisomy 21: Sensitivity to methotrexate. *Annale de Genetique, 29*, 16–19.

Levin, S., Schlesinger, M., Handzel, Z., Hahn, T., Altman, Y., Czernobilsky, B., & Boss, J. (1979). Thymic deficiency in Down's syndrome. *Pediatrics, 63*, 80–87.

Lewis, D.S. (1983). Association between megakaryoblastic leukemia and Down's syndrome [Letter]. *Lancet, ii*, 695.

Lewis, D.S., Thompson, M., Hudson, E., Liberman, M.M., & Samson, D. (1983). Down's syndrome and acute megakaryoblastic leukemia: Case report and review of the literature. *Acta Haematologica, 70*(4), 236–242.

Linderkamp, O., Klose, H., Betke, K., Brodherr-Heberlein, S., Buhlmeyer, K., Kelson, S., & Sengespeik, C. (1979). Increased blood viscosity in patients with cyanotic congenital heart disease and iron deficiency. *Journal of Pediatrics, 95*(4), 567–569.

Linman, J.W., & Bagby, G.C., Jr. (1976). The preleukemic syndrome: Clinical and laboratory features, natural course and management. *Nouvelle Revue Francaise D'Hematologie [New French Review of Blood Cells], 17* (1–2), 11–31.

Little, M., Van Heyningen, V., & Hastie, N. (1991). Dads and disomy and disease. *Nature, 351*, 609–610.

Lott, I.T. (1982). Down's syndrome, aging, and Alzheimer's disease: A clinical review. *Annals of the New York Academy of Sciences, 396*, 15–27.

Lott, I.T., Chase, T.N., & Murphy, D.L. (1972). Down's syndrome: Transport, storage and metabolism of serotonin in blood platelets. *Pediatric Research, 6*(9), 730–735.

Lubiniecki, A.S., Blattner, W.A., Martin, G.R., Fialkow, P.J., Dosik, H., Eatherly, C., & Fraumeni, J.F., Jr. (1979). SV40 T-antigen expression in cultured fibroblasts from patients with Down syndrome and their parents. *American Journal of Human Genetics, 31*(4), 469–477.

Mattei, J.F., Baetman, M.A., & Baret, A. (1982). Erythrocyte superoxide dismutase and redox enzymes in trisomy 21. *Acta Paediatrica Scandinavica, 71*, 589–591.

McCoy, E.E., & Enns, L. (1978). Sodium transport, ouabain binding and Na+/K+ ATPase activity in Down's syndrome platelets. *Pediatric Research, 12*(6), 685–689.

McCoy, E.E., & Sneddon, J.M. (1984). Decreased calcium content and 45Ca2+ uptake in Down's syndrome blood platelets. *Pediatric Research, 18* (9), 914–916.

McWilliams, N.B., & Dunn, N.L. (1982). Aplastic anemia and Down's syndrome. *Pediatrics, 69*, 501–502.

Mellman, W.J., Oski, F.A., Tedesco, T.A., Maciera-Coelho, A., & Harris, H. (1964). Leukocyte enzymes in Down's syndrome. *Lancet, ii*, 674–675.

Mellman, W.J., Raab, S.O., & Oski, F.A. (1967). Abnormal granulocyte kinetics: An explanation of the atypical granulocyte enzyme activities observed in trisomy 21. In *Mongolism* (Ciba Foundation Study Group No. 25, (p. 77). London: Churchill.

Mendelow, B., Krawitz, S., Cohn, R., & Bernstein, R. (1984). "Leukemic" pattern of in vitro growth in a patient with Down syndrome and transient myeloproliferative disorder. *American Journal of Hematology, 16*, 293–296.

Miale, T.D., Nasrallah, A.G., Lobel, S.A., Demian, S., & Bowman, W.P. (1986). Natural killer cell activity and ultrastructure in myeloproliferative reactions in infants with Down's syndrome. *American Journal of Pediatric Hematology/Oncology, 8*, 191–199.

Michelson, A.M., Puget, K., Durosay, P., & Bonneau, I.C. (1977). Clinical aspects of the dosage of erythrocuprein. In A.M. Michelson, J.M. McCord, & I. Firdovich (Eds.), *Superoxide and superoxide dismutase* (pp. 467–499). San Francisco: Academic Press.

Miller, M., & Cosgriff, J.M. (1983). Hematologic abnormalities in newborn infants with Down syndrome. *American Journal of Medical Genetics, 16*(2), 173–177.

Miller, M., Sherrill, J.G., & Hathaway, W.E. (1967). Thrombocythemia in the myeloproliferative disorder of Down's syndrome. *Pediatrics, 40*, 847.

Mills, E.L., & Quie, P.G. (1980). Congenital disorders of the functions of polymorphonuclear neutrophils. *Review of Infectious Diseases, 2*(3), 505–517.

Mitelman, F., Heim, S., & Mandahl, N. (1990). Trisomy 21 in neoplastic cells. *American Journal of Medical Genetics Supplement, 7*, 262–266.

Mittwoch, U. (1964). Frequency of drumsticks in normal women and in patients with chromosomal abnormalities. *Nature, 201*, 317–319.

Morgan, R., Hecht, F., Cleary, M.L., Sklar, J., & Link, M.P. (1985). Leukemia with Down's syndrome: Translocation between chromosomes 1 and

19 in acute myelomonocytic leukemia following transient congenital myeloproliferative syndrome. *Blood*, *66*, 1466–1468.

Murphy, M., & Epstein, L.B. (1990). Down syndrome (trisomy 21) thymuses have a decreased proportion of cells expressing high levels of TCRa,b and CD3. *Clinical Immunology and Immunopathology*, *55*, 453–467.

Murphy, M., Lempert, M.J., & Epstein, L.B. (1990). Decreased level of T cell receptor expression by Down syndrome (trisomy 21) thymocytes. *American Journal of Medical Genetics Supplement*, *7*, 234–237.

Naiman, J.L., Oski, F.A., & Mellman, W.J. (1965). Phosphokinase activity of erythrocytes in mongolism [Letter]. *Lancet*, *i,* (389), 821.

Nakagawa, T., Nishida, H., Arai, T., Yamada, T., Fukuda, M., & Sakamoto, S. (1988). Hyperviscosity syndrome with transient abnormal myelopoiesis in Down syndrome. *Journal of Pediatrics*, *112*(1), 58–61.

Naveh, D., Schwart, J.M., & Pang, K.W. (1971). Neonatal polycythemia and elevated plasma erythropoiten (ESF) in Down syndrome. *Progress American Society of Hematology*, 142–146.

Newburger, P.E., & Ezekowitz, R.A.B. (1988). Cellular and molecular effects of recombinant interferon gamma in chronic granulomatous disease. *Hematology Oncology Clinics of North America*, *2*(2), 267–276.

Noble, R.L., & Warren, R.P. (1987). Altered T-cell subsets and defective T-cell function in young children with Down syndrome (trisomy 21). *Immunological Investigations*, *16*(5), 371–382.

Nordan, U.Z., & Humbert, J.R. (1979). Myelofibrosis and acute lymphoblastic leukemia in a child with Down syndrome. *Journal of Pediatrics*, *94*(2), 253–255.

Oski, F.A., & Naiman, J.L. (1982). Polycythemia and hyperviscosity in the neonatal period. In F.A. Oski & J.L. Naiman (Eds.), *Major problems in clinical pediatrics: Vol. IV. Hematologic problems in the newborn* (3rd ed., pp. 87–96). Philadelphia: W.B. Saunders.

O'Sullivan, M.A., & Pryles, C.V. (1963). A comparison of leukocyte alkaline phosphatase determinations in 200 patients with mongolism and in 200 "familial" controls. *New England Journal of Medicine*, *268*, 1168.

Patterson, D., Graw, S., & Jones, C. (1981). Demonstration by somatic cell genetics of coordinate regeneration of genes for 2 enzymes of purine synthesis assigned to human chromosone 21. *Proceedings of the National Academy of Sciences of the United States of America*, *78*, 405–409.

Pearson, H.A. (1967). Studies of granulopoiesis and granulocyte kinetics in Down syndrome. *Pediatrics*, *40*, 92–95.

Peeters, M., & Poon, A. (1987). Down syndrome and leukemia: Unusual clinical aspects and unexpected methotrexate sensitivity. *European Journal of Pediatrics*, *146*, 416–422.

Phibbs, P.H. (1991). Neonatal polycythemia. In A.M. Rudolph (Ed.), *Rudolph's pediatrics* (19th ed., pp. 206–209). East Norwalk, CT: Appleton and Lange.

Philip, R., Berger, A., McManus, N.H., Warner, N.H., Peacock, M.A., & Epstein, L.B. (1986). Abnormalities of the in vitro cellular and humoral responses to bacterial and viral antigens with concomitant numerical alterations in lymphocyte subsets in Down syndrome (trisomy 21). *Journal of Immunology*, *136*, 1661–1667.

Pochedly, C., & Ente, G. (1968). Disseminated intravascular coagulation in a newborn with Down's syndrome. *Journal of Pediatrics*, *73*(2), 298.

Pottathil, R., & Lang, D.J. (1983). Interferon-induced biochemical changes in cell membranes: Possible role of cellular enzyme superoxide dismutase. In *Developmental pharmacology* (pp. 275–297). New York: Alan R. Liss.

Pueschel, S.M., & Pezzullo, J.C. (1985). Thyroid dysfunction in Down syndrome. *American Journal of Diseases of Children*, *139*(6), 636–639.

Pui, C.H., Williams, D.L., Scarborough, V., Jackson, C.W., Price, R., & Murphy, S. (1982). Acute megakaryoblastic leukemia associated with intrinsic platelet dysfunction and constitutional ring 21 chromosome in a young boy. *British Journal of Haematology*, *50*, 191–200.

Puukka, R., Puukka, M., Leppilampi, M., Linna, S.L., & Kouvalainen, K. (1982). Erythrocyte adenosine deaminase, purine nucleoside phosphorylase and phosphoribosyl-transferase activity in patients with Down's syndrome. *Clinical Chemistry Acta*, *126*(3), 275–281.

Ragab, A.H., Abdel-Mageed, A., Shuster, J.J., Frankel, L.S., Pullen, J., van Eys, J., Sullivan, M.P., Boyett, J., Borowitz, M., & Crist, W. (1991). Clinical characteristics and treatment outcome of children with acute lymphocytic leukemia and Down's syndrome. *Cancer*, *67*(4), 1057–1063.

Reik, W., Collick, A., Norris, M.L., Barton, S.C., & Surani, M.A. (1987). Genomic imprinting determines methylation of parental alleles in transgenic mice. *Nature*, *328*(6127), 248–251.

Robinson, L.L., Nesbit, M.E., Sather, H.N., Level, C., Shahidi, N., Kennedy, A., & Hammond, D. (1984). Down syndrome and acute leukemia in children: A 10-year retrospective survey from Children's Cancer Study Group. *Journal of Pediatrics*, *105*, 235–242.

Roizen, N.J., & Amarose, A.P. (1991). Increased mean corpuscular volume (MCV) in children with Down syndrome (DS). *Pediatric Research*, *29*(4/2), 149/A.

Rosner, F., Kozinn, P.J., & Jervis, G.A. (1973). Leukocyte function and serum immunoglobulins in Down's syndrome. *New York State Journal of Medicine*, 73(5), 672–675.

Rosner, F., & Lee, S.L. (1972). Down's syndrome and acute leukemia: Myeloblastic or lymphoblastic? *American Journal of Medicine*, 53, 203–218.

Rosner, F., Ong, B.H., Mahanand, D., Paine, R.S., & Jacobsen, C.B. (1964). Leukocyte enzymes in Down's syndrome [Letter]. *Lancet, ii*, 1345–1346.

Rowley, J.D. (1981). Down syndrome and acute leukemia: Increased risk may be due to trisomy 21. *Lancet, ii*, 1020–1022.

Rubin, C.M., O'Leary, M., Koch, P.A., & Nesbit, M.E. (1986). Bone marrow transplantation for children with acute leukemia and Down syndrome. *Pediatrics*, 78, 688–691.

Saribam, E., Oliver, C., Corash, L., Cossman, J., Whang-Peng, J., Jaffe, E.S., Grainick, H.R., & Poplack, D.G. (1984). Acute megakaryoblastic leukemia in childhood. *Cancer*, 54, 1423–1428.

Schickler, M., Knobler, H., Avraham, K.B., Elroy-Stein, O., & Groner, Y. (1989). Diminished serotonin uptake in platelets of transgenic mice with increased Cu/Zn-superoxide dismutase activity. *EMBO Journal*, 8(5), 1385–1392.

Scott, M.D., Meshnick, S.R., & Eaton, J.W. (1987). Superoxide dismutase-rich bacteria: Paradoxical increase in oxidant toxicity. *Journal of Biological Chemistry*, 262, 3640–3645.

Scroggin, C.H., & Patterson, D. (1982). Down's syndrome as a model disease. *Archives of Internal Medicine*, 142, 462–464.

Segal, D.J., & McCoy, E.E. (1973). Studies on Down's syndrome in tissue culture: I. Growth rates and protein contents of fibroblast cultures. *Journal of Cellular Physiology*, 83(1), 85–90.

Seibel, N.L., Sommer, A., & Miser, J. (1984). Transient neonatal leukemoid reactions in mosaic trisomy 21. *Journal of Pediatrics* 104(2), 251–254.

Shapiro, B.L. (1983). Down's syndrome: A disruption of homeostasis. *American Journal of Medical Genetics*, 14, 241–269.

Sikand, G.S., Taysi, K., Strandjörd, S.E., Griffith, R., & Vietti, T.F. (1980). Trisomy 21 in bone marrow cells of a patient with prolonged preleukemic phase. *Medical and Pediatric Oncology*, 8(3), 237–242.

Sinet, P.M. (1982). Metabolism of oxygen derivatives in Down's syndrome. *Annals of the New York Academy of Sciences*, 396, 83–94.

Sinet, P.M., Lejeune, J., & Jerome, H. (1979). Trisomy 21 (Down's syndrome) gulathione peroxidase, hexose monophosphate shunt and I.Q. *Life Science*, 24, 29–33.

Smith, A.G., & Willoughby, M.L.N. (1982). Preleukemia in Down's syndrome [Letter]. *Blood*, 59(4), 870.

Spina, C.A., Smith, D., Korn, E., Fahey, J., Herbert, J.G., & Grossman, J. (1981). Altered cellular immune functions in patients with Down's syndrome. *American Journal of Diseases of Children*, 135, 251–255.

Standen, G., Philip, M.A., & Fletcher, J. (1979). Reduced number of peripheral blood granulocytic progenitor cells in patients with Down's syndrome. *British Journal of Hematology*, 42, 417–423.

Stocchi, V., Magnani, M., Cuchiarini, L., Novelli, G., & Dallapiccola, B. (1985). Red blood cell adenine nucleotide abnormalities in Down syndrome. *American Journal of Medical Genetics Supplement*, 20(1), 131–135.

Suarez, C.R., LeBan, M.M., Silberman, S., Fresco, R., & Rowley, J.D. (1985). Acute megakaryoblastic leukemia in Down's syndrome: Report of a case and review of cytogenetic findings. *Medical and Pediatric Oncology*, 13, 225–231.

Suda, J., Eguchi, M., Ozawa, T., Furukawa, T., Hayashi, Y., Kojima, S., Maeda, H., Tadokoro, K., Sato, Y., Miura, Y., Chara, A., & Suda, T. (1988). Platelet peroxidase-positive blast cells in transient myeloproliferative disorder with Down's syndrome. *British Journal of Hematology*, 68, 181–187.

Suda, T., Suda, J., Miura, Y., Hayashi, Y., Eguchi, M., Tadokoro, K., & Saito, M. (1985). Clonal analysis of basophil differentiation in bone marrow cultures from a Down's syndrome patient with megakaryoblastic leukemia. *Blood*, 66, 1278–1285.

Sumi, S., Obayashi, M., Murakami, M., Ito, J., Okada, N., & Shibata, Y. (1990). Acute megakaryoblastic leukemia in Down syndrome following thrombocytopenia with antiplatelet antibody. *Tohoku Journal of Experimental Medicine*, 161, 65–67.

Sunami, S., Fuse, A., Simizu, B., Eguchi, M., Hayashi, Y., Sugita, K., Nakazawa, S., Okimoto, Y., Sato, T., & Nakajima, H. (1987). The c-sis gene expression in cells from a patient with acute megakaryoblastic leukemia and Down's syndrome. *Blood*, 70(2), 368–371.

Sutnick, A.I., London, W.T., Blumberg, B.S., & Gerstley, B.J. (1971). Susceptibility to leukemia: Immunologic factors in Down's syndrome. *Journal of the National Cancer Institute*, 47, 923–933.

Thuring, W., & Tonz, O. (1979). Neonatal thrombocyte values in children with Down's syndrome. *Helvetica Paediatrica Acta*, 34(6), 545–555.

Todaro, G.J., & Martin, G.M. (1967). Increased susceptibility of Down's syndrome fibroblasts to transformation by SV40. *Proceedings of the Society for Experimental Biology and Medicine*, 124(4), 1232–1236.

Tudhope, G.R., & Wilson, G.M. (1960). Anemia in hypothyroidism incidence: Pathogenesis and response to treatment. *Quarterly Journal of Medicine*, 29, 513.

Ueda, K., Kawaguchi, Y., Kodama, M., Tanaka, Y., Usui, T., & Kamada, N. (1981). Primary myelofibrosis with myeloid metaplasia and cytogenetically abnormal clones in 2 children with Down's syndrome. *Scandinavian Journal of Haematology*, *27*, 152–158.

Wachtel, T.J., & Pueschel, S.M. (1991). Macrocytosis in Down syndrome. *American Journal of Mental Retardation*, *95*(4), 417–420.

Weinberg, A.G., Schiller, G., & Windmiller, J. (1982). Neonatal leukemoid reaction: An isolated manifestation of mosaic trisomy 21. *American Journal of Diseases of Children*, *136*, 310–311.

Weinberger, M.M., & Oleinick, A. (1971). Neonatal polycythemia. *Clinical Research*, *29*, 209–213.

Weinblatt, M.E., Higgins, G., & Ortega, J.A. (1981). Aplastic anemia in Down's syndrome. *Pediatrics*, *67*(6), 896–897.

Weinstein, H.J. (1978). Congenital leukemia and the neonatal myeloproliferative syndrome associated with Down's syndrome. *Clinical Haematology*, *7*, 147–154.

Wilson, M.G., Schroeder, W.A., & Graves, D.A. (1968). Postnatal change of hemoglobins F and A_2 in infants with Down's syndrome (G trisomy). *Pediatrics*, *42*(2), 349–353.

Wong, K.Y., Jones, M.M., Srivastava, A.K., & Gruppo, R.A. (1988). Transient myeloproliferative disorder and acute nonlymphoblastic leukemia in Down syndrome. *Journal of Pediatrics*, *112*, 18–22.

Zipursky, A., Peeters, M., & Poon, A. (1987). Megakaryoblastic leukemia and Down's syndrome—A review. In E.E. McCoy & C.J. Epstein (Eds.), *Oncology and immunology of Down syndrome* (pp. 33–56). New York: Alan R. Liss.

CHAPTER 22

Endocrinologic Aspects

Siegfried M. Pueschel and Jo-Ann Blaymore Bier

There were times when Down syndrome was thought to be due to a generalized endocrine disturbance (Benda, 1946). During postmortem examinations, Benda (1946) observed that almost every endocrine gland of the individual with Down syndrome displayed pathologic findings. Because of the observed endocrinologic disturbances, the short stature, and the small hands and feet, Benda (1946) coined the term *congenital acromicria* in analogy to *acromegaly*. Although Benda's (1946) studies never were duplicated, based on his investigations, treatment with pituitary extract and thyroid hormone was advocated and many individuals received these hormonal treatments in the 1940s, 1950s, and 1960s.

During the past few decades, it has been discovered that the majority of persons with Down syndrome do not have significant endocrine disturbances and that the previously recommended hormone therapy for all persons with Down syndrome is not necessary. However, some individuals with Down syndrome have endocrine deficiencies, and those individuals, of course, need specific treatment.

This chapter focuses on hypothalamic-releasing hormones, various hormones produced in the pituitary, and endorgan hormonal functions.

PITUITARY GLAND

Only a few studies on pituitary function in persons with Down syndrome have been reported. Benda and Bixby (1939) found the pituitary gland of persons with Down syndrome to be underdeveloped and to lack secretory cells. In ad-

dition, Benda (1969) observed a reduced number of chromophobic cells and an accumulation of eosinophilic granules and basophilic elements in some areas of the pituitary gland.

According to Schmid (1976), the aberrant development of the central nervous system of children with Down syndrome inevitably will influence the neurosecretory elements in the hypothalamus, with secondary effects on the pituitary gland. Wisniewski, Torrado, and Castello (1989) reported that children with Down syndrome have both anatomic and biochemical derangement of their central nervous system, which also involves the hypothalamus. Moreover, Elroy-Stein and Groner (1988) indicated that neurotransmitter uptake plays an important role in many processes of the central nervous system and that impaired neurotransmitter transport and uptake may in part explain the hypothalamic dysfunction in persons with Down syndrome, which in turn may adversely affect pituitary hormone production.

Growth Hormone

Growth hormone secretion in children with Down syndrome has been studied by several investigators. Milunsky, Lowy, Rubenstein, and Wright (1968) examined carbohydrate tolerance, growth hormone, and insulin levels in children with Down syndrome. They reported normal peaks of plasma growth hormone after insulin-induced hypoglycemia in 7 children with Down syndrome. Pozsony and Friesen (1971) investigated growth hormone secretion after insulin-induced hypoglycemia and arginine infusion in 73 children with a variety of disorders affecting both mental development and physical growth, including 12 children with Down syndrome. One of 4 children in whom growth hormone production was deficient was a 15-year-old girl with Down syndrome whose maximum growth hormone levels after insulin-induced hypoglycemia and arginine stimulation were 4.1 and 2.2 μg/mL, respectively. The growth hormone levels of the remaining 11 children with Down syndrome were normal.

Since synthetic growth hormone became available, several investigators have administered growth hormone to children with Down syndrome. Annerén, Sara, Hall, and Tuvemo (1986) treated 3 girls and 2 boys with Down syndrome with synthetic growth hormone in 6 months. During this time period, the growth velocity doubled and the serum insulin-like growth factor-I levels were restored to normal. Another group of investigators (Wisniewski et al., 1989) reported that growth-retarded children with Down syndrome displayed reduced growth hormone secretion. Subsequent to growth hormone administration, these investigators noted a significant gain in height and head circumference. Pueschel (in press) studied 8 children with Down syndrome with regard to their serum growth hormone levels after L-dopa, clonidine, and growth hormone–releasing factor administration. There was a better response after growth hormone–releasing factor than after L-dopa and clonidine had been given to the children. All children were able to secrete some growth hormone at least during one of the stimulation tests; however, most of the children displayed a reduced or modified response, which also had been observed by Wisniewski et al. (1989).

Corticotropin

Murdoch, Giles, Grant, and Ratcliffe (1979) investigated the hypothalamic-pituitary-adrenocortical function in adults with Down syndrome. They injected synacthen in 19 adults 20–52 years of age and measured their plasma cortisone levels 30 minutes later. The mean peak rise at 30 minutes after synacthen administration was significantly lower in the study group than in the control group, although there was no difference in the basal cortisone levels. The authors concluded that these patients displayed primary adrenal hypofunction. However, since their basal cortisone levels were normal and the corticotropin levels were not significantly elevated, the degree of adrenal hypofunction was relatively modest.

Thyroid-Stimulating Hormone

Murdoch, Gray, McLarty, and Ratcliffe (1978) investigated the pituitary function in 8 males and 8 females with Down syndrome whose ages ranged from 19 to 51 years. According to the authors, these individuals were suspected of having hypothyroidism secondary to pituitary deficiency. Aldenhoff, Waldenmaier, Zabransky, and Helge (1977) studied the response to thyrotropin-releasing hormone in 121 persons with Down syndrome. The authors observed that 101 persons had normal, 11 had increased, and 9 had significantly decreased thyroid-stimulating hormone levels after thyrotropin-releasing hormone stimulation. Another group of investigators (Pozzan et al., 1990) studied thyroid function of 108 home-reared individuals with Down syndrome. They found that 33 of the 108 had high thyroid-stimulating hormone levels with an exaggerated response to thyrotropin-releasing hormone. Also, Sharav, Landau, Zadik, and Einarson (1991) observed in 14 of 47 children with Down syndrome an exaggerated thyroid-stimulating hormone response to thyrotropin-releasing hormone administration. The mean basal thyroid-stimulating hormone levels of individuals with Down syndrome were significantly higher than those of controls for all ages, even though there was a decline in thyroid-stimulating hormone levels in both groups. The authors reported that peak thyroid-stimulating hormone response levels were significantly greater in persons with Down syndrome than in controls. They followed longitudinally 14 children with Down syndrome who had an exaggerated thyroid-stimulating hormone response. It was observed that the response remained exaggerated until the 3rd year of life when it declined to normal levels. The authors suggested that this exaggerated response in the first few years may be due to thyroid dysfunction during the growth spurt of infancy or due to late maturation of the hypothalamic-pituitary-thyroid axis.

Gonadotropin Hormones

In 1978, Horan, Beitins, and Bode reported that baseline follicle-stimulating hormone and luteinizing hormone levels in men with Down syndrome are significantly higher than in controls. Also, Campbell, Lowther, McKenzie, and Price (1982) as well as Hasen, Boyar, and Shapiro (1980) observed elevated levels of follicle-stimulating hormone and luteinizing hormone in males with Down syndrome. In contrast, Pueschel, Orson, Boylan, and Pezzullo (1985) noted lower mean levels of follicle-stimulating hormone and luteinizing hormone of persons with Down syndrome in Tanner stages I and II when compared with normative data. The increase of these hormones from Tanner stage II to Tanner stages III and IV and the decrease from Tanner stage IV to Tanner stage V observed in the study population paralleled the hormonal data reported for normal adolescents during sexual maturation.

The investigation of pituitary hormones of female adolescents also revealed normal concentrations of follicle-stimulating hormone and luteinizing hormone compared with a control population (Pueschel, 1988). The rise of follicle-stimulating hormone and luteinizing hormone during sexual maturation that is ordinarily observed in young females without Down syndrome was also noted in the study population (Pueschel, 1988).

The discrepancy between Pueschel's (1988) studies and previous reports may be due to the fact that other investigators' subjects primarily resided in institutions (it is well known that biologic measurements in institutionalized persons may vary considerably from those individuals living in the community). Moreover, the subjects who were participating in previous studies were older than Pueschel's (1988) patients, which may have contributed in part to the high follicle-stimulating hormone and luteinizing hormone levels. Since senescence is observed at an earlier age in persons with Down syndrome, it is conceivable that the accompanying testicular failure, including germinal cell hypoplasia and decreased Leydig cell function, in these older individuals with Down syndrome may have been responsible for the observed high gonadotropin hormone levels.

ADRENAL GLAND

In contrast to Hirning and Farber (1934), who found a normal appearance of the adrenal cortex of persons with Down syndrome, Benda (1969) observed that the fetal cortex of the adrenal gland in some instances was involuted. Benda (1969) also reported that in older children and adults, the adrenal cortex remained at an infantile level with very little postnatal growth. The zona fasciculata was narrow with considerable degeneration and the zona reticularis varied in size with noticeable fibrosis and hypertrophy. The juxtamedullary zone showed the most startling observation with a broadened area between the zona fasciculata and the zona reticularis that was equal to that of the combined two outer layers. Benda's (1969) histologic investigations have never been replicated.

Whereas Sandrucci and Picotti (1957) reported adrenal deficiency in 50% of individuals with Down syndrome based on 17-ketosteroid and 11-hydroxycorticosteroid urine excretions and the eosinophil response to corticotropin administration, other investigators (Dutton, 1959; O'Sullivan, Reddy, & Farrell, 1961) noted relatively normal adrenal function in persons with Down syndrome. Dutton studied the excretion of neutral 17-ketosteroids and 17-ketogenic steroids in the urine of children with Down syndrome. There was no significant difference in the excretion of these steroids when the Down syndrome group was compared with a control group. Similarly, O'Sullivan et al. (1961), who examined the 17-hydroxycorticosteroid excretion in response to intravenous corticotropin, found essentially normal adrenal function in persons with Down syndrome. Also, Murdoch et al. (1979) did not observe any significant difference in the basal morning plasma cortisone levels between persons with Down syndrome and an age- and sex-matched control group.

Most of the studies on adrenal function of persons with Down syndrome were performed decades ago and are often contradictory. Therefore, new, well-controlled investigations of adrenal functions should be forthcoming.

GONADS

A review of the literature on the subject of gonads in persons with Down syndrome revealed that most reports published prior to 1970 originated from studies carried out in institutions for persons with mental retardation. This needs to be taken into consideration when data from that era are compared with results from more recent investigations.

Male Genitalia

Benda (1969) reported that aberrant sex organ development is common in both males and females with Down syndrome. He indicated that in more than half of the males the testes are either bilaterally or unilaterally undescended and that the scrotum and penis are underdeveloped. Histologically, his examinations noted lack of spermatogenic cells, small seminiferous tubules filled with Sertoli cells, and coarse strands of fibrous tissues separating the tubules (Benda, 1969). Öster (1953) found unilateral or bilateral cryptorchidism (failure of testis to descend) in 27% of his study population. Hanhart (1960) is the only author who reported increased size of genitalia, whereas most other investigators observed the penis and scrotum of males with Down syndrome to be hypoplastic (Schmid, 1976). Also, Rundle and Sylvester (1962) measured the size of testes in 35 adult males with Down syndrome and found them to be significantly reduced in size when compared with those of the control group of males with mental retardation of other etiologies. Stearns, Droulard, and Sahhar (1960) reported reduced sperm counts in semen of men with Down syndrome and Benda (1969) noted a lack of mature sperm cells in 9 older men with Down syndrome.

Investigations on meiosis and spermatogenesis in males with Down syndrome were carried out by Kjessler and de la Chapelle (1971), as well as by Schröder, Lyndecken, and de la Chapelle (1971). These investigators indicated that the extra chromosome may be part of either a trivalent or univalent. Spermatogenic arrest has been reported by Finch, Böök, Finley, Finley, and Tucker (1966), Miller, Mittwoch, and Penrose (1960), and Sasaki (1965). In contrast, Kjessler and de la Chapelle (1971) as well as Schröder et al. (1971) did not observe spermatogenic arrest. The latter investigators reported spermatogenesis, although a decrease in quantity of sperm was noted. On the basis of testicular histology, these researchers could not consider individuals with Down syndrome to be sterile.

Johannisson et al. (1983) investigated the testicular histology in meiosis using both light and electron microscopy in young men with Down syndrome. The electron microscopic studies showed that in most nuclei an extra chromosome 21 was not detectable in the pachytene stage. Univalents or trivalents with segmental pairing structures of an extra chromosome were seen in only a small number of nuclei. In contrast, the great majority of diakinesis figures showed the presence of a supernumerary chromosome 21. The authors concluded that the impairment of fertility or presence of sterility in most individuals with Down syndrome is the effect of the trisomy 21 condition on spermatogenesis and is a consequence of the behavior of the extra chromosome in the meiotic prophase.

Whereas previously it was felt that all males with Down syndrome were infertile, a recent publication by Sheridan Llerena, Natkins, and Debenham (1989) indicated that a person with Down syndrome had fathered a child. This is the first report of confirmed paternity in a male with Down syndrome.

In a study of adolescent development in males with Down syndrome, Pueschel et al. (1985) reported the development of primary and secondary sex characteristics in 45 individuals. These authors observed that the pubic hair development did not differ significantly from that reported in "normal" adolescent males. Young maturing males with Down syndrome initially have darkening of the villous hair at the base of the penis, then hair growth is observed at the groin regions, the mons pubis, the adjacent portion of the lower abdominal wall, and later often extending to the umbilical area, forming the typical male pubic hair pattern. Also, Hsiang, Berkovitz, Bland, Migeon, and Warren (1987) observed that the age of onset and completion of puberty were normal in young men with Down syndrome.

When the size of the genitalia of the males in Pueschel et al.'s (1985) study was contrasted with that of an age-matched "normal" population, there was no statistically significant difference. The testes of Pueschel et al.'s (1985) study population were slightly, but not significantly, larger than reported in a "normal" population (Scholfeld, 1943). This contradicts Benda's (1969) as well as Rundle and Sylvester's (1962) results describing decreased testicular size in males with Down syndrome. The mean penile length of the males with Down syndrome was less and the penile circumference was slightly increased; however, these differences were not statistically significant (Pueschel et al., 1985). Hsiang et al. (1987), however, found the penile length and the mean testicular volume to be significantly below the mean value of "normal" men.

Pueschel et al. (1985) reported serum testosterone levels of adolescents with Down syndrome to be normal. They increased with advancing age, similar to the rise observed in "normal" adolescents (Alsever & Gotlin, 1978). Also, Hsiang et al. (1987) observed normal plasma testosterone levels in males with Down syndrome. A high positive correlation was found between serum hormone concentrations and secondary sex characteristics in Pueschel et al.'s (1985) study population.

Thus, the latter investigations of biologic parameters and specific hormone levels in young maturing males with Down syndrome compared well with normative data obtained from the literature for individuals without Down syndrome (Pueschel et al., 1985). Although Pueschel et al.'s (1985) studies indicate that male adolescents with Down syndrome display normal sequential development of primary and secondary sex characteristics and their pituitary-gonadal axis appears to be intact, there are many unanswered questions relating to the adolescents' sexual function, sperm production, and fertility.

Female Genitalia

With regard to the ovaries of females with Down syndrome, Benda (1969) reported ovarian hypoplasia without activity of the germinal cells and a tendency toward persistence of follicular cysts. He observed a limited number of primordial Graafian follicles with increased degeneration surrounded by fibrous tissue. A study of follicular development in the ovaries of females with Down syndrome was conducted by Hojager, Peters, Byskov, and Faber (1978). These investigators found that all ovaries in females with Down syndrome were abnormal. Forty-two percent of the ovaries of females with Down syndrome were quiescent with small resting follicles and no follicular growth. In addition, the number as well as the size of the antral follicles of young females with Down syndrome differed from those in the normal ovary. The decrease of the number of small follicles occurred earlier in the life of the women with Down syndrome than in those without this chromosome abnormality. Hojager et al. (1978) concluded that the occurrence of binuclear oocytes in small follicles in ovaries of young females with Down syndrome may suggest an endocrine imbalance.

The external genitalia of females with Down syndrome were described by Schmid (1976), who found the labia majora to be hypertrophic and the labia minora to be poorly developed. Bleyer (1937) also noted the oversized labia majora in adult females with Down syndrome; however, he also observed the labia minora to be frequently enlarged and protruding.

Reports by several investigators (Hasen et al., 1980; Hojager et al., 1978; Hsiang et al., 1987) have indicated that women with Down syndrome often have gonadal dysfunction. This has been difficult to reconcile with the following recent clinical observations: 1) occurrence of regular menstrual cycles in many females with Down syndrome, 2) normal levels of estradiol in females with Down syndrome, and 3) documentation of 31 pregnancies in 27 women with Down syndrome (Goldstein, 1988; Rani, Jyothi, Reddy, & Reddy, 1990; Scola & Pueschel, in press).

Öster (1953) reported the mean age of onset of

menstruation in girls with Down syndrome to be 13 years, 9 months, compared to 14 years, 9 months for the control group. In contrast, Benda (1969) mentioned that the menarche of girls with Down syndrome usually occurred at the end of the teen years. Bellone, Tanganelli, LaPlaca, and Daneri (1980) found that the menarche of young women with Down syndrome was at the average age of 13 years, 1 month—1 year later than in control women. In a recent study (Goldstein, 1988), the average age of menarche was 13.6 years for females with Down syndrome and 13.5 years for controls, with an average length of the menstrual cycles being 28.3 and 28.6 days, respectively.

Scola and Pueschel (in press) examined 51 females with Down syndrome over the age of 10 years and observed the average age of menarche of the 38 menstruating women to be 12 years, 6 months (range 10–16 years), whereas the 63 sisters (control group) had an average age of menarche of 12 years, 1 month (range 9–15 years). Of the 13 girls who had never menstruated, 11 were still under the age of 13 years and the remaining 2 were 14 and 26 years of age, respectively. Regular menstrual cycles were reported in 29 of the postmenarcheal females. The lengths of their menstrual cycles varied from 22 to 33 days with the average length of menstrual flow being 4 days. There was average amount of flow in 22, heavy flow in 5, and light flow in 2. Of the 29 young women with regular menstrual cycles, the parents of 16 of them reported that their daughters understood the monthly cyclic nature of menstruation, but only 4 of these parents considered their daughters to be aware of the relationship between menstruation and reproduction (Scola & Pueschel, in press).

In order to assess ovarian function, Tricomi, Valenti, and Hall (1964) examined 13 women with Down syndrome and found evidence of normal ovarian function in 5, possibly adequate ovarian function in 4, and abnormal vaginal smears in the remaining 4. Scola and Pueschel (in press) studied the basal body temperature in 8 women with Down syndrome who had established regular menstrual cycles. Twenty-six basal body temperature curve charts from these 8 women revealed that 23 were clearly biphasic,

2 were possibly biphasic, and 1 had a nonbiphasic menstrual cycle. The 23 biphasic menstrual cycles ranged from 15 to 30 days, with a mean of 25 days, and the length of menstrual flow was 2–6 days, with a mean of 4 days. All 8 women with Down syndrome in this study had at least two biphasic cycles. The preovulatory phase had a mean of 14 days, with a range of 8–21 days, and the postovulatory phase had a mean of 11 days, with a range of 7–15 days (Scola & Pueschel, in press). Thus, the menstrual histories obtained from the study group suggest that many young women with Down syndrome have regular menstrual cycles and the onset of menstruation is at a similar age as other girls who do not have Down syndrome. In addition, the biphasic nature of basal body temperature curves provides presumptive evidence of ovulation in the majority of the menstrual cycles reported (Scola & Pueschel, in press).

There is ample evidence in the literature that some females with Down syndrome are able to reproduce. Pogue (1917) was the first to report that women with Down syndrome were capable of bearing children. As mentioned, a more recent report (Rani et al., 1990) described that 31 pregnancies have occurred so far in 27 women with Down syndrome.

Although earlier reports (Benda, 1969; Hasen et al., 1980; Hojager et al., 1978) indicated hypogonadism and/or ovarian dysfunction in women with Down syndrome, recent investigations (Scola & Pueschel, in press) and a review of reproduction in persons with Down syndrome (Rani et al., 1990) have suggested that there are numerous females with this chromosome disorder who have adequate ovarian function. Since most individuals with Down syndrome now live in the community—with all of the attendant opportunities, freedoms, and risks—it is paramount that further studies concerning sexual development, endocrine concerns, and biologic maturation of the young person with Down syndrome be pursued.

THYROID GLAND

There is a voluminous literature on thyroid abnormalities in persons with Down syndrome.

Whereas a previous review of this subject discussed the results of investigations on thyroid function carried out prior to 1980 (Pueschel et al., 1982), the discussion in this chapter primarily focuses on thyroid dysfunction in individuals with Down syndrome that have been reported since 1977 (Cutler, Benezra-Obeiter, & Brink, 1986; Dinani & Carpenter, 1990; Friedman, Kastner, Pond, & Rice O'Brien, 1989; Lobo, Khan, & Tew, 1980; Murdoch, Ratcliffe, McLarty, Rodger, & Ratcliffe, 1977; Pueschel, Jackson, Giesswein, Dean, & Pezzullo, 1991; Pueschel & Pezzullo, 1985; Quinn, 1980; Vladutiu, Chun, Victor, Gienau, & Bannerman, 1984). The abnormality most commonly found and the one most extensively studied is hypothyroidism (Dinani & Carpenter, 1990; Mani, 1988; Pueschel & Pezzullo, 1985; D.S. Smith, 1988; Tirosh, Taub, Scher, Jaffe, & Hachberg, 1989). The frequency of general thyroid dysfunction in individuals with Down syndrome has been reported to range from 2% to 63% (Friedman et al., 1989) and the prevalence of hypothyroidism in adults with Down syndrome has been found to range from 13% to 54% (D.S. Smith, 1988).

Prevalence of Hypothyroidism

In 1977, Murdoch et al. examined thyroid function in 82 institutionalized adults with Down syndrome and compared them to age- and sex-matched control individuals. They found that adults with Down syndrome had a significantly lower total serum thyroxine level, a lower mean total triiodothyronine level, a lower free thyroxine index, and a higher baseline thyrotropin concentration. Forty-six percent of the 82 adults tested had abnormalities in one or more of the parameters tested. In 1980, Quinn examined 49 persons with Down syndrome for evidence of thyroid dysfunction and observed a statistically increased number of thyroid abnormalities among the individuals with Down syndrome compared to age- and sex-matched controls. Pueschel and Pezzullo studied 151 individuals with Down syndrome in 1985. The thyroid function tests in this group were compared with those of the siblings of these patients. They found that although the mean thyroxine levels did not differ

between the two groups, there was a significant difference in the mean thyrotropin values with the higher values found in the individuals with Down syndrome. Twenty-one percent of individuals with Down syndrome were noted to have a significant increase in their thyrotropin levels.

Kinnell, Gibbs, Teale, and Smith (1987) performed thyroid function tests on 111 institutionalized individuals with Down syndrome. These investigators observed a lower rate of hypothyroidism (9%) in the Down syndrome group as compared to other studies. In 1988, Mani examined the thyroid function of 55 adults with Down syndrome, 12 of whom had some degree of hypothyroidism, resulting in a prevalence rate of 20%. In 1989, Friedman et al. studied 138 individuals with Down syndrome who were living in the community. Twenty-eight of them (20.3%) were noted to have previously unrecognized hypothyroidism. The prevalence of thyroid disorders in individuals with Down syndrome was also investigated in 1990 by Dinani and Carpenter. This study involved 106 adults with Down syndrome (61 male and 45 female) whose average age was 38 years. Abnormal thyroid function tests were found in 40.5% of these individuals; 6% had been diagnosed prior to the study. In a recent report by Percy et al. (1990), the results of thyroid function studies were compared among individuals with Down syndrome who had clinical manifestations of Alzheimer disease as well as with those without Alzheimer disease. Individuals with Down syndrome were noted to have decreased thyroxine and triiodothyronine and increased thyrotropin levels when compared with controls. Pueschel et al. (1991) examined 181 persons with Down syndrome and compared them with 163 control subjects regarding their thyroid function. Sixteen percent (29 of 181) were noted to have some degree of hypothyroidism. The mean thyroxine levels were significantly lower and the triiodothyronine and thyrotropin levels were significantly higher in the study group when compared to the control group.

Age and Sex Influences

The extent to which the age and sex of individuals with Down syndrome influence thyroid function and the potential risk of hypothyroidism has also been investigated. In Mani's (1988) study, 11 of the 12 persons who were diagnosed with hypothyroidism were over 40 years of age and their mean thyroxine and triiodothyronine values were lower when compared to those who were less than 40 years of age. Pueschel and Pezzullo's (1985) results indicated a trend for higher thyrotropin values to occur with advancing age. In a subsequent study, Pueschel et al. (1991) demonstrated a decline of thyroxine and triiodothyronine with increasing age.

Pueschel and Pezzullo (1985) found a significantly higher thyroxine level in the males than in the females. In contrast, Friedman et al. (1989) noted that 78.5% of the individuals in their study with hypothyroidism were females. They confirmed the fact that age seemed to be a risk factor in that most of the individuals diagnosed were between 30 and 50 years of age.

Clinical Features

The difficulty in clinically diagnosing hypothyroidism in individuals with Down syndrome is well known (Criscuolo, Perone, Sinisi, Bellastella, & Fagginio, 1986; Dinani & Carpenter, 1990). The clinical features of untreated congenital hypothyroidism, which overlap to some degree with characteristics of Down syndrome, include short stature, the possibility of a lower activity level, a coarser voice, and dry and rough skin as well as the tendency to gain weight. In Mani's (1988) study, 55 adults were screened for clinical symptoms of hypothyroidism including lethargy, intolerance to cold, coarseness of voice, slowing of motor activity and intellectual functioning, dryness and/or loss of hair, menstrual disturbances, bradycardia, and periorbital edema. The results showed that 7 of the 55 adults had clinical features suggestive of hypothyroidism. Not all of the 7 individuals, however, had abnormal thyroid function tests and, conversely, many of the individuals who had abnormal thyroid function tests did not have clinical features of hypothyroidism. Murdoch et al.'s (1977) study results also showed that clinical features were not a reliable marker in predicting individuals with hypothyroidism. Of 83 patients who

were suspected of having hypothyroidism based on clinical evidence alone, only 1 really did.

Autoimmunity

An autoimmune process as the main etiologic factor causing hypothyroidism in individuals with Down syndrome has been studied extensively (Friedman et al., 1989; Kinnell et al., 1987; Mani, 1988; Murdoch et al., 1977; Pueschel & Pezzullo, 1985; Quinn, 1980). In a review of the literature, Schindler (1989) reported that the prevalence of autoimmune thyroiditis, which is the most common cause of acquired hypothyroidism, is about 30 times higher in individuals with Down syndrome than in the general population. Of 13 individuals studied by Murdoch et al. (1977) in whom thyrotropin-releasing hormone administration showed an exaggerated thyrotropin response, there were 7 (54%) individuals who had thyroid autoantibodies. Lobo et al. (1980) examined the thyroid function of 101 persons with Down syndrome and found that 29% of them had thyroid autoantibodies. Vladutiu et al. (1984) detected thyroid autoantibodies in 16 of 42 (38%) individuals with Down syndrome. Five of the 16 had both thyroglobulin and microsomal autoantibodies, whereas 4 had only thyroglobulin autoantibodies and 7 had only microsomal autoantibodies. It is of note that 5 of 16 patients who had thyroid autoantibodies did not show biochemical evidence of hypothyroidism. Pueschel and Pezzullo (1985) found a significant positive correlation between increased thyrotropin and antimicrosomal antibodies as well as between decreased thyroxine levels and antimicrosomal antibodies. These results suggest that individuals with Down syndrome who have hypothyroidism may have had Hashimoto thyroiditis. It should also be noted, however, that Pueschel and Pezzullo's (1985) results indicated that over half of the individuals who had increased thyrotropin levels did not have an increase in antithyroglobulin or antimicrosomal antibody titers.

Loudon, Day, and Duke (1985) noted that of a total of 116 children, 8 had positive thyroglobulin antibodies and 26 displayed positive microsomal antibodies. Thus, 29% of the entire group had a high titer of at least one of these anti-bodies, whereas only 0%–7% of "normal" children had such antibody titers. The youngest child who had positive thyroid autoantibody titers was 5 years of age, and 20% of children under 10 years of age in this study were found to have positive thyroid autoantibodies. The authors commented that children with Down syndrome have a higher prevalence of thymus-dependent immunologic abnormalities when compared to the general population.

Kinnell et al. (1987) observed thyroid microsomal antibodies present in 29% of 111 institutionalized adults with Down syndrome. Mani's (1988) data support the high prevalence of autoimmune processes in individuals with Down syndrome as 48 of 55 adults screened were found to have increased thyroid cytoplasmic antibodies. Twenty-eight of these persons had enough clinical symptoms to justify thyroid function testing, and it was found that 12 of them had some degree of hypothyroidism. In Friedman et al.'s (1989) study of 66 persons who were tested for thyroid autoantibodies, 26 were noted to have positive antimicrosomal and/or antithyroglobulin antibody titers. In Percy et al.'s (1990) study, antimicrosomal antibody titers were also found to be higher in persons with Down syndrome when compared to controls. Antithyroglobulin antibodies were significantly elevated in adults with Down syndrome without manifestations of Alzheimer disease whereas the antimicrosomal antibody titers were found to be increased in adults with Down syndrome who had Alzheimer disease.

Percy et al. (1990) suggested various theories of why people with Down syndrome have an increased prevalence of autoimmune thyroiditis. He felt that thyroid autoimmune abnormalities may be the result of a triple gene dosage for specific receptors or that there may be an association between particular HLA antigens and autoimmune thyroiditis. Other theories have centered around viral infections, endocrinologic disturbances, and the possibility of a triple gene dosage of superoxide dismutase, increasing the production of hydrogen peroxide. Percy et al. speculated that the latter process may result in an increase in antimicrosomal and antithyroglobulin antibodies as peroxide is a substrate for iodine peroxidases.

Compensated Hypothyroidism

The increased prevalence of compensated hypothyroidism in individuals with Down syndrome has been well documented (Criscuolo et al., 1986; Dinani & Carpenter, 1990; Napolitano et al., 1990; Percy et al., 1990; Pueschel et al., 1991). Compensated hypothyroidism is characterized by a normal or only slightly decreased level of thyroxine and/or triiodothyronine but a significantly higher than normal thyrotropin level and/or an exaggerated thyrotropin response to thyrotropin-releasing hormone. Criscuolo et al. studied 7 children with Down syndrome and although triiodothyronine, thyroxine, and thyrotropin values were normal, these children had a significantly elevated thyrotropin response to thyrotropin-releasing hormone administration. In Pueschel et al.'s (1991) study of 181 individuals with Down syndrome, it was found that 14 (8%) had an increased thyrotropin value but normal thyroxine and triiodothyronine levels. Percy et al. (1990) suggested that compensated hypothyroidism as well as autoimmune thyroiditis are more common in adults with Down syndrome who also have Alzheimer disease. Dinani and Carpenter (1990) observed among 106 individuals with Down syndrome that 6% had normal thyroxine levels but increased thyrotropin concentrations.

In a recent study, Napolitano et al. (1990) investigated the possibility that compensated hypothyroidism was caused by a zinc deficiency. The hypothesis was based upon the fact that early thymic involution is associated with low serum zinc levels, since zinc supplementation had improved thymic function over a short time period. Because thymic function has been reported to be related to normal pituitary-thyroid function, it was felt that zinc treatment may possibly be effective in individuals who demonstrate compensated hypothyroidism. Seventeen patients receiving zinc therapy showed a subsequent decrease in free triiodothyronine; 9 of the 17 had low zinc levels as well as increased thyrotropin values. Zinc supplementation resulted in improved thyroid function.

The possible benefit of thyroid hormone supplementation for individuals with Down syndrome who have low borderline thyroid function was investigated by Tirosh et al. (1989). There was no difference between the thyroxine-treated and the nontreated persons with Down syndrome in this double-blind crossover placebo-controlled study with respect to cognitive performance, medical gains, and personal development.

In 1975, Schmidt et al. examined the prevalence of thyroid dysfunction in children with Down syndrome. The cohort for this study involved 29 noninstitutionalized children with Down syndrome whose ages ranged from 1 to 16 years. Triiodothyronine and thyroxine levels as well as captation of I 131 by the thyroid gland were measured 2 and 24 hours after administration of the I 131. When compared to their normal siblings, significant differences were found 2 hours after administration of I 131, but by 24 hours this difference was no longer present.

Additional studies of thyroid function in newborns, infants, and children have been conducted by Cutler et al. (1986) and Loudon et al. (1985). Loudon et al. (1985) tested 116 children with Down syndrome for biochemical evidence of thyroid dysfunction. The ages of these children ranged from 9 months to 19 years, 10 months. Three of the 116 children showed low thyroxine and increased thyrotropin levels, 1 child was described as being thyrotoxic, and 2 children were found to have low normal thyroxine values, but displayed an exaggerated response of thyrotropin to thyrotropin releasing hormone administration. There were no differences found between males and females.

In 1986, Cutler et al. reported on the thyroid function of 49 children with Down syndrome whose ages ranged from 4 months to 3 years. Of the 49 children, 3 had been diagnosed with congenital hypothyroidism, 2 of whom were found to have an absence of thyroid antibodies as well as a decreased thyroid uptake on radioactive scanning with I 131. The thyroid glands of all 3 of these children were found to be of normal size. Among the remaining 46 children, 1 child

had acquired hypothyroidism presenting at 15 months of age, with a 3-month history of symptoms including lethargy, decreased growth velocity, developmental delay, and constipation. These symptoms resolved after thyroid supplementation. Another child was found to have hyperthyroidism as well as weakly positive antimicrosomal antibodies. Twenty-seven percent (10) of the children displayed increased thyrotropin secretion and normal thyroxine values consistent with compensated hypothyroidism. However, 8 of these 10 were found to have normal thyrotropin values when thyroid function tests were repeated. Excluding the 5 children with definite thyroid dysfunction, there was no difference in mean thyroxine values between the remaining 44 children with Down syndrome and the age-matched control group. Yet, thyrotropin levels were significantly elevated in the infants with Down syndrome compared to age-matched controls. In another retrospective review of 147 children and young adults with Down syndrome whose ages ranged from 4 months to 27 years, it was found that 60% had increased thyrotropin levels (Sharav, Collins, & Baab, 1988). The increased thyrotropin values were found most often in children under 4 years of age and all of these children were noted to be growth retarded compared to "normal" control infants (Sharav et al., 1988).

Congenital Hypothyroidism

The incidence of congenital hypothyroidism in Cutler et al.'s (1986) study was 6% (3 of 49). This incidence figure derived from a select group of persons with Down syndrome differs from the results of a study investigating the incidence of congenital hypothyroidism during newborn screening (Fort et al., 1984). Of 945,000 newborns screened, 1,130 of them had Down syndrome. Of the latter group, 12 infants were positive for hypothyroidism shortly after birth. Follow-up testing of 11 infants confirmed the diagnosis of persistent primary congenital hypothyroidism in 8, and the remaining 3 were described as having transient congenital hypothyroidism. It is of note that the prevalence of persistent primary congenital hypothyroidism of

0.7% and that of transient congenital hypothyroidism of 0.3% is higher than that found in the general population (Fort et al., 1984).

Other Disorders
Associated with Hypothyroidism

The triad of Down syndrome, autoimmune hypothyroidism, and hypoparathyroidism was described by Blumberg and AvRuskin in 1987. Additional concomitant disorders reported in the literature include hypothyroidism and diabetes mellitus and hypothyroidism and precocious sexual development (Pueschel et al., 1985).

Hyperthyroidism

Although hypothyroidism is often seen in individuals with Down syndrome, hyperthyroidism has also been described to occur occasionally. The prevalence of hyperthyroidism in individuals with Down syndrome of 0.87–2.5% has been reported (Cutler et al., 1986; Friedman et al., 1989; Kinnell et al., 1987; Lobo et al., 1980). McCulloch, Clark, and Steele (1982) described a 35-year-old male with Down syndrome who had severe thyrotoxicosis.

CONCLUSION

Most persons with Down syndrome have normal hormone production and the pituitary-endorgan axis of most hormone systems appears to be within normal limits in most individuals. However, there are a number of persons with this chromosome disorder who display endocrinologic disturbances and there is a higher prevalence of specific endocrine disorders in persons with Down syndrome when compared with a "normal" population.

Because of the increased prevalence of thyroid dysfunction, this topic has been discussed in detail. It should be emphasized that if a thyroid disorder is not recognized early, it can further compromise the child's central nervous system function. Since clinical symptoms of hypothyroidism are sometimes interpreted as part of the Down syndrome "Gestalt," thyroid function studies including thyroxine, thyrotropin hormone, and others if indicated should be carried out at regular intervals. When a person with Down syndrome is found to have hypo- or hyperthyroidism, prompt specific treatment should be forthcoming. Optimal thyroid function then will allow normal intracellular processes to take place.

It is assumed that future research of hypothalamic-pituitary-endorgan relationships and other specific hormone investigations will provide us with a greater insight into the complexity of endocrine systems and their aberrations in persons with Down syndrome. In addition, molecular genetic studies may explain why some persons with Down syndrome are at a higher risk of specific hormone dysfunction.

REFERENCES

Aarskog, D. (1969). Autoimmune thyroid disease in children with mongolism. *Archives of Disease in Childhood, 44,* 454–460.

Aldenhoff, P., Waldenmaier, C., Zabransky, S., & Helge, H. (1977). Der TRH-Stimulationstest bei Kindern und Erwachsenen wit Down-syndrom [TRH stimulation in children and adults with Down syndrome]. *Monatsschrift für Kinderheilkunde, 125,* 544–545.

Alsever, R.N., & Gotlin, R.W. (1978). *Handbook of endocrine tests in adults and children.* Chicago: Yearbook Medical Publishers.

Anneren, G., Sara, V.R., Hall, K., & Tuvemo, T. (1986). Growth and somatomedin responses to growth hormone in Down's syndrome. *Archives of Disease in Childhood, 61,* 48–52.

Azizi, F., Chandler, H., Bozorgzadeh, H., & Braverman, L.E. (1974). The occurrence of hyperthyroidism in patients with Down's syndrome. *Johns Hopkins Medical Journal, 134,* 303–306.

Bastedo, D.L.A. (1961). Coexistence of Albright's syndrome and mongolism. *Canadian Medical Association Journal, 84,* 1135–1138.

Bellone, F., Tanganelli, E., LaPlaca, A., & Daneri, C. (1980). Menarca e fisiopatologia menstruale nella sindrome di Down [Menarche and the pathophysiologic aspects of the menstrual cycle in Down syndrome]. *Minerva Ginecologica, 32,* 579–588.

Benda, C.E. (1946). *Mongolism and cretinism.* New York: Grune & Stratton.

Benda, C.E. (1969). *Down's syndrome: Mongolism and its management.* New York: Grune & Stratton.

Benda, C.E., & Bixby, E.M. (1939). Function of the thyroid and the pituitary in mongolism, with a report on the blood groups of American mongoloid defectives and comments on the determination of cholesterol. *American Journal of Diseases of Children, 58,* 1240–1255.

Bhattacharjee, S. (1975). Hyperparathyroidism associated with mongoloid features and atrial septal defect. *Journal of the Indian Medical Association, 44,* 437–438.

Bleyer, A. (1937). Theoretical and clinical aspects of mongolism. *Journal of the Missouri Medical Association, 34,* 222–231.

Blumberg, D., & AvRuskin, T. (1987). Down's syndrome, autoimmune hypothyroidism, and hypoparathyroidism: A unique triad. *American Journal of Diseases of Children, 141,* 1149–1153.

Bock, J.E. (1974). The hypothalmic-pituitary-gonadal and adrenal cortical function in adult women with Down's syndrome. *Acta Obstetrica Gynecologica Scandinavica Supplement, 29,* 69–72.

Campbell, W.A., Lowther, J., McKenzie, I., & Price, W.H.. (1982). Serum gonadotrophins in Down's syndrome. *Journal of Medical Genetics, 19,* 98–99.

Clover, T. (1960). Thyrotoxicosis in a mongoloid child. *American Journal of Diseases of Children, 100,* 950–954.

Criscuolo, T., Perone, L., Sinisi, A.A., Bellastella, A., & Fagginio, M. (1986). Subclinical hypothyroidism in children with Down syndrome. *Minerva Endocrinologica, 11,* 169–171.

Cutler, A.T., Benezra-Obeiter, R., & Brink, S.J. (1986). Thyroid function in young children with Down syndrome. *American Journal of Diseases of Children, 140,* 479–483.

Dallaire, L., & Kingsmill-Flynn, D. (1967). Frequency of antibodies to thyroglobulin in relation to gravidity and to Down's syndrome. *Canadian Medical Association Journal, 97,* 209–212.

Daniels, D.M., & Simon, J.L. (1968). Down's syndrome, hypothyroidism, and diabetes mellitus. *Journal of Pediatrics, 72,* 697–699.

Dinani, S., & Carpenter, S. (1990). Down syndrome and thyroid disorder. *Journal of Mental Deficiency Research, 34,* 187–193.

Dutton, G. (1959). The physical development of mongols. *Archives of Disease in Childhood, 34,* 46–50.

Elroy-Stein, O., & Groner, Y. (1988). Impaired neurotransmitter uptake in PC12 cells overexpressing human Cu/Zn-superoxide dismutase implication for gene dosage effects in Down syndrome. *Cell, 52,* 259–267.

Finch, R.A., Böök, J.A., Finley, W.H., Finley, S.C., & Tucker, C.C. (1966). Meiosis in trisomic Down's syndrome. *Alabama Journal of Medical Science, 3,* 117–125.

Fort, P., Lifshitz, F., Bellisario, R., Davis, J., Lanes, R., Pugliese, M., Richman, R., Post, E.M., & David, R. (1984). Abnormalities of thyroid function in infants with Down syndrome. *Journal of Pediatrics, 104,* 545–549.

Friedman, D.L., Kastner, T., Pond, W.S., & Rice O'Brien, D. (1989). Thyroid dysfunction in individuals with Down syndrome. *Archives of Internal Medicine, 149,* 1990–1993.

Goldstein, H. (1988). Menarche, menstruation, sexual relations and contraception of adolescent females with Down syndrome. *European Journal of Obstetrics, Gynecology and Reproductive Biology, 27,* 343–349.

Hanhart, E. (1960). 800 Fälle von Mongoloidismus in konstitutioneller Betrachtung [The physical description of 800 cases of mongolism]. *Archiv der Julius Klaus-Stiftung, Vererbungsforschung, Sozialanthropologie und Rassenhygiene, 35,* 1–12.

Hasen, J. (1974). Endocrine studies in a patient with a G-21 trisomy. *Steroids Lipids Research, 5,* 179–184.

Hasen, J., Boyar, R.M., & Shapiro, L.R. (1980). Gonadal function in trisomy 21. *Hormone Research, 12,* 345–350.

Hirning, L.C., & Farber, S. (1934). A histological study of the adrenal cortex in mongolism. *American Journal of Pathology, 10,* 435–442.

Hojager, B., Peters, H., Byskov, A.G., & Faber, M. (1978). Follicular development in ovaries of children with Down's syndrome. *Acta Paediatrica Scandinavica, 67,* 637–643.

Horan, R.F., Beitins, I.Z., & Bode, H.H. (1978). LH-RH testing in men with Down's syndrome. *Acta Endocrinologica, 88,* 594–600.

Hsiang, Y.H., Berkovitz, G.D., Bland, G.L., Migeon, C.J., & Warren, A.C. (1987). Gonadal function in patients with Down syndrome. *American Journal of Medical Genetics, 27,* 449–458.

Hubble, D. (1963). Precocious menstruation in a mongoloid child with hypothyroidism-hormonal overlap. *Journal of Clinical Endocrinology, 23,* 1302–1305.

Johannisson, R., Gropp, A., Winking, H., Coerdt, W., Rheder, H., & Schwinger, E. (1983). Down's syndrome in the male. Reproductive pathology and meiotic studies. *Human Genetics, 63,* 132–138.

Kinnell, H.G., Gibbs, N., Teale, J.D., & Smith, J. (1987). Thyroid dysfunction in institutionalized Down syndrome adults. *Psychological Medicine, 17,* 387–392.

Kjessler, B., & de la Chapelle, A. (1971). Meiosis and spermatogenesis in two postpubertal males with Down's syndrome: 47,XY,G+. *Clinical Genetics, 2,* 50–57.

Lobo, E.D., Khan, M., & Tew, J. (1980). Community study of hypothyroidism in Down syndrome. *British Medical Journal, 24,* 1253–1255.

Loudon, M.M., Day, R.E., & Duke, E.M.C. (1985).

Thyroid dysfunction in Down syndrome. *Archives of Disease in Childhood, 60,* 1149–1151.

Mani, C. (1988). Hypothyroidism in Down syndrome. *British Journal of Psychiatry, 153,* 102–104.

McCulloch, A.J., Clark, F., & Steele, N.R. (1982). Graves' disease and Down's syndrome. *Journal of Medical Genetics, 20,* 133–134.

Miller, O.J., Mittwoch, U., & Penrose, L.S. (1960). Spermatogenesis in man with special reference to aneuploidy. *Heredity, 14,* 456–461.

Milunsky, A., Lowy, C., Rubenstein, A.G., & Wright, A.D. (1968). Carbohydrate tolerance, growth hormone, and insulin levels in mongolism. *Developmental Medicine and Child Neurology, 10,* 25–31.

Milunsky, A., & Neurath, P.W. (1968). Diabetes mellitus in Down's syndrome. *Archives of Environmental Health, 17,* 372–378.

Murdoch, J.C., Giles, C.A., Grant, J.K., & Ratcliffe, J.G. (1979). Hypothalamic-pituitary-adreno-cortical function in adults with Down syndrome. *Journal of Mental Deficiency Research, 23,* 157–162.

Murdoch, J.C., Gray, C.A., McLarty, D.G., & Ratcliffe, J.G. (1978). Pituitary function in Down syndrome. *Journal of Mental Deficiency Research, 22,* 273–276.

Murdoch, J.C., Ratcliffe, W.A., McLarty, J.C., Rodger, J.C., & Ratcliffe, J.G. (1977). Thyroid function in adults with Down syndrome. *Journal of Clinical Endocrinology and Metabolism, 44,* 153–158.

Napolitano, G., Palk, G., Lio, S., Bucci, I., De-Remigis, P., Stuppia, L., & Monaco, F. (1990). Is zinc deficiency a cause of subclinical hypothyroidism in Down syndrome? *Annales de Genetique, 33,* 9–15.

O'Sullivan, J.B., Reddy, W.J., & Farrell, M.J. (1961). Adrenal function in mongolism. *American Journal of Diseases of Children, 101,* 37–40.

Öster, J. (1953). *Mongolism: A clinico-geneological investigation comprising 526 mongols living in Seeland and neighboring islands of Denmark.* Copenhagen: Danish Science Press.

Parkin, J.M. (1974). Down's syndrome, hypothyroidism, and diabetes mellitus [Letter]. *British Medical Journal, 2,* 384.

Percy, M.E., Dalton, A.J., Markowitz, V.D., Crapper-McLachlan, D.R., Gera, E., Hummel, J., Rusk, A.C.M., Somerville, M.J., Andrews, D.F., & Walfish, P.G. (1990). Autoimmune thyroiditis associated with mild "subclinical" hypothyroidism in adults with Down syndrome: A comparison of patients with and without manifestation of Alzheimer's disease. *American Journal of Medical Genetics, 36,* 148–154.

Pogue, M.E. (1917). A brief report of twenty-nine cases of mongolian idiocy, with special reference to the etiology from the standpoint of the clinical history with presentation of three cases. *Illinois Medical Journal, 32,* 296–302.

Pozsony, J., & Friesen, H. (1971). Growth hormone investigation in patients with mental dysfunction. *Canadian Medical Association Journal, 104,* 26–29.

Pozzan, G.B., Rigon, F., Girelli, M.E., Rubello, D., Busnardo, B., & Baccichetti, C. (1990). Thyroid function in patients with Down syndrome: Preliminary results from non-institutionalized patients in the Veneto region. *American Journal of Medical Genetics Supplement, 7,* 57–58.

Pueschel, S.M. (1988). The biology of the maturing person with Down syndrome. In S.M. Pueschel (Ed.), *The young person with Down syndrome: Transition from adolescence to adulthood* (pp. 23–34). Baltimore: Paul H. Brookes Publishing Co.

Pueschel, S.M. (in press). Growth hormone response after administration of L-dopa, clonidine, and growth hormone releasing factor in children with Down syndrome. *Journal of Mental Deficiency Research.*

Pueschel, S.M., Jackson, I.M.D., Giesswein, P., Dean, M.K., & Pezzullo, J.C. (1991). Thyroid function in Down syndrome. *Research in Developmental Disabilities, 12,* 287–296.

Pueschel, S.M., Orson, J.M., Boylan, J.M., & Pezzullo, J.C. (1985). Adolescent development in males with Down syndrome. *American Journal of Diseases of Children, 139,* 236–238.

Pueschel, S.M., & Pezzullo, J.C. (1985). Thyroid dysfunction in Down syndrome. *American Journal of Diseases of Children, 139,* 636–639.

Pueschel, S.M., Sassaman, E.A., Scola, P.S., Thuline, H.C., Stark, A.M., & Horrobin, M. (1982). Biomedical aspects in Down syndrome. In S.M. Pueschel & J.E. Rynders (Eds.), *Down syndrome: Advances in biomedicine and the behavioral sciences* (pp. 241–249). Cambridge, MA: Ware Press.

Quinn, M.W. (1980). Down syndrome and hypothyroidism. *Irish Journal of Medical Science, 149,* 19–22.

Rani, A.S., Jyothi, A., Reddy, P.P., & Reddy, O.S. (1990). Reproduction in Down's syndrome. *International Journal of Gynecology and Obstetrics, 31,* 81–86.

Rundle, A.T., & Sylvester, P.E. (1962). Endocrinological aspects of mental deficiency: II. Maturational status of adult males. *Journal of Mental Deficiency Research, 6,* 87–94.

Ruvalcaba, R.H., Ferrier, P.E., & Thuline, H.C. (1969). Incidence of goiter in patients with Down's syndrome. *American Journal of Diseases of Children, 118,* 451–453.

Sandrucci, M., & Picotti, M.L. (1957). The functional condition of the adrenal cortex in mongolism. *Minerva Pediatria, 9,* 1368–1374.

Sare, Z., Ruvalcaba, R.H., & Kelley, V.C. (1978).

Prevalence of thyroid disorder in Down syndrome. *Clinical Genetics, 14,* 154–158.

Sasaki, M. (1965). Meiosis in a male with Down's syndrome. *Chromosoma, 16,* 652–657.

Schindler, S. (1989). Hypothyroidism in a child with Down syndrome. *Hospital Practice, 24,* 231–232.

Schmid, F. (1976). *Das Mongolismus-Syndrom [The mongolism syndrome].* Muensterdorf: Hansen and Hansen.

Schmidt, B.J., Carvalho, N., Ortega, C.C., Leiberman, J., Biazzi, J.M.M., Tapajos, P.M., & Krynski, S. (1975). Studies of the thyroid function in children with Down syndrome. *Arquives de Neuropsyquiatric, 33,* 21–24.

Scholfeld, W.A. (1943). Primary and secondary sexual characteristics: Study of their development in males from birth through maturity, with biometric study of penis and testis. *American Journal of Diseases of Children, 65,* 535–549.

Schröder, J., Lyndecken, K., & de la Chapelle, A. (1971). Meiosis and spermatogenesis in G-trisomic males. *Humangenetik, 13,* 15–24.

Scola, P.S., & Pueschel, S.M. (in press). Menstrual cycles and basal body temperature curves in women with Down syndrome. *Obstetrics and Gynecology.*

Shaheed, W.A., & Rosenbloom, L. (1973). Down's syndrome with diabetes mellitus and hypothyroidism. *Archives of Disease in Childhood, 48,* 917–918.

Sharav, T., Collins, R.M., & Baab, P.J. (1988). Growth studies in infants and children with Down syndrome and elevated levels of thyrotropin. *American Journal of Diseases of Children, 142,* 1302–1306.

Sharav, T., Landau, H., Zadik, Z., & Einarson, T.R. (1991). Age-related patterns of thyroid-stimulating hormone response to thyrotropin releasing hormone stimulation in Down syndrome. *American Journal of Diseases of Children, 145,* 172–175.

Sheridan, R., Llerena, J., Jr., Natkins, S., & Debenham, P. (1989). Fertility in a male with trisomy 21. *Journal of Medical Genetics, 26,* 294–298.

Smith, D.S. (1988). Hypothyroidism in children with Down syndrome. *American Journal of Diseases of Children, 142,* 127.

Stearns, P.E., Droulard, K.E., & Sahhar, F.H. (1960). Studies bearing on fertility of male and female mongoloids. *American Journal of Mental Deficiency, 65,* 37–41.

Tirosh, E., Taub, Y., Scher, A., Jaffe, M., & Hachberg, Z. (1989). Short-term efficacy of thyroid hormone supplementation for patients with Down syndrome and low borderline thyroid function. *American Journal of Mental Retardation, 93,* 652–656.

Tricomi, V., Valenti, C., & Hall, J.E. (1964). Ovulatory patterns in Down's syndrome. *American Journal of Obstetrics and Gynecology, 89,* 651–656.

Vladutiu, A.O., Chun, T.C., Victor, A., Gienau, L., & Bannerman, R.M. (1984). Down syndrome and hypothyroidism: A role for thyroid autoimmunity? *Lancet, i,* 14–16.

Williams, J.D., Summitt, R.L., & Camacho, A.M. (1971). Hypothyroidism in children with the Down syndrome: Report of three cases. *Birth Defects Original Article Series, 7,* 43–47.

Wisniewski, K.E., Torrado, C., & Castello, S. (1989). Treatment in growth hormone deficient Down syndrome children with recombinant human growth hormone. *Down's Syndrome Papers & Abstracts for Professionals, 12,* 1–2.

CHAPTER 23

Metabolic and Biochemical Concerns

Siegfried M. Pueschel and Göran Annerén

Since the early 1950s, we have witnessed an increased activity in biochemical and metabolic investigations relating to Down syndrome. In particular, after Lejeune, Gautier, and Turpin (1959) reported the discovery of a supernumerary small acrocentric chromosome in the cells of children with Down syndrome, investigators became interested in the teleologic function of the extra genetic material on chromosome 21 in biochemical and metabolic terms. A thorough literature search uncovered that many of the studies on this subject were done prior to the 1980s, and, in fact, very few metabolic and biochemical investigations with regard to carbohydrate and protein metabolism in persons with Down syndrome were carried out from 1980 to 1990. The focus has now shifted toward the molecular genetic arena where most of the exciting research is forthcoming. However, the literature that has accumulated is voluminous, and only certain aspects thereof can be discussed within the context of this chapter.

CARBOHYDRATES

In 1928, Brousseau and Brainard pointed to the abnormal response of individuals with Down syndrome to a glucose challenge. A few years later, O'Leary (1931) reported both abnormally high and low blood sugar levels during oral glucose tolerance tests in persons with Down syndrome. Similarly, Benda (1960) found variations in response to oral glucose administration: Some subjects had late peaks, some displayed flat glucose tolerance curves, and others had a slow return of the blood sugar to the fasting level.

Runge (1959) employed intravenous glucose

tolerance tests, which were abnormal in more than 50% of patients. Some persons had an initial high peak and a fast return to baseline. Others had a high peak after intravenous glucose administration, followed by a gradual decline to the fasting level, whereas a third group did not display the initial high peak, but had a delayed return to normal levels. Runge also found that persons with Down syndrome had low normal fasting blood sugar levels; in 13% of the individuals studied, hypoglycemic levels were recorded.

During insulin tolerance tests, Runge (1959) noted insulin hypersensitivity in individuals with Down syndrome. The epinephrine tolerance test yielded a normal increase of blood glucose, although there was a delay in the return to fasting glucose levels. The galactose tolerance test was abnormal in the majority of those persons with Down syndrome who also had had an abnormal glucose tolerance test. Unfortunately, Runge did not use a control group of subjects matched for sex, age, and environmental circumstances, nor did she provide a statistical analysis of her results, making the interpretation of her data difficult.

Milunsky, Lowy, Rubenstein, and Wright (1968) studied 7 children with Down syndrome between the ages of 2–6 years. These investigators performed both glucose and insulin tolerance tests and compared the results with 8 "normal" control children. They found low plasma insulin levels in response to a glucose load in both the study and the control groups.

Raiti, Lifshitz, Trias, and Sigman (1974) examined 8 small adolescents with Down syndrome. The authors found 3 of the 8 had inadequate plasma insulin response to glucose or to arginine infusions. The glucose disappearance rate in one of the adolescents followed a "diabetic pattern." According to these authors, the abnormalities in insulin production and glucose disappearance in a few of the individuals suggest a possible "diabetic tendency."

Yasuda et al. (1979) investigated carbohydrate metabolism in 8 persons with Down syndrome, ages 8–18 years. A diabetic glucose tolerance curve was observed in 1 of the individuals who was significantly overweight. This impaired glucose tolerance improved significantly with a weight-reduction program. Two others displayed a flat glucose tolerance curve and normal glucose tolerance curves were observed in the remaining 5. The insulin response and free fatty acid levels during oral glucose load were within the range of normal, except for the 1 person with the diabetic glucose tolerance curve. According to Yasuda et al., the results obtained in this study suggest that obesity might be partially responsible for the impaired glucose tolerance in some individuals with Down syndrome.

Diabetes mellitus has been noted to coexist with Down syndrome (Cone, 1954; Farquhar, 1969; Milunsky & Neurath, 1968). Farquhar and Milunsky and Neurath studied the frequency of diabetes mellitus in persons with Down syndrome and concluded that carbohydrate metabolic disturbances are seen at a higher frequency in individuals with Down syndrome than in the general population. Groenberg, Larsson, and Jung (1967) found that the prevalence of diabetes mellitus was substantially increased in children with Down syndrome when compared with children without this chromosome disorder.

There have been several studies indicating the presence of an abnormal carbohydrate metabolism in many persons with Down syndrome, and there may be a slightly increased prevalence of diabetes mellitus individuals with this chromosome disorder. However, the majority of persons with Down syndrome are asymptomatic with regard to carbohydrate metabolism.

LIPIDS

Bixby (1940) and Benda (1960) reported normal levels of serum cholesterol in persons with Down syndrome. In contrast, Stern and Lewis (1957a) found a significant difference in mean cholesterol levels in persons with Down syndrome (181.7 mg/dL) when compared with controls (176.5 mg/dL). These investigators observed higher cholesterol levels in the younger age groups between 2 and 6 years than in children from 6 to 12 years in both the study and control groups. Stern and Lewis (1957b) suggested that the neuroendocrine control of lipid metabolism is probably disturbed in persons with Down syndrome.

McCoy and Nance (1971) examined the lipid composition and synthesis of isolated lymphocytes obtained from persons with Down syndrome. The authors did not find any significant difference between the study and control groups in concentration of phospholipids, triglycerides, cholesterol, and cholesterol ester. Also, Nishida, Akaoka, Nishizawa, and Maruki (1977) did not observe any significant difference between persons with Down syndrome and those in the control group with regard to serum total cholesterol, phospholipids, and free fatty acids. Persons with Down syndrome, however, had a significant increase in plasma triglyceride level when compared with those in the control group (224 mg/dL and 173 mg/dL, respectively). Also, Strynadka and McCoy (1978) studied the phospholipid composition in the platelets of persons with Down syndrome and in "normal" controls and found the total amount of phospholipids was similar in both groups. The amount and composition of the phosphatidyl choline and sphingomyelin were also similar in persons with Down syndrome and in those without this chromosome disorder. This report indicates that there is no major difference in phospholipid composition in the platelets of persons with Down syndrome that could account for the observed decrease of sodium-potassium ATPase activity (Strynadka & McCoy, 1978). However, other investigators (Nelson, 1961; Simon, Ludwig, Gofman, & Crook, 1954; Stern & Lewis, 1959) found lipoproteins to be significantly increased in individuals with Down syndrome when compared with persons from a control group.

Murdoch, Rodger, and Rao (1977) reported that fasting serum cholesterol and triglyceride levels did not differ between 70 persons with

Down syndrome and 70 age- and sex-matched controls. However, Salo, Solakivi-Jaakkolo, and Kivimäki (1979) found that plasma triglycerides, low-density lipoprotein cholesterol, and apolipoprotein B levels were significantly higher, and the apolipoprotein AI:B ratio was significantly lower in 20 individuals with Down syndrome when compared to the control group. Similarly, Dörner, Gaethke, Tolksdorf, Schumann, and Gustmann (1984) reported decreased cholesterol and an increased beta:alpha lipoprotein ratio in individuals with Down syndrome.

In a recent study, Pueschel, Craig, and Haddow (in press) examined lipids and lipoproteins in 23 persons with Down syndrome and contrasted the results with those obtained from 23 individuals without this chromosome disorder. The authors reported significantly higher triglyceride levels in the persons with Down syndrome than in the controls. However, serum high-density lipoprotein, cholesterol, apolipoprotein AI and the ratio of high-density lipoprotein cholesterol to total cholesterol were all significantly decreased in the study population relative to controls. There were no significant differences in serum total cholesterol, low-density lipoprotein cholesterol, apolipoprotein B, and the apolipoprotein AI:B ratio between the two groups. Pueschel et al. (in press) concluded that a decreased prevalence of coronary artery disease in individuals with Down syndrome, which had been reported previously (Murdoch et al., 1977), cannot be explained by lipids and lipoprotein levels observed in their study population.

PROTEIN

A review of the literature on serum proteins in persons with Down syndrome could leave the reader with the impression that the subject matter has been well covered, with a high degree of agreement among the various investigators. Yet, a diligent study of the pertinent literature indicates that many of these reports present conflicting results and various interpretations. Many of the studies were done during the time period from the 1950s to the 1970s and very few papers have been published since then.

Many investigators reported that the serum albumin level in persons with Down syndrome is decreased, whereas the globulin concentration is increased (Donner, 1954; Nelson, 1961; Sobel, Strazzulla, Sherman, & Elkan, 1958; Stern & Lewis, 1957b; Stiehm & Fudenberg, 1966; Torre, 1958). Nelson reported higher than normal γ-globulin levels for all children with Down syndrome over 2 years old. Also, Greene, Shenker, and Karelitz (1968) found a statistically significant increase of γ-globulin in adults only. Pritham, Appleton, and Fluck (1963) observed high γ-globulin levels in persons living in residential facilities, but not in noninstitutionalized persons with Down syndrome. Likewise, Donner found increased γ-globulin concentrations in long-term institutionalized individuals with Down syndrome, but not in those persons who had recently been admitted. These data suggest that environmental circumstances, including recurrent infections and dietary and/or other aspects specific to residential facilities, are probably responsible for the increased γ-globulin levels in institutionalized individuals, and that the elevated γ-globulin levels probably do not have any direct association with Down syndrome.

Appleton and Pritham (1967) studied the influence of age and sex on plasma proteins. They found no significant difference between the sexes within or between the group with Down syndrome and a control group for any of the protein fractions studied. Also, total protein did not show variations for sex and age when samples were compared either within or between the groups. Appleton and Pritham noted a tendency for the concentration of albumin to decrease and for γ-globulin to increase with advancing age. They pointed out that their most significant finding was a persistently high concentration of γ-globulin and a low concentration of albumin. There was a significant difference in the relative percentages of albumin, α1- and α2-globulins, in the albumin:globulin ratio, as well as in the mobilities of the γ-globulin fractions when the entire group with Down syndrome was compared with the control group. Appleton and Pritham felt that these data lent validity to the hypothesis that an increase in quantity of γ-globulin in persons with Down syndrome represents an attempt to compensate for poor quality of antibody production.

Greene et al. (1968) examined 101 sera of 88 persons with Down syndrome. They found that the increase in γ-globulin observed in persons with Down syndrome was mainly due to the IgG fraction of the immunoglobulin system. Levels of IgA were increased in the older population with Down syndrome, whereas IgM values tended to be in the normal range. Griffiths, Sylvester, and Baylis (1969) found no difference between persons with Down syndrome and controls for levels of IgA or IgG; only IgA was found to be significantly elevated in males. Rundle, Atkin, and Clothier's (1973) investigations of the serum protein in persons with Down syndrome revealed significant reductions in the levels of total protein, albumin, α2-globulins, and β-globulins, as well as in the α1- and β-glycoproteins. Significant elevations were found, however, in the α1-glycoproteins and in the IgA and IgD fractions. These researchers failed to uncover any structural differences in 30 individual proteins studied by both double-diffusion and immunoelectrophoresis techniques.

Ingenito, Prier, Booth, Fan, and Litzenberg (1968) studied the serum protein in persons with Down syndrome by employing gel electrophoresis. They found some individuals with distinct protein bands between the β- and γ-globulin position, which the authors called the X1 protein factor.

The sera from 187 persons with Down syndrome and from 93 individuals with mental retardation due to other etiologies were studied by Nelson and Gholz (1962) for quantitative and qualitative differences in serum glycoproteins by paper electrophoresis. A small but significant decrease was noted in the β-globulin fraction of the serum glycoproteins in persons with Down syndrome when compared with controls. This reduction of the β-globulins was found to be more marked in younger than in older children. The difference was not significant in adults. Also, no significant difference was noted among persons with Down syndrome and controls in the albumin or the α1-, α2-, and γ-globulin fractions of serum glycoprotein. Nelson and Gholz reported the incidental finding of a significant increase in glycoprotein in the albumin and γ-globulin fractions and the corresponding significant decrease in the α2 fraction. A double

band in the γ-globulin range of the serum glycoprotein was found in many of the persons with Down syndrome, but in only a few of the controls.

Klose, Zeindl, and Sperling (1982) analyzed the protein patterns in two-dimensional gels of cultured human cells with trisomy 21. The authors found clearly visible differences in the staining intensity of corresponding polypeptide spots between cell lines of persons with trisomy 21 and those of controls. A few quantitatively variant polypeptides occurred in all trisomic cell lines, but no variants were consistently present in all of the 13 cell lines investigated. However, the total number of variants was considerably higher in the trisomic cells than in normal cells. In another study, Devine-Gage, Brown, Jenkins, Dutkowski, and Sammons (1987), using two-dimensional gel electrophoresis, observed several proteins in which synthesis was altered by the presence of chromosome 21 and identified six proteins as being specific to chromosome 21. These gene products may be involved in the pathogenesis of Down syndrome and may be related to the neurologic defects and premature aging seen in persons with this chromosome disorder (Devine-Gage et al., 1987).

AMINO ACIDS

A few abnormal results of amino acid metabolism have been reported in persons with Down syndrome involving β-amino acids, such as β-aminoisobutyric acid and taurine, and tryptophan and its metabolites. Wright and Fink (1957) noted an increased prevalence (34%) of high excretors of β-aminoisobutyric acid in persons with Down syndrome. In contrast, only 7% of "normal" controls and 17% of persons with mental retardation of other etiologies had increased β-aminiosobutyric acid urine output. Lundin and Gustavson (1962) discussed the increased amount of urinary β-aminoisobutyric acid. These authors felt that the high β-aminoisobutyric acid excretion is probably a "physiologic deviation" similar to those observed in other areas of biochemical dysfunction in Down syndrome. Perry, Shaw, and Walker (1959) used the same method (paper chromotography) as Wright and Fink in identifying amino acids, but they did not find an increase in the number of high excretors of β-aminosobutyric acid in persons with Down syndrome when compared with controls.

King, Goodman, and Thomas (1966) investigated the urinary excretion of amino acids in persons with Down syndrome by using semiautomatic ion exchange chromotography. The authors found that β-aminoisobutyric acid excretion was more variable among persons with Down syndrome than among the controls. There was no significant difference between the mean excretion of β-aminoisobutyric acid in these two groups, however.

Goodman, King, and Thomas (1964) and Wainer, King, Goodman, and Thomas (1966) demonstrated low urinary taurine excretion in persons with Down syndrome. Also, McCoy and Wehrle (1966) observed a reduced 24-hour urine output of taurine in persons with Down syndrome when compared with a control population. King, Goodman, Wainer, and Thomas (1968) studied the effect of a variety of experimental conditions on urinary taurine excretion in a "normal" population and in persons with Down syndrome. They found that in "normal" subjects, taurine excretion was increased by ingestion of sulphur-rich proteins, cysteamine, hypotaurine, and prednisone. Yet, little effect was noted on intake of cysteic acid and cysteine, and no effect was observed with cysteine sulfinic acid and pyridoxine. Loading studies (4 mg/kg/day), as well as long-term administration (6 weeks) of pyridoxine, did not correct the subnormal excretion of taurine in persons with Down syndrome, and there was no correlation between serum and urine taurine values.

Priscu, Moraru, Albu, and Sichitiu (1974) studied free amino acid levels in the cerebral spinal fluid of infants with Down syndrome. The authors reported elevated dicarboxylic acid levels and significant changes in the ratios of phenylalanine:tyrosine and glycine:alanine. In addition, abnormal levels of lysine, histidine, valine, and methionine were found. These data suggested to Priscu et al. that there is a need for increased intraneural synthesis and augmented transport across the blood–brain barrier.

Since Gershoff, Hegsted, and Trulson (1958) first reported abnormalities in tryptophan metabolism of persons with Down syndrome, there have been numerous reports indicating derangements in various pathways of tryptophan metabolism in children with this chromosome disorder (Jerome, Lejeune, & Turpin, 1960; McCoy & Chung, 1964; O'Brien & Groshek, 1962; Pare, Sandler, & Stacey, 1960; Rosner, Ong, Paine, & Mahanand, 1965; Tu & Zellweger, 1965). A constant finding was the markedly reduced serotonin levels in peripheral blood of the children with Down syndrome (Bazelon et al., 1967; Berman, 1965; Rosner et al., 1965; Tu & Zellweger, 1965).

Many investigators have attempted to provide a suitable explanation for this metabolic deviation, and many hypotheses have been generated throughout the years. Diminished or delayed intestinal absorption of tryptophan compounds was postulated by Careddu, Tenconi, and Sacchetti (1963). Tu and Zellweger's (1965) investigations indicated that there was no increase in blood serotonin levels in children with Down syndrome after an oral tryptophan load, and Bazelon (1967) felt that this was due to a faulty transport mechanism. Bennett and Giarman (1965) suggested that the decreased serotonin level could result from a reduced capacity to hydroxylate tryptophan to 5-hydroxytryptophan, particularly since this step has been described as rate limiting in the serotonin pathway. Also, McCoy, Rostafinsky, and Fishburn (1968) hypothesized a block in the hydroxylation reaction. In the next step along the serotonin pathway, defective decarboxylation could lead to a low blood serotonin concentration in children with Down syndrome. Three mechanisms could be involved: There may be a limited amount of coenzyme (pyridoxine) available, the apoenzyme (5-hydroxytryptophan decarboxylase) could be deficient, or there may be a combination of both (Tu & Zellweger, 1965).

Other researchers have investigated the storage and uptake of serotonin (Boullin & O'Brien, 1973; Jerome & Kamoun, 1970; Karki, Kuntzman, & Brodie, 1962; McCoy & Bayer, 1973; McCoy & England, 1968; McCoy, Segal, & Strynadka, 1975). Another defect observed by several investigators concerns ATP concentrations in platelets and the ability to bind and store 5-hydroxytryptamine (Airaksinen, 1974; Airaksinen & Airaksinen, 1972; Boullin, Coleman, & O'Brien, 1969; Boullin & O'Brien, 1973; Jerome & Kamoun, 1970; Lott, Chase, & Murphy, 1972; McCoy & Bayer, 1973). Many of the authors considered the low serotonin content to be due to a defective transport mechanism and impaired binding because of reduced amounts of ATP available in platelets. Hence, it was concluded that the primary defect was a deficiency of ATP in platelets, resulting in abnormal uptake and binding of serotonin.

CATECHOLAMINES

The catecholamines in Down syndrome have been studied by several investigators (Bergsman, 1959; Gustavson, Wetterberg, Bäckström, & Ross, 1973; Keele, Richards, Brown, & Marshall, 1969; Perry, 1962; Wetterberg, Gustavson, Bäckström, Ross, & Froden, 1972). Bergsman found the urinary excretion of epinephrine in children with Down syndrome to be low, yet Perry observed the urinary normetanephrine to be normal in these children. Keele et al. examined the catecholamine concentrations in the urine and plasma of children with Down syndrome and appropriate controls. The urinary dopamine, 3-methoxy-4-hydroxymandelic acid, 3,4-dehydroxymandelic acid, metanephrine, normetanephrine, and norepinephrine levels were not statistically different in children with Down syndrome when compared with controls. The urinary epinephrine levels, however, were statistically significantly lower in the children with Down syndrome, whereas plasma epinephrine and norepinephrine concentrations did not differ from those found in controls.

Wetterberg et al. (1972) reported decreased dopamine-β-hydroxylase in the plasma of children with Down syndrome, which they interpreted as an expression of abnormal catecholamine metabolism. Since catechol-O-methyltransferase is involved in the inactivation of catecholamines, Gustavson et al. (1973) investigated this enzyme system. They found an increase in catechol-O-methyltransferase activity in the erythrocytes of children with Down syndrome and their mothers.

Udeschini, Casati, Bassani, Picotti, and Culotta (1985) compared 5 women with Down syndrome with 5 age-matched controls in the standing and cold pressure tests. No significant differences were observed between the two groups in heart rate, systolic and diastolic blood pressure, and plasma adrenaline and dopamine concentrations. The plasma adrenaline levels, however, tended to be higher in the women with Down syndrome, both in standing and in the cold pressure tests. A more recent investigation on biochemical changes in catecholamine responses in adolescents with Down syndrome was reported by Eberhard, Eterradossi, and Therminarias (1991). Adolescents with Down syndrome and controls were participating in an incremental exercise test lasting 10 minutes. The authors found a slightly lower maximal value of catecholamines in the adolescents with Down syndrome, suggesting a reduced sympathetic response to maximal exercise.

URIC ACID

During the past decades, many reports have appeared in the literature concerning uric acid concentrations in various tissues of persons with Down syndrome. Some investigators indicated that the serum uric acid level was in the normal range (Rosner et al., 1965; Sobel et al., 1958). However, the majority of studies reported a markedly increased uric acid level in individuals with Down syndrome (Appleton, Haab, Burti, & Orsulak, 1969; Appleton et al., 1964; Chapman & Stern, 1964; Fuller, Luce, & Mertz, 1962; Goodman, Lofland, & Thomas, 1966; Kaufman & O'Brien, 1967; Mertz, Fuller, & Concon, 1963; Pant, Moser, & Krane, 1968; Winer & Feller, 1972).

Although increased serum uric acid levels are frequently reported in persons with Down syndrome, only a few persons with coexisting gout have been described in the literature. Ciompi et al. (1984) reported two persons with Down syndrome and concomitant gout. These authors also studied the purine salvage pathway and turnover of uric acid. The results, according to the authors, were consistent with the metabolic findings observed in persons with gout.

There has been much speculation concerning

the pathogenetic mechanisms responsible for the increase of uric acid in persons with Down syndrome. Since serum uric acid levels are also raised in persons with leukemia, it has been suggested that the immature leukocytes prevalent in persons with Down syndrome and the increased prevalence of leukemia in persons with Down syndrome might be related to the elevated serum uric acid levels. In addition, the rapid turnover of leukocytes, which was reported by Mellman, Raab, and Oski (1967), could in part explain the elevated serum uric acid levels in persons with Down syndrome. However, Kaufman and O'Brien (1967) felt that hyperuricemia in persons with Down syndrome is probably not the result of a preleukemic state, since the total leukocyte count did not correlate with uric acid levels; moreover, the leukocyte counts were similar in the study and control groups. These authors offered an alternative explanation. They hypothesized that the hyperuricemia may be due to some gene localized at chromosome 21 that is responsible for the overexpression of an enzyme that either causes overproduction of uric acid or its inadequate renal excretion.

Pant et al. (1968) also noted the serum creatinine levels in hyperuricemic persons with Down syndrome to be slightly higher than in "normal" individuals with normal levels of uric acid. The authors questioned whether this was a primary "immaturity" of kidney function or whether it presented renal damage due to high uric acid load. Since multiple enzymes are known to be increased in persons with Down syndrome, the high uric acid excretion suggested to Pant et al. that overproduction of uric acid might be a contributing factor in the hyperuricemia of persons with Down syndrome. Appleton et al. (1969) felt that the high uric acid levels could affect the conversion of hypoxanthine and xanthine to uric acid via the xanthine oxidase system.

Puukka, Puukka, Perkkilä, and Kouvalainen (1986) showed that the increased uric acid levels in persons with Down syndrome are due to an increase of adenosine deaminase activity in both erythrocytes and lymphocytes. In all persons with Down syndrome, positive correlations between erythrocyte adenosine deaminase activity, lymphocyte adenosine deaminase or deoxyadenosine activity, and plasma uric acid concentrations were found. The authors suggested that the increased activities of some purine-metabolizing enzymes found in both erythrocytes and lymphocytes may contribute to the increased purine degradation and hyperuricemia in persons with Down syndrome.

Although alternative explanations for the increased uric acid concentrations in the blood of persons with Down syndrome have been offered, at this time we do not fully understand the underlying pathogenetic mechanisms. It remains to be determined whether overproduction, diminished excretion, increased purine biosynthetic enzyme activity, or a combination thereof may be responsible for the hyperuricemia.

OXYGEN METABOLISM RELATING TO SUPEROXIDE DISMUTASE

The mechanism whereby specific genes on chromosome 21 contribute to the pathology of Down syndrome remains elusive. Since Down syndrome is a gene-dosage disorder, overproduction of certain proteins encoded by the otherwise normal genes on the extra chromosome 21 distorts the delicate balance of some biochemical pathways that are important for proper development and function of the organs affected in Down syndrome (Epstein, 1988). One of the genes assigned to chromosome 21 is the superoxide dismutase-1 (SOD-1) gene. The SOD-1 gene is mapped at 21q22.1 (Sinet, Coutrier, & Dutrillaux, 1976). This is outside the chromosome segment responsible for the phenotype of Down syndrome, the "Down syndrome specific segment" (Korenberg et al., 1990, p. 238). SOD-1 is a scavenger enzyme in the antioxidative system and overproduction of SOD-1 in Down syndrome has been proposed to result in increased lipid peroxidation of the brain.

Three isoenzymes of SOD have been identified. The cytoplasmic Cu/Zn-SOD (SOD-1) is encoded by chromosome 21 as mentioned above (Sinet et al., 1976; Tan, Tischfield, & Ruddle, 1973). The mitochondrial Mn-SOD (SOD-2) is mapped on chromosome 6 (Creagen, Tischfield, Ricciuti, & Ruddle, 1973). A third, extracellular

SOD is not yet assigned to any chromosome. The SODs catalyze the dismutation of the superoxide anion (O_2-) to hydrogen peroxide (H_2O_2), which in turn is reduced to water. H_2O_2 is metabolized mainly by two enzymes: the soluble catalase (CAT) and the cytoplasmic and mitochondrial glutathione peroxidase (GSH-Px). Catalase reduces H_2O_2 and GSH-Px has the ability to catalyze the degradation of both H_2O_2 and organic hydrogen peroxides. The GSH-Px gene is assigned to chromosome 3 (Donald, Wang, & Hamerton, 1979; Winjen, Monteba-vanHeuvel, Pearson, & Meera Kahn, 1978). GSH-Px has a molecular weight of 81,000, with 4 atoms of selenium present as selenocystein (Wendel, Kerner, & Graupe, 1978), and is the only human protein known to contain selenium. Mitochondrial glutathione peroxidase is selenium dependent and the activity of GSH-Px reflects the selenium status (Smith, Tappel, & Chow, 1974). An excess of SOD relative to the peroxidase might result in the build-up of hydrogen peroxide, whereas a relative deficiency of SOD might lead to the build-up of the superoxide radical. Both these events result in an increase of oxygen radicals and cell damage.

Because of the central role of SOD-1 in the generation of H_2O_2 and OH, it has been suggested that the enhanced SOD-1 activity in human trisomy 21 could result in an increased generation of H_2O_2 and in increased lipid peroxidation (Annerén, Edqvist, Gebre-Medhin, & Gustavson, 1985; Brooksbank & Balazs, 1984; Frischer, Chu, Ahmad, Justice, & Smith, 1981; Kedziora & Bartosz, 1988; Percy et al., 1990; Sinet, Lejeune, & Jerome, 1979). It has been proposed that the presenile dementia in persons with Down syndrome, at least partly, may be due to increased lipid peroxidation of the brain.

Individuals with Down syndrome have a 1.5-fold elevation of the SOD-1 activity, as a primary gene-dosage effect, in all cells and tissues: erythrocytes (Sichitiu, Sinet, Lejeune, & Frézal, 1974), fibroblasts (Annerén & Epstein, 1987; Feaster, Kwok, & Epstein, 1977), platelets (Sinet, Michelson, Bazin, Lejeune, & Jerome, 1975), lymphocytes (Feaster et al., 1977), and fetal brain (Brooksbank & Balazs, 1984). In some types of cells, however, the activities of

SOD-1 and SOD-2 have been found to be regulated coordinately (Crosti et al., 1985). An increase in SOD-1 might thus be accompanied by a decrease in SOD-2.

The generation of O_2- in the polymorphonuclear leukocytes (PMNs) of persons with Down syndrome is decreased to 75% of that in the PMNs of controls (Annerén & Björkstén, 1984; Kedziora, Blaszczyk, Sibinska, & Bartosz, 1990). The activity of CAT has been found to be normal in the cells of individuals with Down syndrome (Mattei et al., 1982; Pantelakis, Karaklis, Alexiou, Vardas, & Valaes, 1970). Also supporting the theory, Annerén, Edqvist, et al. (1985), and Annerén and Epstein (1987), Frischer et al., (1981), Sinet et al., (1975), and Sinet et al. (1979) found an increased activity of GSH-Px in the erythrocytes, lymphoid cells, and fibroblasts in persons with trisomy 21. The increased GSH-Px activity is proposed to be a secondary gene-dosage effect of SOD-1, secondary to an increased basal production of H_2O_2 in cells with trisomy 21.

As GSH-Px is a selenium-dependent enzyme, the concentrations of selenium in erythrocytes and plasma have been studied in persons with Down syndrome and compared with "normal" individuals. The concentration of selenium in individuals with Down syndrome compared to controls was found to be increased intracellularly in relation to the extracellular concentration (Annerén, Gebre-Medhin, Gustavson, & Plantin, 1985). This finding has been explained by an increased demand of intracellular selenium caused by increased GSH-Px activity. The hypothesis has also been confirmed by the results of Brooksbank and Balazs (1984) of a 50% increase in lipid peroxidation of human fetal brains with trisomy 21 as compared with controls. The experiment was repeated on matched human trisomy 21 and diploid fibroblast strains. In human trisomic fibroblasts, the level of lipid peroxidation was increased, the SOD-1 activity was 150% of controls, and the GSH-Px activity was also slightly elevated. Furthermore, Annerén, Gardner, and Lundin (1986) found that the GSH-Px activity in the erythrocytes of persons with Alzheimer disease was elevated compared to that in "normal" controls. The activity of SOD-1 in persons with Alzheimer disease has, however, been found to be normal (Marklund, Adolfsson, Gott-fries, & Winblad, 1985). In has also been shown that the manifestation of premature aging in individuals with Down syndrome is associated with changes in the red cell oxygen-scavenging processes. Persons with Down syndrome and Alzheimer disease manifestation had significantly lower SOD levels than matched control individuals (Percy et al., 1990; see also Lai, chap. 17, this volume). Finally, Elroy-Stein and Groner (1988) reported that L cells and HeLa cells transfected with a cloned human SOD-1 gene were more resistant to the lethal effect of paraquat (an agent that generates superoxide in vivo) than were control cells. The degree of in vitro lipid peroxidation in the transfected cells overexpressing the human SOD gene was significantly enhanced.

All of these studies have thus supported the notion that an abnormal oxygen metabolism, due to the unbalanced SOD-1 gene in persons with Down syndrome, might result in increased lipid peroxidation in brain cells, which partly could be responsible for the presenile dementia in persons with Down syndrome. Some questions, however, remain to be solved. It is difficult to understand why no secondary increase in the GSH-Px activity was found in the most vulnerable organ, the brain (Brooksbank & Balazs, 1984). Also, it seems unlikely that SOD-1 is present in rate-limiting amounts. The pattern of polyunsaturated lipids is quite different in fetal brains with trisomy 21 as compared to control fetal brains. In trisomic brains, there are significantly more of the n-3 (linolenic series) than the n-6 (linolic series) fatty acids (Brooksbank, Martinez, & Balazs, 1985). Since the n-3 fatty acids are more vulnerable to lipid peroxidation, the question arises whether the structural differences in the brain, and not the gene-dosage effects of the SOD-1 gene, could explain the increased lipid peroxidation in persons with Down syndrome.

Since this could not be studied in humans, investigations using an animal model, the trisomy 16 mouse, were pursued (Annerén & Epstein, 1987). In contrast to what had been observed in human trisomic erythrocytes and lymphocytes

(Annerén, Gebre-Medhin, et al., 1985; Sinet et al., 1975), but similar to what was found in trisomy 21 fetal brain (Brooksbank & Balazs, 1984), no increase of the GSH-Px activity was noted in trisomy 16 mouse brains. Furthermore, the level of lipid peroxidation measured by malonaldehyde production was unexpectedly decreased in mouse trisomy 16 fetal brains compared with the fetal brains of diploid mice. This series of experiments thus supported the idea that increased lipid peroxidation in Down syndrome is not only a dosage effect of the SOD-1 gene, but also an effect of abnormalities of the brain structure. A 1.5-fold increase in SOD-1 activity in the brain is thus not necessarily accompanied by either an enhancement of GSH-Px activity or an increase in lipid peroxidation.

Elroy-Stein and Groner (1988) reported that increased SOD-1 activity interferes with the transport of biogenic amines into chromaffin granules. Since neurotransmitter uptake plays an important role in many processes of the central nervous system, SOD-1 gene dosage may contribute to the neurobiologic abnormalities of Down syndrome (Yates et al., 1983). Reduced levels of the neurotransmitter serotonin in blood platelets is characteristic of individuals with Down syndrome. It has been found that platelets of transgenic SOD-1 animals that overexpress the transgene contain lower levels of serotonin than nontransgenic littermate mice (Groner et al., 1990). The reduction in the content of neurotransmitters in persons with Down syndrome thus might be a secondary gene-dosage effect of SOD-1.

In order to determine if selenium is a rate-limiting trace element for the selenium-dependent GSH-Px activity, 48 children with Down syndrome were treated with organic selenium (10 ug/kg of body weight/day) for 6 months (Annerén, Gebre-Medhin, & Gustavson, 1989). The selenium supplementation was tolerated well and no side effects were observed. The supplementation resulted in increased concentrations of selenium both in plasma and erythrocytes, but unexpectedly decreased GSH-Px activity in erythrocytes. This means, concerning the GSH-Px activity, that children with Down syndrome are not selenium deficient and do not have any beneficial effect from selenium supplementation. According to spontaneous reports by their parents, 34 of the 48 children had fewer infections during and after the selenium supplementation period. The serum pattern of the four immunoglobulin G (IgG) subclasses has been found to be abnormal in individuals with Down syndrome, with low levels of IgG2 and IgG4, but normal or increased concentrations of IgG1 and IgG3 (Anneren, Magnusson, Lilja, & Nordvall, in press; Avanzini et al., 1988). The IgG subclass concentrations were measured in the serum of 29 of the selenium-supplemented children with Down syndrome in samples obtained before and immediately after the period of supplementation, and 1 year after it was terminated. Selenium had a significant augmentative effect on the serum concentrations of IgG2 and IgG4, but not of IgG1 and IgG3, and the concentrations of IgG2 and IgG4 decreased significantly 1 year after the treatment had been terminated (Anneren, Magnusson, & Nordvall, 1990). This study thus suggested that selenium is not only important for the selenium-dependent scavenger enzyme GSH-Px, but also has an immunoregulatory effect on children with Down syndrome.

In summary, as a primary gene-dosage effect, the SOD-1 activity is 1.5-fold enhanced in all cells with trisomy 21. A direct secondary effect from the overproduction of SOD-1 is the reduction of the concentration of superoxide in PMNs. A subsequent direct secondary effect of that is an increase in the GSH-Px activity, but without change in the CAT activity. Increased lipid peroxidation is found in fetal brains and fibroblasts with trisomy 21, but this is not necessarily an effect from the increased SOD-1 activity. However, in transfected cells, which overexpress the human SOD-1 gene, enhanced lipid peroxida-

tion is found. These results indicate that, at least in part, the increased SOD-1 activity in persons with Down syndrome is responsible for the premature aging that is often seen. The exact mechanism is still unclear. The increased SOD-1 activity in persons with Down syndrome might also lead to reduced levels of neurotransmitters, such as serotonin. Although the oxygen metabolism in persons with Down syndrome has been studied more than any other metabolic system, the effects from overproduction of SOD-1 are still not well defined and will require further study.

CONCLUSION

Although the majority of individuals with Down syndrome have no significant abnormalities with regard to carbohydrate, lipid, and protein metabolism, some minor deviations have been observed. For example, previous studies noted slight derangements in carbohydrate metabolism and an increased prevalence of diabetes in individuals with Down syndrome. Also, minor abnormalities have been reported in persons with Down syndrome concerning lipid and protein metabolism, as just noted. Most consistent derangements have been noted in uric acid levels, which may be due to the increased activity of some purine-metabolizing enzymes found in both erythrocytes and lymphocytes that may contribute to the increased purine degradation resulting in hyperuricemia. In addition, much has been learned about the oxygen metabolism relating to superoxide dismutase activity in recent years. It has been reported that the abnormal oxygen metabolism due to the unbalanced SOD-1 gene in persons with Down syndrome might result in increased lipid peroxidation in brain cells.

REFERENCES

Airaksinen, E.M. (1974). Tryptophan treatment of infants with Down's syndrome. *Annals of Clinical Research, 6,* 33–39.

Airaksinen, E.M., & Airaksinen, M.M. (1972). The binding of tryptophan to plasma proteins and the rate of the inactivation of 5-HT released from plate-

lets in Down's syndrome. *Annals of Clinical Research, 4,* 361–365.

Anneren, G., & Björksten, B. (1984). Low superoxide levels in blood phagocytic cells in Down's syndrome. *Acta Paediatrica Scandinavica, 73,* 345–348.

Annerén, G., Edqvist, L-E., Gebre-Medhin, M., & Gustavson, K-H. (1985). Glutathione peroxidase activity in erythrocytes in Down syndrome (abnormal variation in relation to age and sex through childhood and adolescence). *Trisomy, 21*(1), 9–17.

Annerén, G., & Epstein, C.J. (1987). Lipid peroxidation and superoxide dismutase-1 and glutathione peroxidase activities in trisomy 16 fetal mice and human trisomy 21 fibroblasts. *Pediatric Research, 21*, 88–92.

Annerén, G., Gardner, A., & Lundin, T. (1986) Increased glutathione peroxidase activity in patients with Alzheimer's disease/senile dementia of Alzheimer's type. *Acta Neurologica Scandinavica, 73*, 586–589.

Annerén, G., Gebre-Medhin, M., & Gustavson, K-H. (1989). Increased plasma and erythrocyte selenium concentrations but decreased erythrocyte glutathione peroxidase activity after selenium supplementation in children with Down syndrome. *Acta Paediatrica Scandinavica, 78*, 879–884.

Annerén, G., Gebre-Medhin, M., Gustavson, K-H., & Plantin, L-O. (1985). Selenium in plasma and erythroctyes in Down's syndrome and healthy controls: Variation in relation to age, sex, and glutathione peroxidase activity in erythrocytes. *Acta Paediatrica Scandinavica, 74*, 508–514.

Annerén, G., Magnusson, C.G.M., Lilja, G., & Nordvall, S.L. (in press). Abnormal serum IgG subclass pattern in children with Down's syndrome. *Archives of Disease in Childhood.*

Annerén, G., Magnusson, C.G.M., & Nordvall, S.L. (1990). Increase in serum concentrations of IgG2 and IgG4 by selenium supplementation in children with Down's syndrome. *Archives of Disease in Childhood, 65*, 1353–1355.

Appleton, M.D., Haab, W., Burti, U., & Orsulak, P.J. (1969). Plasma urate levels in mongolism. *American Journal of Mental Deficiency, 74*, 196–199.

Appleton, M.D., Haab, W., Casey, P.J., Castellino, F.J., Schorr, J.M., & Miraglia, R.J. (1964). Role of vitamin A in gamma globulin biosynthesis and uric acid metabolism of mongoloids. *American Journal of Mental Deficiency, 69*, 324–327.

Appleton, M.D., & Pritham, G.H. (1967). Biochemical studies in mongolism: II. The influence of age and sex on the plasma proteins. *American Journal of Mental Deficiency, 67*, 521–525.

Avanzini, M.A., Söderström, T., Wahl, M., Plebani, A., Burgio, G.R., & Hansson, A. (1988). IgG subclass deficiency in patients with Down's syndrome and aberrant hepatitis B vaccine response. *Scandinavian Journal of Immunology, 28*, 467–470.

Bazelon, M. (1967). Serotonin metabolism in Down's syndrome. *Clinical Proceedings of the Children's Hospital National Medical Center, 23*, 58–63.

Bazelon, M., Paine, R.S., Cowie, V.A., Hunt, P., Houch, J.C., & Mahanand, D. (1967). Reversal of hypotonia in infants with Down's syndrome by administration of 5-hydroxytryptophan. *Lancet, i*, 1130.

Benda, C.E. (1960). *The child with mongolism.* New York: Grune & Stratton.

Bennett, D.S., & Giarman, G.Y. (1965). Schedule of appearance of serotonin (5HT) and associated enzymes in developing rat brain. *Journal of Neurochemistry, 12*, 911–916.

Bergsman, A. (1959). The urinary output of adrenalin and noradrenalin in some mental diseases. *Acta Psychiatrica et Neurologica Scandinavica, 34*, 100–107.

Berman, J.L. (1965). The metabolism of 5-hydroxytryptamine (serotonin) in the newborn. *Journal of Pediatrics, 67*, 603–609.

Bixby, E.M. (1940). Further biochemical studies in mongolism. *American Journal of Mental Deficiency, 45*, 201–206.

Boullin, D.J., & O'Brien, R.A. (1973). The metabolism of 5-hydroxytryptamine by blood platelets from children with mongolism. *Biochemical Pharmacology, 22*, 1647–1651.

Boullin, D.J., Coleman, M., & O'Brien, R.A. (1969). Defective binding of 5-HT by blood platelets from children with trisomy 21 form of Down's syndrome. *Journal of Physiology, 204*, 128–129.

Brooksbank, B.W.L., & Balázs, R. (1984). Superoxide dismutase, glutathione peroxidase and lipoperoxidation in Down's syndrome fetal brain. *Developmental Brain Research, 16*, 37–44.

Brooksbank, B.W.L., Martinez, M., & Balázs, R. (1985). Altered composition of polyunsaturated fatty acyl groups in phosphoglycerides of Down's syndrome fetal brain. *Journal of Neurochemistry, 44*, 869–877.

Brousseau, K., & Brainard, H.G. (1928). *Mongolism: A study of the physical and mental characteristics of mongolian imbeciles.* London: Bailliere, Tindall, and Cox.

Careddu, P., Tenconi, L.T., & Sacchetti, G. (1963). Transmethylation in mongols. *Lancet, i*, 828.

Chapman, M.J., & Stern, J. (1964). Uric acid in Down's disease. *Journal of Mental Deficiency Research, 8*, 119–124.

Ciompi, M.L., Bazzichi, L.M., Bertolucci, D., Mazzoni, M.R., Barbieri, P., Mencacci, S., Macchia, D., & Mariani, G. (1984). Uric acid metabolism in two patients with coexistent Down's syndrome and gout. *Clinical Rheumatology, 3*, 229–233.

Cone, T.E. (1954). Diabetes mellitus in a mongoloid. *Journal of the Medical Society of New Jersey, 51*, 66.

Creagen, R.P., Tischfield, J.A., Ricciuti, F., & Ruddle, F.H. (1973). Chromosome assignments of genes in man using mouse-human somatic hybrids: Mitochondrial superoxide dismutase (indophenoloxydase-B, tetrameric) to chromosome 6. *Humangenetik, 20*, 203–209.

Crosti, N., Bajer, J., Serra, A., Rigo, A., Scarpa, M., & Viglino, P. (1985). Coordinate expression of MnSOD and CuZn SOD in human fibroblasts. *Experimental Cell Research*, *160*, 396–402.

Devine-Gage, E.A., Brown, W.T., Jenkins, E.C., Dutkowski, R., & Sammons, D. (1987). Assignment of proteins to human chromosome 21 using two-dimensional gel electrophoresis and somatic cell genetic: An approach to the study of Down syndrome. *Journal of Neurogenetics*, *4*, 215–216.

Donald, L.J., Wang, H.S., & Hamerton, J.L. (1979). Confirmation of the assignment of a glutathione peroxidase locus to chromosome 3 in man. *Cytogenetics and Cell Genetics*, *23*, 141–143.

Donner, M. (1954). An investigation into immunological reactions and antibody production in mongolism. *Annales Medicinae Experimentalis et Biologiae Fenniae*, *32*, 9–15.

Dörner, K., Gaethke, A.S., Tolksdorf, M., Schumann, K.P., & Gustmann, H. (1984). Cholesterol fractions and triglycerides in children and adults with Down's syndrome. *Clinica Chimica Acta*, *142*, 307–311.

Eberhard, Y., Eterradossi, J., & Therminarias, A. (1991). Biochemical changes and catecholamine responses in Down's syndrome adolescents in relation to incremental maximal exercise. *Journal of Mental Deficiency*, *35*, 140–146.

Elroy-Stein, E., & Groner, Y. (1988). Impaired neurotransmitter uptake in PC12 cells overexpressing human Cu/Zn-superoxide dismutase—Implication for gene dosage effects in Down syndrome. *Cell*, *52*, 259–267.

Epstein, C.J. (1988). Specificity versus nonspecificity in the pathogenesis of aneuploid phenotypes [Invited editorial comment]. *American Journal of Medical Genetics*, *29*, 161–165.

Farquhar, J.W. (1969). Early-onset diabetes in the general and the Down's syndrome population. *Lancet*, *ii*, 323–324.

Feaster, W.W., Kwok, L.W., & Epstein, C.J. (1977). Dosage effects for superoxide dismutase-1 on nucleated cells aneuploid for chromosome 21. *American Journal of Human Genetics*, *29*, 563–570.

Frischer, H., Chu, L.K., Ahmad, T., Justice, P., & Smith, G.F. (1981). Superoxide dismutase and glutathione peroxidase abnormalities in erythrocytes and lymphoid cells in Down syndrome. In G.J. Brewer (Ed.), *The red cell: Fifth Ann Arbor Conference* (pp. 269–283). New York: Alan R. Liss.

Fuller, R.W., Luce, M.W., & Mertz, E.T (1962). Serum uric acid in mongolism. *Science*, *137*, 868–869.

Gershoff, S.N., Hegsted, D.M., & Trulson, M.F. (1958). Metabolic studies of mongoloids. *American Journal of Clinical Nutrition*, *6*, 526–532.

Goodman, H.O., King, J.S., & Thomas, J.J. (1964). Urinary excretion of beta-aminoisobutyric acid and taurine in mongolism. *Nature*, *204*, 650–652.

Goodman, H.O., Lofland, H.B., & Thomas, J.J. (1966). Serum uric acid levels in mongolism. *American Journal of Mental Deficiency*, *71*, 437–442.

Greene, E.L., Shenker, I.R., & Karelitz, S. (1968). Serum protein fractions in patients with Down's syndrome (mongolism). *American Journal of Diseases of Children*, *115*, 599–602.

Griffiths, A.W., Sylvester, P.E., & Baylis, E.M. (1969). Serum globulins and infection in mongolism. *Journal of Clinical Pathology*, *22*, 76–78.

Groenberg, A., Larsson, T., & Jung, J. (1967). Diabetes in Sweden. A clinico-statistical, epidemiological and genetic study of hospital patients and death certificates. *Acta Medica Scandinavica*, *477*(Suppl. 5), 1–7.

Groner, Y., Elroy-Stein, O., Avraham, K.B., Yarom, R., Schickler, M., Knobler, H., & Rotman, G. (1990). Down syndrome clinical symptoms are manifested in transfected cells and transgenic mice overexpressing the human Cu/Zn-superoxide dismutase gene. *Journal of Physiology*, *84*, 53–77.

Gustavson, K.H., Wetterberg, L., Bäckström, M., & Ross, S.B. (1973). Catechol-O-methyltransferase activity in erythrocytes in Down's syndrome. *Clinical Genetics*, *4*, 279–280.

Ingenito, E.F., Prier, J.E., Booth, E., Fan, E., & Litzenberg, M. (1968). Serum proteins in Down's syndrome. *Lancet*, *i*, 979.

Jerome, H., & Kamoun, P. (1970). Platelet binding of serotonin. *Annals of the New York Academy of Science*, *171*, 543–550.

Jerome, H., Lejeune, J., & Turpin, R. (1960). Study of the urinary excretion of some tryptophan metabolites in mongoloid children. *Comptes Rendus Hebdomadaires des Seances de L'Academie des Sciences*, *251*, 474–476.

Karki, N., Kuntzman, R., & Brodie, B.B. (1962). Storage, synthesis, and metabolism of monoamines in the developing brain. *Journal of Neurochemistry*, *9*, 53–59.

Kaufman, J.M., & O'Brien, W.M. (1967). Hyperuricemia in mongolism. *New England Journal of Medicine*, *276*, 953–956.

Kedziora, J., & Bartosz, G. (1988). Down's syndrome: A pathology involving the lack of balance of reactive oxygen species. *Free Radical Biology & Medicine*, *4*, 317–330.

Kedziora, J., Blaszczyk, J., Sibinska, E., & Bartosz, G. (1990). Down's syndrome: Increased enzymatic antioxidative defense is accompanied by decreased superoxide anion generation in blood. *Hereditas*, *112*, 73–75.

Keele, D.K., Richards, C., Brown, J., & Marshall, J. (1969). Catecholamine metabolism in Down's syndrome. *American Journal of Mental Deficiency*, *74*, 125–129.

King, J.S., Jr., Goodman, H.O., & Thomas, J.J. (1966). Urinary amino acid excretion in mongolism. *Acta Geneticae Medicae et Gemettiologiae (Roma)*, *16*, 132–154.

King, J.S., Jr., Goodman, H.O., Wainer, A., &

Thomas, J.J. (1968). Factors influencing urinary taurine excretion by normal and mongoloid subjects. *Journal of Nutrition, 94*, 481–489.

Klose, J., Zeindl, E., & Sperling, K. (1982). Analysis of protein patterns in two-dimensional gels of cultured human cells with trisomy 21. *Clinical Chemistry, 28*, 987–992.

Korenberg, J.R., Kawashima, H., Pulst, S.M., Ikeuchi, T., Ogasawara, N., Yamamoto, K., Schonberg, S.A., West, R., Allen, L., Magenis, E., Ikawa, K., Taniguchi, N., & Epstein, C.J. (1990). Molecular definition of a region of chromosome 21 that causes features of the Down syndrome phenotype. *American Journal of Human Genetics, 47*, 236–246.

Lejeune, J., Gautier, M., & Turpin, R. (1959). Études des chromosomes somatiques de neuf enfants mongoliens [Study of somatic chromosomes of nine mongoloid children]. *Comptes Rendus Hebdomadaires des Seances de L'Academie des Sciences, Paris, 248*, 602–603.

Lott, I.T., Chase, T.N., & Murphy, D.L. (1972). Down's syndrome: Transport, storage, and metabolism of serotonin in blood platelets. *Pediatric Research, 6*, 730–735.

Lundin, L.G., & Gustavson, K.H. (1962). Urinary BAIB excretion in Down's syndrome (mongolism). *Acta Genetica, 12*, 156–163.

Marklund, S.L., Adolfsson, R., Gottfries, C.G., & Winblad, B. (1985). Superoxide dismutase isoenzymes in normal brains and in brains from patients with dementia of Alzheimer type. *Journal of Neurological Science, 67*, 319–325.

Mattei, J.F., Baeteman, M.A., Baret, A., Ardissone, J.P., Rebuffel, P., & Giraud, F. (1982). Erythrocyte superoxide dismutase and redox enzymes in trisomy 21. *Acta Paediatrica Scandinavica, 71*, 589–591.

McCoy, E.E., & Bayer, S.M. (1973). Decreased serotonin uptake and ATPase activity in platelets from Down's syndrome patients. *Clinical Research, 21*, 304–309.

McCoy, E.E., & Chung, S.I. (1964). The excretion of tryptophan metabolites following deoxypyridoxine administration in mongoloid and nonmongoloid patients. *Journal of Pediatrics, 64*, 227–235.

McCoy, E.E., & England, J. (1968). Excretion of 4-pyridoxic acid during deoxypyridoxine and pyridoxine administration to mongoloid and nonmongoloid subjects. *Journal of Nutrition, 96*, 525–528.

McCoy, E.E., & Nance, J.L. (1971). Lipid composition and synthesis of isolated polymorphonuclear leukocytes in Down's syndrome. *Journal of Mental Deficiency Research, 15*, 1–11.

McCoy, E.E., Rostafinsky, M.J., & Fishburn, C. (1968). The concentration of serotonin by platelets in Down's syndrome. *Journal of Mental Deficiency Research, 12*, 18–21.

McCoy, E.E., Segal, D.J., & Strynadka, K. (1975). Decreased ATPase, increased Na+ and decreased K+ in Down's syndrome platelets. In R. Koch & F. De La Cruz (Eds.), *Down's syndrome (mongolism): Research, prevention, and management* (pp. 125–129). New York: Brunner/Mazel.

McCoy, E.E., & Wehrle, H. (1966). The excretion of taurine during deoxytyridoxine administration in Down's syndrome patients and controls. *Proceedings of the Society for Experimental Biology and Medicine, 123*, 170–174.

Mellman, W.J., Raab, S.O., & Oski, F.A. (1967). Abnormal granulocyte kinetics: An explanation for the atypical granuloctye enzyme activities observed in trisomy 21. In G.E. Wolstenholme & R. Porter (Eds.), *Ciba Foundation Study Group No. 25* (pp. 77–84). Boston: Little, Brown.

Mertz, E.T., Fuller, R.W., & Concon, J.M. (1963). Serum uric acid in young mongoloids. *Science, 141*, 535–536.

Milunsky, A., Lowy, C., Rubenstein, A.H., & Wright, A.D. (1968). Carbohydrate tolerance, growth hormone and insulin levels in mongolism. *Developmental Medicine and Child Neurology, 10*, 25–31.

Milunsky, A., & Neurath, P.W. (1968). Diabetes mellitus in Down's syndrome. *Archives of Environmental Health, 17*, 372–378.

Murdoch, J.C., Rodger, C.J., & Rao, S.S. (1977). Down's syndrome: An atheroma-free model? *British Medical Journal, ii*, 226–228.

Nelson, T. (1961). Serum protein and lipoprotein fractions in mongolism. *American Journal of Diseases of Children, 102*, 369–374.

Nelson, T., & Gholz, B. (1962). Serum glycoproteins in mongolism. *American Journal of Mental Deficiency, 66*, 551–554.

Nishida, Y., Akaoka, I., Nishizawa, T., & Maruki, M. (1977). Synthesis and concentration of 5-phosphoribosyl-1-pyrophosphate in erythrocytes from patients with Down's syndrome. *Annals of the Rheumatic Diseases, 36*, 361–363.

O'Brien, D., & Groshek, A. (1962). The abnormality of tryptophan metabolism in children with mongolism. *Archives of Disease in Childhood, 37*, 17–20.

O'Leary, W.D. (1931). Carbohydrate metabolism in mongolian idiots as evidence of endocrine dysfunction. *American Journal of Diseases of Children, 41*, 544–551.

Pant, S.S., Moser, H.W., & Krane, S.M. (1968). Hyperuricemia in Down's syndrome. *Journal of Clinical Endocrinology and Metabolism, 28*, 472–478.

Pantelakis, S.N., Karaklis, A.G., Alexiou, D., Vardas, E., & Valaes, T. (1970). Red cell enzymes in trisomy 21. *American Journal of Human Genetics, 22*, 184–193.

Pare, C.M.B., Sandler, M., & Stacey, R.S. (1960). 5-Hydroxyindoles in mental deficiency. *Journal of Neurology, Neurosurgery and Psychiatry, 23*, 341–347.

Percy, M.E., Dalton, A.J., Markovic, A.D., Crapper-

McLachlan, D.R., Hummel, J.T., Rusk, A.C.M., & Andrews, D.F. (1990). Red cell superoxide dismutase, glutathione peroxidase and catalase in Down syndrome patients with and without manifestations of Alzheimer disease. *American Journal of Medical Genetics*, *35*, 459–467.

Perry, T.L. (1962). Urinary excretion of amines in phenylketonuria and mongolism. *Science*, *136*, 879–880.

Perry, T.L., Shaw, K.N.F., & Walker, D. (1959). Urinary excretion of beta-amino-isobutyric acid in mongolism. *Nature*, *184*, 1970–1971.

Priscu, R., Moraru, I., Albu, A., & Sichitiu, S. (1974). Les taux des amino-acides libres dans le liquide cerebro-spinal chez les nourrissons trisomiques 21 [The concentration of free amino acids in the cerebrospinal fluid in infants with trisomy 21]. *Human Genetics*, *21*, 63–68.

Pritham, G.E., Appleton, M.D., & Fluck, E.R. (1963). Biochemical studies in mongolism: I. The influence of the environment on the concentrations and mobilities of plasma proteins. *Journal of Mental Deficiency*, *67*, 517–520.

Pueschel, S.M., Craig, W.Y., & Haddow, J.E. (in press). Lipids and lipoproteins in persons with Down syndrome. *Journal of Mental Deficiency Research*.

Puukka, R., Puukka, M., Perkkilä, L., & Kouvalainen, K. (1986). Levels of some purine metabolizing enzymes in lymphocytes from patients with Down's syndrome. *Biochemical Medicine and Metabolic Biology*, *36*, 45–50.

Raiti, S., Lifshitz, F., Trias, E., & Sigman, B. (1974). Down's syndrome: Study of carbohydrate metabolism. *Acta Endocrinologica*, *76*, 506–512.

Rosner, F., Ong, B.H., Paine, R.S., & Mahanand, D. (1965). Biochemical differentiation of trisomic Down's syndrome (mongolism) from that due to translocation. *New England Journal of Medicine*, *273*, 1356–1361.

Rundle, A.T., Atkin, J., & Clothier, B. (1973). Serum proteins in Down's syndrome. *Developmental Medicine and Child Neurology*, *15*, 736–747.

Runge, G.H. (1959). Glucose tolerance in mongolism. *American Journal of Mental Deficiency*, *63*, 822–828.

Salo, M.K., Solakivi-Jaakkolo, T., & Kivimäki, T. (1979). Plasma lipids and lipoproteins in Down's syndrome. *Scandinavian Journal of Clinical Laboratory Investigation*, *39*, 485–490.

Sichitiu, S., Sinet, P.M., Lejeune, J., & Frézal, J. (1974). Surdosage de la forme dimérque de l'indophénoloxydase dans la trisomie 21, secondaire au surdosage génique [Triple dose of the dimeric form of indolphenoloxidase in trisomy 24 secondary to the increased genetic material]. *Humangenetik*, *23*, 65–72.

Simon, A., Ludwig, G., Gofman, J.W., & Crook, G.H. (1954). Metabolic studies in mongolism. Serum protein-bound iodine, cholesterol and lipoprotein. *American Journal of Psychiatry*, *3*, 139–145.

Sinet, P.M., Coutrier, J., & Dutrillaux, B. (1976). Trisomie 21 et superoxide dismutase-1 (IPO-A): Tentative de localisation sur la sous-bande 21q22.1 [Trisomy 21 and superoxide dismutase-1 (IPO-A): Tentative localization on band 21q22.1]. *Experimental Cell Research*, *97*, 47–55.

Sinet, P.M., Lejeune, J., & Jerome, H. (1979). Trisomy 21 (Down syndrome) glutathione peroxidase, hexose monophosphate shunt and IQ. *Life Science*, *24*, 29–35.

Sinet, P.M., Michelson, A.M., Bazin, A., Lejeune, J., & Jerome, H. (1975). Increase in glutathione peroxidase activity in erythrocytes from trisomy 21 subjects. *Biochemical and Biophysical Research Communication*, *67*, 910–915.

Smith, P.J., Tappel, A.L., & Chow, C.K. (1974). Glutathione peroxidase activity as a function of dietary selenomethionine. *Nature*, *247*, 392–398.

Sobel, A.E., Strazzulla, M., Sherman, B.S., & Elkan, B. (1958). Vitamin A absorption and other blood composition studies in mongolism. *American Journal of Mental Deficiency*, *62*, 642–656.

Stern, J., & Lewis, W.H.P. (1957a). The serum cholesterol level in children with mongolism and other mentally retarded children. *Journal of Mental Deficiency Research*, *1*, 96–106.

Stern, J., & Lewis, W.H.P. (1957b). Serum proteins in mongolism. *Journal of Mental Science*, *103*, 222–226.

Stern, J., & Lewis, W.H.P. (1959). The serum lipoproteins of mentally retarded children. *Journal of Mental Science*, *105*, 1012–1016.

Stiehm, E.R., & Fudenberg, H.H. (1966). Serum levels of immune globulins in health and disease: A survey. *Pediatrics*, *37*, 715–721.

Strynadka, K., & McCoy, E.E. (1978). Phospholipid composition of Down's syndrome and normal platelets. *Clinical Biochemistry*, *11*, 35–37.

Tan, Y.H., Tischfield, J., & Ruddle, F.H. (1973). The linkage of genes for human interferon-induced antiviral protein and indophenol oxidase B traits to chromosome G-21. *Journal of Experimental Medicine*, *137*, 1041–1044.

Torre, M. (1958). Investigations on the humoral syndrome of mongolism-pathogenetic aspects. *Giornale di Psichiatrie, Neuropatologia*, *86*, 17–63.

Tu, J., & Zellweger, H. (1965). Blood serotonin deficiency in Down's syndrome. *Lancet*, *ii*, 715.

Udeschini, G., Casati, G., Bassani, F., Picotti, G.B., & Culotta, P. (1985). Plasma catecholamines in Down's syndrome, at rest and during sympathetic stimulation. *Journal of Neurology, Neurosurgery and Psychiatry*, *48*, 1060–1061.

Wainer, A., King, J.S., Jr., Goodman, H.O., & Thomas, J.J. (1966). S35 taurine metabolism in normal and mongoloid individuals. *Proceedings of the Society for Experimental Biology and Medicine*, *121*, 212–216.

Wendel, A., Kerner, B., & Graupe, K. (1978). The selenium moiety of glutathione peroxidase. *Hoppe-Seylers Zeitschrift für Physiologische Chemie*, *359*, 1035–1043.

Wetterberg, L., Gustavson, K.H., Bäckström, M., Ross, S.B., & Froden, I. (1972). Low dopamine-beta-hydroxylase activity in Down's syndrome. *Clinical Genetics*, *3*, 152–153.

Winer, R.A., & Feller, R.P. (1972). Composition of parotid and submandibular saliva and serum in Down's syndrome. *Journal of Dental Research*, *51*, 449.

Winjen, L.M.M., Monteba-vanHeuvel, M., Pearson, P.L., & Meera Kahn, P. (1978). Assignment of a gene for glutathione peroxidase (GPX) to human chromosome 3. *Cytogenetics and Cell Genetics*, *22*, 232–235.

Wright, S.W., & Fink, K. (1957). The excretion of beta-aminoisobutyric acid in normal, mongoloid, and nonmongoloid defective children. *American Journal of Mental Deficiency*, *61*, 530–533.

Yasuda, K., Sakurada, T., Yamamoto, M., Kikuchi, M., Okuyama, M., & Miura, K. (1979). Carbohydrate metabolism in Down's syndrome. *Tohoku Journal of Experimental Medicine*, *129*, 367–372.

Yates, C.M., Simpson, J., Gordon, A., Maloney, A.F.J., Allison, Y., Ritchie, J.M., & Urguhart, A. (1983). Catecholamine and cholinergic enzymes in presenile and senile Alzheimer-type dementia and Down's syndrome. *Brain Research*, *280*, 119–126.

CHAPTER
24

General Health Care
and Therapeutic Approaches

Siegfried M. Pueschel

In past centuries, and even up to the 1960s and early 1970s, most individuals with Down syndrome were usually not afforded appropriate medical care and adequate educational services. Children with Down syndrome were frequently institutionalized and they were often deprived of even the most elementary medical services. Immunizations were incomplete, nutrition was substandard, infections were rampant, and congenital heart disease as well as other medical problems were rarely treated effectively. Hence, a high mortality rate was noted and only about 50% of children with Down syndrome survived the 1st decade of life.

In the 1970s and 1980s, unforeseen progress has been made in both the biomedical and behavioral sciences relating to Down syndrome. The emergence of molecular genetics and novel investigations in epidemiology and pathogenesis, as well as recent biomedical studies, have provided us with a better understanding of the biology of the person with Down syndrome. In spite of the progress we have witnessed over the past decades, there is still no effective medical treatment available for individuals with Down syndrome that would significantly improve their cognitive function. Yet, we have learned that the quality of life of persons with Down syndrome can be enhanced if we pay attention to the numerous medical issues that have been detailed in this volume and if we effectively treat those conditions that have been observed to occur at a higher frequency in individuals with Down syndrome.

The first section of this chapter deals with regular health care issues and focuses on effective therapeutic approaches of specific medical concerns in youngsters with Down syndrome. Next, this chapter elaborates on numerous unconventional treatments that have been advocated over the past years. Although such therapeutic approaches have been found to be ineffective and in general are not helpful to persons with Down syndrome, it is important that professionals be aware of them so they will be able to respond to questions asked by parents of children with Down syndrome in regard to these issues. Some of the more recent therapeutic modalities that have been published in the medical literature then are briefly reviewed and some of the issues concerning facial plastic surgery are discussed. The chapter concludes with a look into the future, proposing therapeutic approaches based on molecular genetic concepts.

GENERAL PRINCIPLES OF HEALTH CARE

In this section, the importance of optimal health maintenance by fostering the well-being of persons with Down syndrome in all areas of human functioning is emphasized. If provided with appropriate health services, individuals with Down syndrome can live a more meaningful life and can contribute more fully to society.

Routine Newborn Care

One of the important general principles of health care includes the active pursuit of optimal well-being in persons with Down syndrome. The cornerstone of such a principle must be a comprehensive health maintenance program for these individuals.

As do all newborns, infants with Down syndrome need a thorough physical examination in the neonatal period—with particular focus on those systems that are frequently affected in children with this chromosome disorder. The newborn examination should include neurologic and neurobehavioral assessments. Routine screening tests should be carried out in the newborn period, such as screening for certain inborn errors of metabolism and hypothyroidism. Although most inborn errors of metabolism are rare, congenital hypothyroidism has been reported to occur more often in infants with Down syndrome than in the general population (Fort et al., 1984).

Counseling of Parents

It is well known that parents who are told that their child has Down syndrome frequently experience profound emotional distress. Although there is no completely satisfactory way to counsel parents in this initial traumatic experience, the physician's positive approach, tact, compassion, and truthfulness can have a vital influence on the parents' subsequent adjustment and the child's overall progress. The physician's style and manner of counseling is of utmost importance inasmuch as it will set the tone for the atmosphere that will prevail in future years. The critical role of parenthood should be stressed as well as the chance for the infant to be nurtured and loved by caring parents. In emphasizing that the infant with Down syndrome is, first and foremost, a human being with inherent rights, the physician shows genuine concern and thus endows the infant with significance and worth.

Specific Concerns in the Newborn Period

Due to the increased frequency of specific congenital anomalies in infants with Down syndrome, there are a number of neonatal concerns that require immediate attention. Some of these conditions may be life threatening and need to be corrected immediately, whereas others may become apparent during the first few weeks and months subsequent to the child's birth.

For example, congenital cataracts occur in approximately 3%–4% of newborns with Down syndrome. It is important to identify those children with dense congenital cataracts, as these must be extracted. Appropriate corrections with glasses or contact lenses must then be made in order to ensure adequate vision. (See also Catalano, chap. 6, this volume.)

Of primary concern are congenital anomalies of the gastrointestinal tract. If esophageal or duodenal atresia or other bowel obstructions are present, nutrients and fluids cannot be absorbed and the infant will starve to death if not operated on promptly. Previously, surgical intervention of such congenital anomalies was not always recommended. Such a decision is clearly unethical and inhumane. Generally speaking, no medical or surgical treatment should be withheld from a child with Down syndrome that would be provided unhesitatingly to a child without this chromosome disorder. (See also Levy, chap. 11, this volume.)

Congenital heart disease, when not diagnosed early, may result in cardiac failure, with life-threatening complications in some children. Others may thrive poorly and/or develop early pulmonary artery hypertension. Therefore, it is recommended that shortly after birth, a pediatric cardiologist examine the child with Down syndrome. In addition to the clinical evaluation, an echocardiogram and other diagnostic procedures should be done. If a significant cardiac defect is identified, appropriate medical management, including administration of digitalis and diuretics and surgical repair of the heart defect at an optimal time, will improve the quality of life of the infant with Down syndrome. (See also Marino, chap. 9, this volume.)

Well-Baby Care

After discharge from the hospital, routine infant care encompasses regular well-baby check-ups, when physical growth, developmental progress, and the general well-being of the child can be assessed. During these well-baby visits, the pediatrician or other health care provider should also be concerned with nutritional, environmental, and behavioral issues as well as with other aspects that may affect the physical and emotional well-being of the child. In addition, the parents should be informed of accident prevention, general safety in the home, and avoidance of any environmental hazards that potentially might compromise the child's health.

Another important aspect of preventive medicine relates to the immunization of infants. In addition to the immunization program as recommended by the American Academy of Pediatrics, some children with Down syndrome who have frequent lower respiratory infections will benefit from additional vaccines against influenza virus and pneumococcal infections. If children with Down syndrome are diagnosed to have specific infections, they, of course, should be treated appropriately. Although those children with significant congenital heart disease, nutritional deficiencies, and immunologic impairments generally have more respiratory infections, the vast majority of home-reared children with Down syndrome do not have these health concerns and usually do not have more respiratory infections than do children without this chromosome disorder. Skin infections are more often observed in adolescents with Down syndrome, in particular at the thighs, buttocks, and the perigenital area. Regular hygiene, frequent sitz baths, and topical antibiotic treatment usually help.

Nutritional Aspects

On the one hand, feeding problems may be encountered in some infants with Down syndrome, which may result in poor weight gain. On the other hand, increased weight gain often becomes apparent in many youngsters with Down syndrome as they grow older (see also Cronk & Annerén, chap. 3, this volume). Therefore, it is important to educate parents concerning an appropriate caloric intake concomitant with physical exercise, in order to avoid undernutrition or excessive weight gain. Good eating habits, a balanced diet, avoidance of high caloric foods, and regular physical activities can prevent the child with Down syndrome from becoming obese (see also Pipes, chap. 4, this volume).

Specific Medical
Concerns During Childhood

In addition to the following few selected conditions, there are numerous other frequently occurring conditions in persons with Down syndrome that need to be recognized and treated. Many of these concerns, such as seizure disorders, hematologic diseases, and sleep apnea, have been well covered in previous chapters (see Florez, chap. 16; Howenstine, chap. 10; Lubin, Kahn, & Scott, chap. 21, this volume).

Sensory Impairments Sensory impairments, including visual and hearing deficits, have been described to occur at a higher frequency in individuals with Down syndrome. Thus, particular attention should be paid to these sensory modalities. For example, hearing deficits have been found to be present in 50–80% of children with Down syndrome (Balkany, Downs, Jafek, & Krajicek, 1978; Schwartz & Schwartz, 1978). Since the significance of a hearing impairment lies in its effect on all phases of psychological and emotional development, proper assessment of audiologic functions and remediation, if a hearing loss is uncovered, are of paramount importance. It has been well documented that even a mild conductive hearing deficit can lead to a reduced rate of language development and secondary interpersonal problems. (See also Dahle & Baldwin, chap. 7, this volume.)

Likewise, optimal visual acuity is important for any child and, of course, also for the child with Down syndrome. For children with mental retardation, an additional handicap of sensory impairment may further limit cognitive functioning, which may prevent them from participating in significant learning processes. Therefore, regular ophthalmologic follow-up and appropriate treatment if a visual impairment is identified are strongly recommended. (See also Catalano, chap. 6, this volume.)

Thyroid Dysfunction If children with Down syndrome are noted to have thyroid dysfunction, particularly if hypothyroidism has been identified, appropriate treatment should be forthcoming. Since hypothyroidism may compromise normal central nervous system functioning and because clinical symptoms of hypothyroidism may be insidious and are sometimes interpreted as being part of the "Down syndrome Gestalt," thyroid function studies including thyroid-stimulating hormone, thyroxine, and triiodothyronine should be obtained at regular (probably annual) intervals. Optimal thyroid function will allow normal learning processes to take place. (See also Pueschel & Blaymore Bier, chap. 21, this volume.)

Atlantoaxial Instability   It is of importance to identify children with atlantoaxial instability early because of its relatively high prevalence and its potential for remediation. Some individuals with Down syndrome may have difficulties verbalizing specific complaints relating to neck discomfort and neuromotor difficulties. Also, sometimes their motor dysfunction and broad-based gait may conceal significant neurologic concerns. Thus, it is important to diagnose those children with atlantoaxial instability and provide appropriate treatment. A delay in recognizing this condition may result in irreversible spinal cord damage. (See also Pueschel & Solga, chap. 14, this volume.)

UNCONVENTIONAL TREATMENTS

During the past decades, numerous treatment procedures and therapeutic modalities for children with Down syndrome have been proposed by professionals in the attempt to enhance intellectual functioning. Despite the large number of reports that claim success in their treatment efforts (Benda, 1960; Gadson, 1951; Harrell, Capp, Davis, Peerless, & Ravitz, 1981; Haubold, 1967; Turkel, 1975), at the present time there are no known medical therapies available that would significantly improve the cognitive abilities of children with Down syndrome. Many workers in the field who indicated that their specific treatment approach resulted in improvements of the child's intellectual functioning often did not provide scientific evidence of their claims and frequently there were flaws in study design and statistical analysis. In many instances, subsequent studies that attempted to replicate specific investigations negated the original results (Black, Kato, & Walker, 1966; Bumbalo, Morelewicz, & Berens, 1964; Koch, Share, & Graliker, 1965; Van Dyke, Lang, van Duyne, Heide, & Chang, 1990).

It is often difficult for parents to evaluate the scientific (or sometimes pseudoscientific) aspects of various treatment approaches that have come to the public's attention. In particular, just after the birth of a child with Down syndrome,

many parents try to obtain any help they can get. During this vulnerable time, many parents may "grasp for straws." Therefore, parents should be informed of unconventional treatment approaches and should be told that there is no cure for Down syndrome, nor is there any effective medical treatment available at the present time that would significantly improve their child's mental development.

Numerous treatment approaches have been advocated—too many to be reviewed in detail in this section of the chapter. Instead, this section focuses on the therapies most publicized in the United States.

Pituitary Extract

The use of pituitary extract has been suggested by Benda (1960) and Goldstein (1956) on the premise that panhypopituitarism was a contributing factor in Down syndrome. Although claims of marked improvement in children have been made after pituitary extract administration, Berg, Kirman, Stern, and Mittwoch (1961), Diamond and Moon (1961), and Freeman (1970) found that pituitary extract given to children with Down syndrome did not benefit their intellectual and social developments.

Glutamic Acid

Glutamic acid and its derivatives have been employed in the treatment of children with Down syndrome. Some workers have reported good results with such therapy (Gadson, 1951; Goldstein, 1956). Other investigators (Astin & Ross, 1960; Lombard, Gilbert, & Donofrio, 1955), however, reported no significant improvement after glutamic acid administration to children with Down syndrome.

Thyroid Hormone

Since T.T. Smith introduced thyroid hormone treatment for children with Down syndrome in 1896, this form of therapy has been used by many professionals. Benda's (1969) histopathologic examinations of thyroid glands from diseased persons with Down syndrome, which revealed many microscopic structural abnormalities, encouraged the use of thyroid hormone for children with Down syndrome. Benda's

(1969) studies, however, have never been duplicated and most investigators would disagree that thyroid abnormalities are universally present in persons with Down syndrome.

In order to investigate whether thyroid hormone is beneficial to children with Down syndrome, Koch et al. (1965) followed 73 noninstitutionalized children with Down syndrome in a 6-year longitudinal double-blind study. The children were randomly assigned to one of three groups: Children in the first group were placed on sodium lyothyronine, those in the second group were given a placebo, and children in the third group received neither thyroid hormone nor placebo. Height, bone age, protein-bound iodine, and intellectual functioning were assessed on all of the children. At the end of the 6-year study period, no significant differences were found among the three groups in terms of their intellectual functioning. Thus, although thyroid dysfunction is reportedly more common in persons with Down syndrome (Pueschel & Pezzullo, 1985) and thyroid hormone supplementation should be administered to those persons with documented hypothyroidism, thyroid hormone has not been found to improve intellectual function in euthyroid persons with Down syndrome.

5-Hydroxytryptophan

The finding by Tu and Zellweger (1965) of low blood levels of the neuroregulatory amine, 5-hydroxytryptamine (serotonin), in persons with Down syndrome stimulated interest in the use of 5-hydroxytryptophan, a serotonin precursor, in the treatment of children with this chromosome disorder. 5-hydroxytryptophan was reported by Bazelon et al. (1967) to improve muscle tone, decrease tongue protrusion, and increase the activity level in infants with Down syndrome. In a subsequent study, Coleman (1973) compared a group of children with Down syndrome who had received 5-hydroxytryptophan with a placebo group and found no significant difference in cognitive development between the children in the two groups. In 1971, Partington, MacDonald, and Tu described a controlled trial of 5-hydroxytryptophan administered to children with Down syndrome. These investigators did not detect any

improvement in motor, behavioral, or neurologic functions. Similarly, Weise, Koch, Shaw, and Rosenfeld (1974) gave 5-hydroxytryptophan to young children with Down syndrome. They also observed that this compound was not effective in accelerating the children's rate of development and no discernable behavioral differences were found between the treated and untreated children. Moreover, Pueschel, Reed, Cronk, and Goldstein (1980) studied the effects of 5-hydroxytryptophan and pyridoxine, singly and in combination, administered to 89 children with Down syndrome during the first 3 years of life. The results of this longitudinal study revealed that there was no significant improvement in motor, mental, or social development with administration of these compounds. Although there exists a good rationale for the use of 5-hydroxytryptophan in children with Down syndrome, the above-mentioned studies did not detect any beneficial effects.

Dimethyl Sulfoxide

Dimethyl sulfoxide, a solvent that is extracted from lignin found in wood pulp, has been used to treat many conditions, including Down syndrome. Chilean investigators (Aspillaga, Morizon, Avendano, Sanchez, & Capdeville, 1975) reported improvement in the overall functioning of children with Down syndrome following treatment with dimethyl sulfoxide. Unfortunately, there were many methodologic inadequacies in this study. Another investigation was carried out in Oregon to assess the effects of orally administered dimethyl sulfoxide on behavior and learning in individuals with mental retardation, including children with Down syndrome (Gabourie, Becker, & Bateman, 1975). Sixty-seven subjects were paired by age, level of functioning, and diagnosis, and assigned to either a high-dose or a low-dose group. Twenty-three additional children received no treatment. On standardized normative intelligence tests and language instruments, no significant differences were noted among the three groups.

Sicca Cell

Sicca cell treatment, also known as cell, dry cell, or fetal cell therapy, was introduced in the

1930s. It was first used to treat children with mental retardation, including youngsters with Down syndrome, in the 1950s (Fröhlich & Prokop, 1977). Sicca cell treatment consists of injection of freeze-dried cells from various organs of fetal cattle and sheep. Proponents of sicca cell therapy hypothesize that the injected fetal cells migrate to corresponding target organs in the individual where the biochemical substrates and enzymes of the injected cells revitalize the target organ.

Schmid (1976) reported an average height of 161 cm in treated males and of 146 cm in treated females compared to the height of 148 cm–150 cm for untreated males and 138 cm–140 cm for untreated females with Down syndrome. Head circumference measurements of males treated over a long term were between those of untreated subjects with Down syndrome and the general population. According to Schmid, sicca cell therapy started in early infancy will normalize the brain volume index to a large extent and will raise the IQ of children with Down syndrome significantly. In terms of academic achievement, Schmid concluded that with sicca cell treatment, it is definitely possible to teach the majority of children with Down syndrome to speak, read, and write. The interpretation of the results of Schmid's sicca cell therapy is difficult since there is a lack of information concerning study design and specific confounding conditions that may have influenced the results. In addition, it is impossible to know whether or not the reported improvements are specific to sicca cell therapy or whether other components of Schmid's therapeutic regimen are contributing factors.

Two controlled investigations to evaluate the efficacy of sicca cell therapy were conducted independently in the 1960s. Bardon (1964) studied 10 children with Down syndrome with a mean chronologic age of 3.3 years and assigned them to five pairs matched for age, sex, physical development, and intelligence. One child in each pair received sicca cell injections and the other did not. At the end of 1 year, the observers recorded an increase of intellectual function in all children, with no significant difference between the pair members. These results were confirmed

during a 2nd year of observations and assessments. Another study (Black et al., 1966) involved 59 individuals with mental retardation, ages 5–25 years, 36 of whom had Down syndrome. The subjects were randomly assigned to two groups, a treatment group that received three injections of sicca cells over a period of 9 months and a control group that was given placebo injections. Statistical analysis of the results indicated that there was no evidence that treated individuals benefited from sicca cell treatment when compared with the control group. In a retrospective study, Van Dyke et al. (1990) examined 21 subjects who had received cell therapy abroad. Comparing the treated subjects with those in the control group matched for age, sex, socioeconomic status, and cardiac history, there was no statistically significant difference for all developmental and growth variables measured.

Thus, there is no evidence that sicca cell therapy has any beneficial effect on persons with Down syndrome. However, there are several potential adverse effects, including allergic and anaphylactic reactions as well as the potential risk of transmission of slow viruses by injection of fetal animal tissues (National Down Syndrome Congress, 1986).

Vitamins, Minerals, and Other Compounds

There have been numerous therapeutic approaches using various combinations of vitamins, minerals, hormones, and enzymes. In Germany, Haubold (1955, 1967) recommended a mixture of vitamins, hormones, and minerals that he termed "basis therapy." Although Haubold reported a beneficial effect of this treatment regimen, White and Kaplitz (1964), who treated children with Down syndrome according to Haubold's instructions, did not detect any significant improvement.

In the United States, Turkel (1975) has treated hundreds of children with Down syndrome during the past decades with the so-called U-series, which contains about 50 different compounds, including thyroid hormone, vitamins, minerals, enzymes, and medications such as aminophylline and chlorpheniramine maleate. Turkel reported numerous case studies where he has seen improvement of physical features and intellectual functioning after the administration of the U-series.

To date, there has been only one controlled study that investigated the effects of the U-series in children with Down syndrome (Bumbalo et al., 1964). Twenty-four children with Down syndrome were randomly assigned to treatment and placebo groups. After the data were analyzed without knowledge of the subject's group assignment, no objective improvement was observed on most biologic measurements in children who received the U-series. On initial psychologic testing, 1 child had an IQ of 50 and the other 23 children had IQs of less than 50. At the end of the study, all children in both groups had IQs of less than 50.

Further interest in the use of vitamins and minerals in the treatment of children with mental retardation including those with Down syndrome was generated by Harrell et al. (1981). This study was undertaken after Harrell et al. had noted a remarkable improvement in intellectual functioning in a 7-year-old boy with mental retardation following treatment with specific nutritional supplements. According to Harrell et al., this child could not speak and had an IQ of 25–30. However, after the administration of the vitamin and mineral mixture, the child had normal speech, read and wrote at an elementary school level, played ball and the flute, and had an IQ of 90.

Prompted by this experience and an interest in the "genotrophic concept" of disease, Harrell et al. (1981) initiated a study. Twenty-two children with mental retardation, including 5 children with Down syndrome, were assigned to two groups matched primarily on the basis of IQ. For the first 4 months of the study, one group received the vitamin and mineral treatment, which included 11 vitamins and 8 minerals in doses ranging from 1.2 to 333 times the recommended daily allowance. The other group of children received a placebo. During the second 4 months of the study, both groups received the vitamin and mineral treatment. Intelligence testing was done at the beginning of the study and at the end of both 4-month treatment periods by Harrell and

several other psychologists. In the first 4-month period, the treated subjects made an average IQ gain of 9.6 points and in the second 4-month period, they made additional gains. The group receiving the vitamin and mineral supplementation in the second period alone increased their IQ by an average of 10.2 points. In particular, 3 of the 5 children with Down syndrome had increases of 10–25 IQ points. Although a placebo control group was used and the evaluators were blind to group assignment, some problems remain with Harrell et al.'s study. In particular, there was no random assignment to study and control groups; no attempt was made to match the two groups on the basis of other variables, such as educational experience and socioeconomic status; and during the total study period of 8 months, many of the children were administered an IQ test six times, suggesting that a practice effect needs to be taken into consideration.

Subsequently, several investigations were carried out to replicate Harrell et al.'s (1981) study and to evaluate the administration of the vitamin and mineral supplementation on various functions in children with Down syndrome. Weathers (1983) treated 6- to 17-year old children for 4 months with the same dose of vitamins and minerals used by Harrell and co-workers. Measures of IQ, visual-motor integration, height, weight, and vision, as well as behavior ratings provided by parents, failed to show any significant differences between the two groups.

Bennett, McClelland, Kriegsmann, Brazee, and Sells (1983) also evaluated the vitamin and mineral supplement as used by Harrell et al. (1981) in a double-blind case-controlled study involving 20 home-reared children with Down syndrome. Following an 8-month period, no significant differences between placebo and treatment groups were found in IQ, school achievement, speech and language acquisition, and neuromotor functioning. The beginning mean IQ in the treatment group was 53.1, and the mean IQ at the end of the study was 52.5; the beginning mean IQ in the placebo group was 45.2, and the mean IQ at the end of the study was 46.

In 1984, Smith, Spiker, Peterson, Cicchetti,

and Justine reported their double-blind clinical trial using Harrell et al.'s (1981) vitamin and mineral mixture. The study involved 56 home-reared children, 7–15 years of age. Pairs were formed that were matched for IQ, age, sex, socioeconomic status, and type of educational program. Membership in either treatment or placebo group was randomly assigned. The vitamin and mineral mixture was used in the treatment group for the first 4 months. During the second 4-month study period, the vitamin A dose was decreased from 15,000 IU to 5,000 IU. No significant differences were found between treatment and placebo groups at the 4- or 8-month test periods. Further, no changes over time were observed in either group on the Visual Motor Integration Test (Smith et al., 1984).

Recent reports by Bidder, Gray, Newcombe, Evans, and Hughes (1989) as well as by Pruess, Fewell, and Bennett (1989) again demonstrated that vitamin therapy is not useful for children with Down syndrome. In particular, Bidder et al. noted that treatment with vitamins and minerals was associated with decreased developmental progress and various side effects.

Children with Down syndrome, in fact, all children, are in need of vitamins, minerals, and other nutrients. However, well-controlled studies show that megadoses of such compounds do not improve intellectual and other functions of children with Down syndrome.

ADMINISTRATION OF ZINC AND SELENIUM

Recently, some investigators have reported that the administration of compounds such as zinc sulphate and selenium may benefit children with Down syndrome. In a study by Napolitano et al. (1990), it was observed that 15 of 22 children who received zinc sulphate for a 6- to 9-month period reached a higher percentile in their growth rate, whereas the remaining 7 children showed no change. The average height velocity changed from 23.84 mm ± 7.98 mm per 6 months to 40.8 mm ± 7.68 mm per 6 months. Growth hormone as well as somatomedin serum levels also increased during the treatment period. The authors concluded that zinc sulphate

therapy provided to children with Down syndrome not only affects their immune system positively but also can accelerate longitudinal growth.

Selenium therapy also has been suggested for persons with Down syndrome. Antila, Nordberg, Syväoja, and Westermarck (1990) studied 24 children with Down syndrome with regard to their response to selenium in a double-blind approach. The selenium supplementation increased the erythrocyte glutathione peroxidase activity in youngsters with Down syndrome. This, however, was not observed in the control group. Therefore, the authors concluded that in spite of the heterogeneity of the population, children with Down syndrome benefit from selenium supplementation through optimization of their antioxidant protection by glutathione peroxidase.

In contrast, Annerén, Gebre-Medhin, and Gustavson (1989) observed a decrease of glutathione peroxidase activity in erythrocytes after supplementation with selenium-rich yeast tablets. The plasma and erythrocyte selenium concentrations, however, increased during the experiment. An interesting finding was that many of the parents spontaneously reported a reduced rate of infections among their children after treatment with selenium. In another investigation, Annerén, Magnusson, and Nordvall (1990) studied the concentration of four IgG subclasses of 29 children with Down syndrome. They found that selenium had a significant augmentative effect on the serum concentration of IgG2 and IgG4, but not on IgG1 and IgG3. The authors suggested that selenium indeed has an immunoregulatory effect that might be of importance in clinical practice.

There is a need for further controlled studies that will either confirm or disagree with the results and conclusions of the above-cited investigations. Until then, the decision of whether to use zinc and selenium therapy will have to be made on a case-by-case basis.

FACIAL PLASTIC SURGERY

Since Höhler (1977) described a child with Down syndrome and her changes in facial expression as a result of facial plastic surgery, this subject has been discussed in both the lay press and in the medical literature. In particular, in Germany and Israel, and only sporadically in Canada, Australia, the United States, and other countries, plastic surgeons have operated on persons with Down syndrome in order to improve their facial appearance during the 1980s.

Although the surgical procedures may vary according to the child's individual needs and the surgeon's preferential approach, surgery usually involves the removal of epicanthal folds; straightening out the oblique palpebral fissures; implants of silicone or cartilage at the nasal bridge, cheeks, and chin; reduction of the lower lip; and a wedge resection of the tongue (Lemperle, 1985; Lemperle & Radu, 1980; Olbrisch, 1982, 1983). Proponents of facial plastic surgery suggest that because the child's tongue is too large, surgery will enhance the child's speech and language abilities (Lemperle, 1985; Olbrisch, 1983). In addition, proponents claim that after surgery, children with Down syndrome are better accepted by society, they drool less and have less difficulty chewing solid food and drinking liquids, and they have less frequent respiratory infections.

Subjective observations have been made by parents of children with Down syndrome on how facial plastic surgery improves the lives of people with Down syndrome. Olbrisch (1982) reported the results of a questionnaire that had been completed by parents whose children had undergone facial plastic surgery. According to these data, postoperatively, 85% of the children kept their mouths closed, and 78% had fewer or no upper respiratory infections; 83% of the parents said the smaller tongue improved both eating and speech, 78% felt that their child's facial features had improved, and 28% observed a change of attitude toward their child by others. However, it is probable that most parents of children who had undergone facial plastic surgery were motivated from the very beginning to have this procedure done and thus expected positive results.

Other reports have discussed the results of facial plastic surgery in a more critical way.

Arndt, Lefebvre, Travis, and Munro (1986) examined 24 children with Down syndrome after they had undergone facial plastic surgery. These investigators reported that independent observers had reviewed photographs taken preoperatively and postoperatively and found that the children's appearance postoperatively was slightly less attractive than the preoperative appearance. The parents of these children, however, reported that their children's appearance was noticeably improved with facial plastic surgery. The investigators concluded that positive psychologic consequences may be largely the result of the parents' satisfaction with the surgical results.

Two other studies focused on articulation and speech intelligibility after partial glossectomy in children with Down syndrome. Parsons, Iacono, and Rozner (1987) assessed the articulation of 18 children with Down syndrome before and after tongue-reduction surgery. They found no significant difference in the number of articulation errors before and after the operation, nor at the 6-month follow-up examination. Another group of investigators (Margar-Bacal, Witzel, & Munro, 1987) examined the speech intelligibility of 23 children with Down syndrome after partial glossectomy. Preoperative and postoperative audiotaped samples of spoken words and connected speech were rated by three lay people and three professionals on a 5-point intelligibility scale. When the data were analyzed statistically, there was no significant difference between preoperative and postoperative acoustic speech intelligibility.

There are numerous issues concerning facial plastic surgery that have not yet been investigated and evaluated and many questions remain unanswered:

- For whom is the facial surgery performed— for the child, for the parents, or for society?
- Will the child be involved in the decision-making process of whether or not facial plastic surgery should be performed?
- What are the true indications for facial plastic surgery?
- How will the surgical trauma affect the child?

- Can one remove societal prejudice by improving the physical characteristics of the child with Down syndrome?
- What will the results of facial plastic surgery mean to the child's identity and self-image?
- Should the degree of mental retardation be a criterion for who should and who should not have facial plastic surgery?

Other concerns relate to possible inappropriate expectations for normality after surgery that may lead to denial of the child's underlying disorder. Belfer (1980) mentioned that the assumption of perfect normality following any craniofacial procedure, especially if it is an assumption arrived at too readily and too early, leaves the youngster potentially vulnerable to a more severe disappointment in later life and may not, in fact, give persons with Down syndrome an opportunity to integrate their changed bodily appearance.

At the present time, facial plastic surgery in Down syndrome is controversial. Instead of anecdotal reports, well-designed and well-controlled studies, with proper rationale and sound objectives, should be conducted. Whether or not facial plastic surgery will be beneficial and will improve the achievement and acceptance in society of people with Down syndrome can only be determined from the results of such studies.

FUTURE THERAPEUTIC APPROACHES

One can categorically state that at the present time no cure and no medical or surgical treatments exist that will significantly improve the overall development and function of children with Down syndrome. However, recent research in molecular biology has supported the hypothesis that the primary effect of an extra chromosome 21 in people with Down syndrome is an increase in transcriptional RNA coded for by genes on this chromosome (Kurnit, 1979). The challenge for the future, then, is to isolate, map, and characterize further the gene sequences on chromosome 21. If we would be able to identify the genes, their respective functions, and their interference in normal developmental processes, and if we would be able to counteract specific actions of those genes and/or their products, a rational approach to medical treatment could evolve.

Although no effective therapeutic modalities are available, people with Down syndrome should be afforded all medical and surgical services that are offered to children without this chromosome disorder. If this principle is followed without exception, then the quality of life of individuals with Down syndrome can be improved significantly and they will be able to function as productive citizens in society.

REFERENCES

Annerén, G., Gebre-Medhin, M., & Gustavson, K-H. (1989). Increased plasma and erythrocyte selenium concentrations but decreased erythrocyte glutathione peroxidase activity after selenium supplementation in children with Down syndrome. *Acta Paediatrica Scandinavica, 78,* 879–884.

Annerén, G., Magnusson, C.G.M., & Nordvall, S.L. (1990). Increase in serum concentrations of IgG2 and IgG4 by selenium supplementation in children with Down's syndrome. *Archives of Disease in Childhood, 65,* 1353–1355.

Antila, E., Nordberg, L., Syväoja, E., & Westermarck, T. (1990). Selenium therapy in Down syndrome (DS): A theory and a clinical trial. In I. Emerit (Ed.), *Antioxidants in therapy and preventive medicine* (pp. 183–186). New York: Plenum.

Arndt, E.M., Lefebvre, A., Travis, F., & Munro, I.R. (1986). Fact and fantasy: Psychosocial consequences of facial surgery in 24 Down syndrome children. *British Journal of Plastic Surgery, 39,* 498–504.

Aspillaga, M.J., Morizon, G., Avendano, I., Sanchez, M., & Capdeville, L. (1975). Dimethyl sulfoxide therapy in severe retardation in mongoloid children. In S. Jacob & R. Herschler (Eds.), *Biological actions of dimethyl sulfoxide* (pp. 421–431). New York: New York Academy of Science.

Astin, A.W., & Ross, S. (1960). Glutamic acid and human intelligence. *Psychological Bulletin, 57,* 429–434.

Balkany, T.J., Downs, M.P., Jafek, B.W., & Krajicek, M.J. (1978). Otologic manifestations of Down's syndrome. *Surgical Forum, 29,* 582–585.

Bardon, L.M. (1964). Sicca cell treatment in mongolism. *Lancet, ii,* 234–235.

Bazelon, M., Paine, R.S., Cowie, V.A., Hunt, P., Houch, J.C., & Mahanand, D. (1967). Reversal of hypotonia in infants with Down syndrome by administration of 5-hydroxytryptophan. *Lancet, i.* 1130–1132.

Belfer, M. (1980). [Discussion: Lemperle, G., & Radu, D. Facial plastic surgery in children with Down syndrome]. *Plastic and Reconstructive Surgery, 66,* 343–344.

Benda, C.E. (1960). *The child with mongolism.* New York: Grune & Stratton.

Benda, C.E. (1969). *Mongolism and cretinism* (2nd ed.). New York: Grune & Stratton.

Bennett, F.C., McClelland, S., Kriegsmann, F.A., Brazee, A., & Sells, C.J. (1983). Vitamin and mineral supplementation in Down syndrome. *Pediatrics, 72,* 707–713.

Berg, J.M., Kirman, B.H., Stern, J., & Mittwoch, U. (1961). Treatment of mongolism. *Journal of Mental Sciences, 107,* 475–480.

Bidder, R.T., Gray, P., Newcombe, R.G., Evans, B.K., & Hughes, M. (1989). The effects of multivitamins and minerals on children with Down syndrome. *Developmental Medicine and Child Neurology, 31,* 532–537.

Black, D.B., Kato, J.G., & Walker, G.W.H. (1966). A study of improvement in mentally retarded children accruing from sicca cell therapy. *American Journal of Mental Deficiency, 70,* 499–508.

Bumbalo, T.S., Morelewicz, H.V., & Berens, D.L. (1964). Treatment of Down's syndrome with the "U" series of drugs. *Journal of the American Medical Association, 5,* 187.

Coleman, M. (1973). *Serotonin in Down's syndrome.* New York: Elsevier/North-Holland.

Diamond, E.F., & Moon, M.S. (1961). Neuromuscular development in mongoloid children. *American Journal of Mental Deficiency, 66,* 218–226.

Fort, P., Lifshitz, F., Bellisario, R., Davis, M.D., Lanes, R., Pugliese, M., Richman, R., Post, D.R., & David, R. (1984). Abnormalities of thyroid function in infants with Down syndrome. *Journal of Pediatrics, 104,* 545–549.

Freeman, R. (1970). Psychopharmacology and the retarded child. In F. Menolascino (Ed.), *Psychiatric approaches to mental retardation* (pp. 77–89). New York: Basic Books.

Frölich, C., & Prokop, O. (1977). Die Zellulartherapie [Sicca cell therapy]. In O. Prokop (Ed.), *Medizinischer Okkultismus* (pp. 153–174). New York: Gustav Fischer Verlag.

Gabourie, J., Becker, J., & Bateman, B. (1975). Oral dimethyl sulfoxide in mental retardation. Part I. Preliminary behavioral and psychometric data. In S. Jacob & R. Herschler (Eds.), *Biological actions of dimethyl sulfoxide* (pp. 449–459). New York: New York Academy of Sciences.

Gadson, E.J. (1951). Glutamic acid and mental deficiency. *American Journal of Mental Deficiency, 55,* 521–528.

Goldstein, H. (1956). Treatment of congenital acro-

micria syndrome in children. *Archives of Pediatrics, 13,* 153–156.

Harrell, R.F., Capp, R.H., Davis, D.R., Peerless, J., & Ravitz L.R. (1981). Can nutritional supplements help mentally retarded children? An exploratory study. *Proceedings of the National Academy of Sciences of the United States of America, 78,* 574–578.

Haubold, H. (1955). Neue therapeutische Möglichkeiten beim Mongolismus, Vorschlag einer Nachreif ungsbehandlung [New therapeutic possibilities in mongolism, suggestions for specific treatments]. *Arzeneimittel Forschung, 9,* 211–228.

Haubold, H. (1967). Beeinflussung des Phenotyps mongoloider Kinder durch eine früheinsetzende Dauerbehandlung [Influencing the phenotype of mongoloid children using early and continuing therapy]. *Asthetische Medizin, 13,* 3–12.

Höhler, H. (1977). Changes in the facial expression as a result of plastic surgery in mongoloid children. *Aesthetic Plastic Surgery, 1,* 245–251.

Koch, R., Share, J.B., & Graliker, B. (1965). The effects of Cytomel on children with Down's syndrome —A double-blind longitudinal study. *Pediatrics, 66,* 776–778.

Kurnit, D.M. (1979). Down syndrome: Gene dosage at the transcriptional level in skin fibroblasts. *Proceedings of the National Academy of Sciences of the United States of America, 76,* 2372–2375.

Lemperle, G. (1985). Plastic surgery. In D. Lane & B. Stratford (Eds.), *Current approaches to Down's syndrome* (pp. 131–145). Sidney, Australia: Holt, Rinehart & Winston.

Lemperle, G., & Radu, D. (1980). Facial plastic surgery in children with Down's syndrome. *Plastic and Reconstructive Surgery, 66,* 337–342.

Lombard, J.P., Gilbert, J.G., & Donofrio, A.F. (1955). The effects of glutamic acid upon the intelligence, social maturity, and adjustment of a group of mentally retarded children. *American Journal of Mental Deficiency, 60,* 122–132.

Margar-Bacal, F., Witzel, M.A., & Munro, I.R. (1987). Speech intelligibility after partial glossectomy in children with Down's syndrome. *Plastic and Reconstructive Surgery, 79,* 44–47.

Napolitano, G., Palka, G., Grimaldi, S., Giuliani, C., Laglia, G., Calabrese, G., Satta, M.A., Neri, G., & Monaco, F. (1990). Growth delay in Down syndrome and zinc sulphate supplementation. *American Journal of Medical Genetics Supplement, 7,* 63–65.

National Down Syndrome Congress. (1986). Issues statement on sicca cell therapy. *Down Syndrome News, 10,* 4.

Olbrisch, R.R. (1982). Plastic surgical management of children with Down's syndrome: Indications and results. *British Journal of Plastic Surgery, 35,* 195–200.

Olbrisch, R.R. (1983). Plastic surgery in 250 children with Down's syndrome: Indications and results. *Transactions of the 8th International Congress on Plastic and Reconstructive Surgery, 702–703.*

Parsons, C.L., Iacono, T.A., & Rozner, L. (1987). Effect of tongue reduction on articulation in children with Down syndrome. *American Journal of Mental Deficiency, 91,* 328–332.

Partington, M.W., MacDonald, M.R.A., & Tu, J.B. (1971). 5-hydroxytryptophan (5-HTP) in Down's syndrome. *Developmental Medicine and Child Neurology, 13,* 362–372.

Pruess, J.B., Fewell, R.R., & Bennett, F.C. (1989). Vitamin therapy and children with Down syndrome: A review of research. *Exceptional Children, 55,* 336–341.

Pueschel, S.M., & Pezzullo, J.C. (1985). Thyroid dysfunction in Down syndrome. *American Journal of Diseases of Children, 139,* 636–639.

Pueschel, S.M., Reed, R.B., Cronk, C.E., & Goldstein, B.I. (1980). 5-hydroxytryptophan and pyridoxine. *American Journal of Diseases of Children, 134,* 834–844.

Schmid, F. (1976). *Das Mongolismus-Syndrom* [The mongolism syndrome]. Munsterdorf, Germany: Verlag Hansen & Hansen.

Schwartz, D., & Schwartz, R. (1978). Acoustic impedance and otoscopic findings in young children with Down's syndrome. *Archives of Otolaryngol-ogy, 104,* 652–656.

Smith, G.F., Spiker, D., Peterson, C.P., Cicchetti, D., & Justine, P. (1984). Use of megadoses of vitamins with minerals in Down syndrome. *Journal of Pediatrics, 105,* 228–234.

Smith, T.T. (1896). A peculiarity in the shape of the hand of idiots of the mongol type. *Pediatrics, 2,* 315–318.

Tu, J., & Zellweger, H. (1965). Blood serotonin deficiency in Down's syndrome. *Lancet, ii,* 715–716.

Turkel, H. (1975). Medical amelioration of Down's syndrome incorporating the orthomolecular approach. *Journal of Orthomolecular Psychiatry, 4,* 102–115.

Van Dyke, D.C., Lang, D.J., van Duyne, S., Heide, F., & Chang, H. (1990). Cell therapy in children with Down syndrome: A retrospective study. *Pediatrics, 85,* 79–84.

Weathers, C. (1983). Effects of nutritional supplementation on IQ and certain other variables associated with Down syndrome. *American Journal of Mental Deficiency, 88,* 214–217.

Weise, P., Koch, R., Shaw, K.N., & Rosenfeld, M.J. (1974). The use of 5-HTP in the treatment of Down's syndrome. *Pediatrics, 54,* 165–168.

White, D., & Kaplitz, S.E. (1964). Treatment of Down's syndrome with a vitamin-mineral preparation. *International Copenhagen Congress of the Scientific Study of Mental Retardation, 1,* 224–228.

Index

Hormones—*continued*
  premenstrual syndrome and, 143
  secondary sex characteristics and, 29
  see also Endocrine disorders; *specific hormones*
Human growth hormone therapy, 33
Human leukocyte antigen (HLA), thymus and, 219
Hydration, postoperative, after adenotonsillectomy,
      77–78
Hydrocephalus, dementia in, Alzheimer disease
      versus, 187
Hydrops, keratoconus and, 60, 61
11-Hydroxycorticosteroid excretion, 261
5-Hydroxyindolacetic acid, 162
5-Hydroxytryptamine, 162, 163, 277
5-Hydroxytryptophan, 277
  administration of, 293
Hygiene
  hepatitis A virus and, 127
  menstrual, 142
  oral, *see* Oral hygiene
Hypercarbia, in obstructive sleep apnea, 112
Hypercarotenemia, 40, 41, 214
Hyperkeratosis, in Norwegian scabies, 213, 214
Hyperkinetic conduct disorder, attention deficit hy-
      peractivity disorder and, 202
Hypermenorrhea, 141–142
  intrauterine contraceptive device and, 144
Hypertelorism, 5, 6
Hypertension, pulmonary, 93, 94, 95, 110–112
Hyperthyroidism, 60, 269
Hyperuricemia, 279
Hyperviscosity syndrome, 235
Hypodontia, dental caries and, 86–87
Hypogenitalism, 135
Hypoglycemia, insulin-induced, growth hormone
      and, 259–260
Hypogonadism, 264
Hypoparathyroidism, 269
Hypoplastic nose, 6, 69
Hypospadias, distal, 135
Hypotelorism, 5–6, 69
Hypothalamic dysfunction
  growth retardation and, 32
  pituitary gland and, 259
Hypothyroidism, 260
  age and, 265–266
  Alzheimer disease and, 184
  autoimmunity and, 266–267
  carotenemia and, 214
  clinical features of, 266
  compensated, 267–268
  congenital, 268–269
  dementia in, Alzheimer disease versus, 187
  disorders associated with, 269
  growth and, 34
  hypermenorrhea and, 141
  macrocytosis versus, 236–237
  prevalence of, 265
  sex and, 265–266

  treatment of
    in childhood, 291–292
    thyroid hormone in, 292–293
Hypotonia
  acoustic reflexes and, 76
  congestive heart failure and, 95
  overweight and, 31
Hypoxemia, in obstructive sleep apnea, 112
Hypoxia, pulmonary hypertension and, 112
Hysterectomy
  in hypermenorrhea, 142
  for sterilization, 145

ICAM-1, *see* intercellular adhesion molecule-1
Ichthyosis, 214
Idiopathic thrombocytopenic purpura, 241
Ig, *see* Immunoglobulins
Immittance audiometry, 76
Immune function, 217–227
  antibody-mediated immunity and, 224–226
  chronic active hepatitis and, 129
  granulocyte abnormalities and, 240
  granulocyte defects and, 238–239
  infections and, 70–71
  leukemia and, 244–245
  monocytes and, 226–227
  natural killer cells and, 223–224
  neutrophils and, 226–227
  Norwegian scabies and, 213–214
  nutrient effects on, 40
  periodontal disease and, 84, 85
  T-cell–mediated immunity and, 219–223
  thymus in, 218–219
  see also Thymus
Immunization, *see* Vaccine(s)
Immunoglobulins, 224–226, 276
  selenium and, 282, 296
Incus, 71
Independent living, nutrition and, 43–44
Infant(s)
  birth length of, 19–20, 21, 22
    gestational age and, 25
  birth weight of, 19, 20, 21, 22
    gestational age and, 25
  growth of, 21–25
    see also Growth
  newborn
    congenital hypothyroidism in, 268–269
    routine care of, 289–290
    specific concerns with, 290
    transient myelodysplasia in, 247–249
  well-baby care for, 290–291
Infantile autism, 201
Infantile glaucoma, 60–61
Infantile spasms, 169
Infarctions, cerebral, Alzheimer disease versus, 187
Infection(s)